Fundamentals of Phonetics
A Practical Guide for Students

Fourth Edition

Larry H. Small
Bowling Green State University

Boston   Columbus   Indianapolis   New York   San Francisco   Upper Saddle River
Amsterdam   Cape Town   Dubai   London   Madrid   Milan   Munich   Paris   Montréal   Toronto
Delhi   Mexico City   São Paulo   Sydney   Hong Kong   Seoul   Singapore   Taipei   Tokyo

Vice President and Editorial Director: Jeffery W. Johnston
Executive Editor: Ann Castel Davis
Editorial Assistant: Janelle Criner
Executive Field Marketing Manager: Krista Clark
Marketing Manager: Christopher Barry
Project Manager: Kerry Rubadue
Program Manager: Joe Sweeney
Procurement Specialist: Deidra Skahill
Senior Art Director: Diane Ernsberger
Cover Designer: Carie Keller

Cover Image: Shutterstock
Media Producer: Autumn Benson
Media Project Manager: Tammy Walters
Full-Service Project Management: S4Carlisle
  Publishing Services
Composition: S4Carlisle Publishing Services
Printer: Edwards Brothers Malloy
Binder: Edwards Brothers Malloy
Cover Printer: Edwards Brothers Malloy
Text Font: Charis SIL

Library of Congress Cataloging-in-Publication Data
Small, Larry H.
    Fundamentals of phonetics: a practical guide for students / Larry H.
Small.—4th ed.
        p. cm.
    Includes bibliographical references and index.
    ISBN-13: 978-0-13-389572-8
    ISBN-10: 0-13-389572-6
    1. English language—Phonetics—Problems, exercises, etc.   I. Title.
    PE1135.S49 2016
    421'.58—dc23

                                        2014043769

                                 10 9 8 7 6 5 4 3
                Traditional Book ISBN-13: 978-0-13-389572-8
                                 ISBN-10:   0-13-389572-6

                             E-text ISBN-13: 978-0-13-389573-5
                                 ISBN-10:   0-13-389573-4

PEARSON

for
dB
and
ZB

Preface

I began the manuscript for the first edition of *Fundamentals of Phonetics: A Practical Guide for Students* in 1996 when I could not find the "perfect" phonetics textbook that aligned with my lectures. I was hard-pressed to find a phonetics textbook that provided an abundance of practice exercises for students to become proficient in the skill of phonetic transcription of American English. Therefore, I was determined to create such a textbook. I would never have believed that almost 20 years later I would be writing a preface to the fourth edition of this book. I hope that this new edition continues to provide students with the tools they need to become skilled experts in phonetic transcription.

The fourth edition is similar in its basic format to the previous three editions. Each chapter has been revised with updated material and new exercises. A couple of the chapters have been reorganized in terms of content.

Recordings of many of the exercises in the text are available on supplemental audio CDs from Pearson. These recordings are essential in helping students learn the subtleties of pronunciation, both in relation to the segmental and suprasegmental characteristics of speech. A list of the recordings appears in the Appendix of this text.

New to This Edition

- Additional information relating to the use of computer fonts in phonetic transcription has been added to Chapter 1, *Phonetics: A "Sound" Science.*

- More exercises have been added to Chapter 3, *Anatomy and Physiology of the Speech Mechanism.* Information relating to resonance of the vocal tract has been restored to this chapter from previous editions.

- The information relating to the acoustics of speech sounds has been removed from Chapter 4, *Vowels,* and Chapter 5, *Consonants,* from the third edition, and has been incorporated into the new Chapter 6, *Acoustic Characteristics of Vowels and Consonants.* This new chapter provides expanded information relating to the acoustic characteristics of speech sounds; several new figures have been added as well.

- Chapter 9, *Dialectal Variation,* has been greatly revised. Updated information reflects current census data as it relates to the population demographics of the United States. The section on *regional dialects* has been expanded, and the section on East Asian languages has been reworked.

- A new section on Asian Indian English has been added to Chapter 9.

- Learning Objectives have been updated in each chapter to reflect new changes in content.

- Online Resources have been updated to include additional websites that should prove beneficial to students' understanding of phonetics.

- All references have been updated to reflect current philosophies and best practices in the speech, language, and hearing professions.

- The supplemental audio CDs contain new recordings to accompany some of the exercises in Chapter 7, *Connected Speech*, and Chapter 9, *Dialectal Variation.* The recordings for Chapter 7 emphasize the suprasegmental aspects of speech utilizing both adults and children as speakers. Chapter 9 incorporates new recordings of a female speaker from New Delhi to complement the new section on Asian Indian English.

Acknowledgments

I would like to express my sincere appreciation to several individuals who have helped in the creation of this fourth edition. First, I would like to thank my mentor and friend, Zinny Bond, who sparked my interest in phonetics when I was still a doctoral student at Ohio University. Without her inspiration and guidance, the first edition of this book would never have been made possible. It is especially gratifying that she continues to use my book in the classroom.

Also, I would like to thank Rob Fox and Ewa Jacewicz at Ohio State University for their continued assistance in the creation of recordings for the supplemental audio CDs. A big thank you goes to Mark Bunce at Bowling Green State University for his work in creating the actual CD masters.

I must thank Nandhu Radhakrishnan of Lamar University and Vijayachandra Ramachandra of Marywood University (both previous doctoral students at Bowling Green State University), who provided invaluable information relating to the new section on Asian Indian English in Chapter 9, *Dialectal Variation.* Additionally, I would like to thank Sethu Karthikeyan of Pace University for her comments and suggestions for this chapter.

A very special thank you goes to Kerry Rubadue, my Project Manager at Pearson. She has helped me transition to a completely new editorial team for this revision. I would also like to give a special thank you to my other Production Manager, Roxanne Klaas of S4 Carlisle, who made the editing process truly enjoyable and hassle-free. Without Kerry and Roxanne's support and encouragement, I am not sure I could have made it through the revision process. A final thank you goes to the reviewers for this fourth edition whose contributions assisted me in the editing process: Troy Clifford Dargin, University of Kansas; Sania Manuel-Dupont, Utah State University; and Sandra B. O'Reilly, C.W. Post College of Long Island University.

Brief Contents

Contents

CHAPTER

1

Phonetics:
A "Sound" Science

Learning Objectives

After reading this chapter you will be able to:

1. Explain the importance of the study of phonetics.
2. Explain the importance of the *International Phonetic Alphabet (IPA)* in phonetic transcription.
3. State reasons for variation in phonetic transcription practice.
4. State the benefits of using a Unicode font for phonetic transcription.

As adults, you are all familiar with the speaking process. Speaking is something you do every day. In fact, most people find speech to be quite automatic. It is safe to say that most of us are experts at speaking. We probably have been experts since the time we were 3 or 4 years old. Yet we never really think about the process of speech. We do not, as a rule, sit around thinking about how ideas are formed and how their encoded forms are sent from the brain to the speech organs, such as the teeth, lips, and tongue. Nor do we think about how the speech organs can move in synchrony to form words. Think about the last party you attended. You probably did not debate the intricacies of the speech process while conversing with friends. Speaking is something we learned during infancy, and we take the entire process for granted. We are not aware of the speech process; it is involuntary—so involuntary that we often are not conscious of what we have said until after we have said it. Those of you who have "stuck your foot in your mouth" know exactly how automatic the speech process is. Often we have said things and we have no idea why we said them.

Phonetics is the study of the production and perception of speech sounds. During your study of phonetics, you will begin to think about the process of speech production. You will learn how speech is formulated by the speech organs. You also will learn how individual speech sounds are created and how they are combined during the speech process to form syllables and words. You will need to learn to *listen* to the speech patterns of words and sentences to become familiar with the sounds of speech that comprise spoken language. A large part of any course in phonetics also involves how speech sounds are transcribed, or written. Therefore, you also will be learning a new alphabet that will enable you to transcribe speech sounds. This alphabet, the **International Phonetic Alphabet (IPA)**, is different from most alphabets because it is designed to represent the *sounds* of words, not their spellings. Without such a systematic phonetic alphabet, it would be virtually impossible to capture on paper an accurate representation of the speech sound disorders of individuals seeking professional remediation. Using the IPA also permits consistency among professionals in their transcription of typical or atypical speech.

Another "sound" science related to phonetics is **phonology**. Phonology is the systematic organization of speech sounds in the production of language. The major distinction between the fields of phonetics and phonology is that *phonetics* focuses on the study of speech sounds, their acoustic and perceptual characteristics, and how they are produced by the speech organs. *Phonology* focuses on the linguistic (phonological) rules that are used to specify the manner in which speech sounds are organized and combined into meaningful units, which are then combined to form syllables, words, and sentences. Phonological rules, along with syntactic/morphological rules (for grammar), semantic rules (for utterance meaning), and pragmatic rules (for language use), are the major rule systems used in production of language.

The idea of studying speech sounds may be an odd idea to understand at first. We generally think about words in terms of how they appear in print or how they are spelled. We usually do not take the time to stop and think about how words are spoken and how spoken words sound to a listener. Look at the word "phone" for a moment. What comes to mind? You might consider the fact that it contains the five letters: p-h-o-n-e. Or you might think of its definition. You probably did not say to yourself that there are only three speech sounds in the word ("f"-"o"-"n"). The reason you do not consider the sound patterns of words when reading is simple—it is not something you do daily. Nor is it something you were taught to do. In fact, talking about the sound patterns of words and being able to transcribe them is an arduous task; it requires considerable practice.

As you soon will find out, the way you believe a word sounds may not be the way it sounds at all. First, it is difficult to forget our notions of how a word is spelled. Second, our conception of how a word sounds is usually wrong. Consider the greeting "How are you doing?" We rarely ask this question with such formality. Most likely, we would say "How ya doin'?" What happens to the word "are" in this informal version? It disappears! Now examine the pronunciation of the words "do" and "you" in "Whatcha want?" (the informal version of "What do you want?"). Neither of these words is spoken in any recognizable form. Actually, these words become the non-English word "cha" in "whatcha." With these examples, you can begin to understand the importance of thinking about the sounds of speech in order to be able to discuss and transcribe speech patterns.

EXERCISE 1.1

The expressions below are written two separate ways: (1) formally and (2) casually. Examine the differences between the two versions. What happens to the production of the *individual* words in the casual version?

Formal	Casual
1. Are you going to eat now?	Ya gonna eat now?
2. Can't you see her?	Cantcha see 'er?
3. Did you go?	Ja go?

Phonetics is a skill-based course much like taking a foreign language or sign language course. In many ways, it *is* like learning a new language because as you learn the IPA, you will be learning new symbols and new rules to represent spoken language. However, the new symbols you will be learning will be representative of the *sounds* of English, *not their spelling*. As with the learning of any new language, phonetics requires considerable practice in order for you to become proficient in its use when transcribing speech patterns. This textbook is designed to promote practice of phonetic transcription principles.

At the beginning of each chapter, several *Learning Objectives* will be listed. By reading through the Learning Objectives, you will have a clear idea of the material contained in each chapter and what you should expect to learn as you read through the text and complete the exercises.

By now, you have noticed that exercises are embedded in the text. It is important that you complete the exercises as you go along instead of waiting until after you have completed the chapter. These exercises emphasize particular points, highlighting the material you just completed, assisting in the learning process. If you are unsure of an answer, simply look in the back of the book for assistance in completing the embedded exercises.

At the end of each chapter, you will find a series of *Review Exercises* so that you may gain expertise with the material presented. The Review Exercises help drive home much of the material discussed in each chapter. All of the answers to the Review Exercises are located at the back of the book. Similar to the embedded exercises, providing the correct answers for the Review Exercises will provide you with immediate feedback, helping you learn from your mistakes. There is no better way to learn! To aid in the learning process, all new terms will be in bold letters the first time they are used. In addition, all new terms can be found in the *Glossary* at the back of the book.

Study Questions at the end of each chapter will help you explore the major concepts presented. *Online Resources* also are provided to supplement the material presented in the text. *Assignments* at the end of the chapters were designed to be collected by your instructor to test your comprehension of the material. Therefore, the answers for Assignments are not given in the text.

There are several conventions that will be adopted throughout the text. When there is a reference to a particular Roman alphabet letter, it will be enclosed with a set of quotation marks: for example, the letter "m." Likewise, references to a particular word will also be enclosed with quotation marks: for example, "mail." Individual speech sounds will be referenced with the traditional slash marks: for example, the /m/ sound. When a word and its transcription are given together, they will appear in the following format: "mail" /meɪl/.

A set of three optional audio CDs provide listening exercises to accompany the text. Clinical practice generally requires phonetic transcription of recorded speech samples. Reading words on paper and transcribing them is not the same as transcribing spoken words. The audio CDs are designed to increase your listening skills and your ability to transcribe spoken English. Exercises requiring the audio CDs will be indicated with a CD icon in the margin of the text. There also will be a notation indicating the CD track number where the recorded exercise may be found. A complete listing of the audio tracks is given in the Appendix.

Variation in Phonetic Practice

Although the IPA was developed for consistency, not everyone transcribes speech in the same manner. The IPA does allow for some flexibility in actual practice. If you were to pick up another phonetics textbook, you would find some definite differences in transcription symbols. Therefore, alternate transcription schemes will be introduced throughout this text.

One reason transcription practice differs from individual to individual is due to personal habit or the method learned. For instance, the word "or" (or "oar") could be transcribed reliably in all of the following ways:

/ɔr/, /or/, /ɔɚ/, /oɚ/, /ɚ/

All of these forms have appeared in other phonetics textbooks and have been adopted by professionals through the years.

Several years ago, I was assigned to a jury trial that lasted two weeks. Due to the length of the trial, the judge allowed us to take notes. So that no one could read my notes, I decided to use the IPA! Because I had to write quickly, my transcription habits changed. At the beginning of the trial, I transcribed the word "or" as /ɔɚ/ due to personal preference. By the middle of the trial, I had switched to /ɔr/, simply because it was easier to write and was more time efficient.

Another difference in ease of use of transcription symbols involves the symbol /r/, traditionally used to transcribe the initial sound in the word "red." According to the IPA, this sound actually should be transcribed with the symbol /ɹ/. The IPA symbol /r/ represents a *trill*, a sound found in Spanish and other languages, but not part of the English speech sound system. Because /r/ and /ɹ/ both do not exist in English, /r/ routinely has been substituted simply because it is easier to write. Since most speech and hearing professionals have continued to use the symbol /r/ instead of /ɹ/ in written transcription, the tradition will be continued in this textbook.

As future speech and hearing professionals, you will be using the IPA to transcribe clients with speech sound disorders. Because the IPA was not originally designed for this purpose, clinicians have varied in their choice of symbols in transcription of speech sound disorders. In 1990, an extended set of phonetic symbols (known as the extIPA) was created as a supplement to the IPA to provide a more standard method for transcription of speech sound disorders (see Chapter 8). Similar to the original IPA, the extIPA has not been used consistently among phoneticians, linguists, and speech and hearing professionals.

Is one method of transcription "better" or more correct than another? Some linguists and phoneticians might argue that one form is superior to another based on linguistic, phonological, or acoustic theory. The form of transcription you adopt is not important as long as you understand the underlying rationale for your choice of symbols. In addition, you need to make sure that you are consistent and accurate in the use of the symbols you adopt. Throughout this book, variant transcriptions will be introduced to increase your familiarity with the different symbols you may encounter in actual clinical practice in the future.

The IPA and Unicode Fonts

Historically, the typical typewriter or computer did not lend itself well to the IPA. Some keyboard symbols were routinely substituted for IPA symbols simply because typewriters and computer keyboards did not have keys for many of the IPA symbols. For example, the word "dot" was typically transcribed (i.e., typed) as /dat/ instead of the correct form /dɑt/ because it simply was not possible to type the vowel symbol /ɑ/.

You may not know it, but you already may have the ability to type IPA symbols with one of the fonts located on your computer. In Microsoft Windows 7 or 8, these include Times New Roman, Arial, Tahoma, and Lucida Sans Unicode. Mac OS X users can select from Helvetica, Lucida Grande, and Monaco. In 1991, the Unicode Consortium was established to develop a universal character set that would represent all of the world's languages. The Consortium continues to publish the Unicode Standard, which in its most recent version, version 7.0.0, covers virtually all of the characters of all the languages of the world, including several character sets for the IPA. In addition, there are character sets for currency symbols, braille patterns, geometric shapes, musical symbols, mathematical symbols, and even emoticons.

The current version of the Standard allows for over 110,000 characters, each mapped to a unique alphanumeric sequence called a *code point.* A code point is a hexadecimal sequence of numbers (0 through 9) and/or letters ("a" through "f") that uniquely identify each of the characters in the set. Each character also has a unique name. For instance, the code point for the Roman letter "j" is *006A*, and its name is "Latin small letter j." Similarly, the code point for the Greek letter "θ" is *03B8*, and its name is "Greek small letter theta." Since each character in the universal set is linked to an alphanumeric sequence, the word processor and font you select will determine the "look" of each individual character, that is, what appears on your monitor and what is reproduced by your printer. Keep in mind that any one particular Unicode font does not contain all of the code points from the universal set.

The nice thing about Unicode fonts is that they can be used on multiple platforms (e.g., Macintosh, Windows, Linux), and can be used with all word processing software packages. Unicode fonts also can be used when creating HTML documents for online use. In the past, cross-platform fonts did not exist. Also, there was a limit to the number of characters contained in any one font package; most fonts were limited to 256 characters. Fonts of different languages existed separately as well, making it difficult to switch between writing systems in the same document.

Another advantage of using a Unicode font with IPA symbols is that once the symbols have been typed into a particular document, you can switch to a different Unicode font and all of the symbols will remain intact. The only difference in appearance between fonts would be related to a particular font's size and shape, and whether it is a serif or sans serif font. Prior to the utilization of Unicode, it was not possible to switch fonts without obliterating all of the IPA symbols in a document. Trust me, I know!

A number of Unicode phonetic fonts are available online. Many are available for free and are really quite easy to download and use. The phonetic symbols in this book were created with *Charis SIL*, a Unicode font available from SIL International (see "Online Resources" at the end of this chapter). This font contains over 2000 characters. *Doulos SIL* and *Gentium* are two other Unicode phonetic fonts available for free from the SIL International website.

There are three ways to enter IPA symbols from a Unicode font into a document: (1) make use of software that creates an alternate keyboard layout; (2) enter the code point for each IPA symbol; or (3) insert each symbol individually by using character maps available as part of the Windows and Macintosh operating systems.

The easiest method is to use an alternate keyboard layout. I obtained a specialized keyboard for entering the IPA symbols in this text from the website of the Speech, Hearing and Phonetic Sciences Department at the University College London (UCL) (see "Online Resources" at the end of the chapter). Once the keyboard was installed, all I had to do to enter the symbol /ʃ/ was to simply type SHIFT + "s." Without such a keyboard, it would be necessary to type the unique code point for each character (which is a tedious and time-consuming task). In Microsoft Word (Windows), you would have to type the four-character code point, followed by the sequence ALT + "x," for entry of a particular symbol. For instance, typing the sequence "0283" followed by ALT + "x" will yield the IPA symbol /ʃ/ (without the slash marks). With Mac OS X, you would need to go to *System Preferences,* and select either the *International* or *Language and Text* icon, depending on your version of the operating system. Then, click on the *Input* or *Input Sources* tab, and select the keyboard titled *Unicode Hex Input.* Once you have done this, you would hold down the OPTION key and then type the code point for the phonetic symbol you want. Alternatively, you also could use the "insert symbol" function (Windows) or use the "character palette" (Macintosh) to enter the symbols individually from a character map that shows all of the symbols associated with a particular font. This process is also very tedious and time-consuming.

EXERCISE 1.2

Configure your computer so that you can enter code points into a text document (see "Online Resources" at the end of the chapter for help). Then, enter the following code points and write the corresponding IPA symbol in the blanks provided.

Code Point	IPA Symbol
1. 0259	_____
2. 03B8	_____
3. 028A	_____
4. 0271	_____
5. 0279	_____

A Note on Pronunciation and Dialect

As you read this book, and as you attempt to answer the various exercises, please keep in mind that English pronunciation varies depending upon individual speaking style as well as on **dialect**. A dialect is a variation of speech or language based on geographical area, native language background, and social or ethnic group membership. Dialect involves not only pronunciation of words but also grammar (syntax) and vocabulary usage. As you will see in Chapter 9, there is no one fixed standard of English in the United States as is the case in other countries. Instead, Americans speak several different varieties of English depending upon the region of the country in which they live. Additionally, dialects such as African American English and Chicano English have particularly strong ties to ethnic group membership even though regional variations do exist among these dialects. The population of the United States contains many foreign-born residents who have learned English as a second language. The dialect of English spoken by a foreign-born individual is affected, at least in part, by her native language. This is because foreign languages have a different set of speech sounds than those we use in English. There are sounds that are present in English that are not present in the foreign language, and vice versa. For example, English has 14 vowels, whereas Spanish has only 5 vowels. Therefore, when a native Spanish speaker is learning English, it is not uncommon for the speaker to substitute one of the 5 Spanish vowels for an English vowel that does not exist in the Spanish vowel system, contributing to the person's "accent."

Knowledge of dialects is extremely important when establishing a treatment plan for individuals with a communication deficit and whose speech patterns reflect regional or ethnic dialectal variation. Because a dialect should not be considered a substandard form of English, a speech-language pathologist should be concerned only with remediation of clients' speech sound errors, not their dialects.

The pronunciations used in this book often reflect the author's Midwest (northern Ohio) pronunciation patterns. This does not mean that alternate pronunciations are wrong! The numerous text and recorded examples, as well as the answer key, may not be indicative of the way *you* pronounce a particular word or sentence. Always check with your instructor for alternate pronunciations of the materials found in this book and on the supplemental CDs.

Study Questions

1. What is a *phonetic alphabet*?
2. Why is it important to use a phonetic alphabet in transcription of individuals with speech sound disorders?
3. Why is there variation in phonetic transcription from professional to professional?
4. What is the difference between *phonetics* and *phonology*?
5. What is a Unicode font? What are the advantages of using such a font?
6. What are three ways you can enter phonetic symbols into a document using a Unicode font?

Online Resources

Penn State Teaching and Learning with Technology. (2013). *Computing with accents, symbols and foreign scripts—Typing with non-English keyboards.* Retrieved from
http://symbolcodes.tlt.psu.edu/keyboards
(information regarding phonetic font keyboards)

SIL International. (2014). *IPA Unicode keyboards.* Retrieved from
http://scripts.sil.org/cms/scripts/page.php?site_id = nrsi&id = UniIPAKeyboard
(keyboarding information)

SIL International. (2014). *Welcome to computers and writing systems.* Retrieved from
http://scripts.sil.org/Home
(phonetic fonts)

The Unicode Consortium. (1991–2014). Retrieved from
http://www.unicode.org
(information regarding the most current Unicode standard; access to character code charts for all the world's languages, the IPA, and many different symbol and character sets)

University College London (UCL) Speech, Hearing and Phonetic Sciences. (2013). *Phonetic symbols, keyboards and transcription.* Retrieved from
http://www.phon.ucl.ac.uk/resource/phonetics.php
(phonetic font keyboard)

Wells, John. (2013). *The International Phonetic Alphabet in Unicode.* University College London (UCL) Speech, Hearing and Phonetic Sciences. Retrieved from
http://www.phon.ucl.ac.uk/home/wells/ipa-unicode.htm
(Unicode code points for the IPA symbols)

Wood, Alan. (2013). *Alan Wood's Unicode resources: Unicode and multilingual support in HTML, fonts, web browsers and other applications.* Retrieved from
http://www.alanwood.net/unicode/
(information about Unicode fonts)

CHAPTER
2

Phonetic Transcription of English

> **Learning Objectives**
>
> *After reading this chapter you will be able to:*
>
> 1. Contrast the differences between spelling and sound in English.
> 2. Describe the various sections of the IPA chart.
> 3. Define and contrast the terms *phoneme, allophone,* and *morpheme.*
> 4. Define and describe the components of a syllable.
> 5. Identify primary stress in words.
> 6. Describe the differences between broad and narrow transcription.

As you begin your study of phonetics, it is extremely important to think about words in terms of how they sound and *not* in terms of how they are spelled. As you begin your study of phonetics, it is extremely important to think about words in terms of how they sound and *not* in terms of how they are spelled. *The repetition of this first sentence is not a typographical error.* The importance of this concept cannot be stressed enough. You *must* ignore the spelling of words and concentrate only on speech sounds. If you have been troubled in the past with your inability to spell, do not fear—phonetics is the one course where spelling is highly discouraged.

For many, ignoring spelling and focusing only on the sounds of words will be a difficult task. Most of us started to spell in preschool or in kindergarten as we learned to read. It was drilled into our heads that "cat" was spelled C-A-T and "dog" was spelled D-O-G. Consequently, we learned to connect the spoken (or printed) words with their respective spellings. Imagine the following fictitious scenario between a parent and a child reading along together before bedtime:

> "OK, Mary. Now, let's think about the word 'cat.' It's spelled C-A-T, but the first speech sound is a /k/ as in 'king,' the second sound is an /æ/ as in 'apple,' and the third sound is a /t/ as in 'table.' Notice that the first sound is really a /k/ even though the word begins with the letter 'c.' When 'c' begins a word, it may sound like /k/ or may sound like /s/, as in the word 'city.' Actually, Mary, there is no phonetic symbol in English that uses the printed letter 'c.'"

Obviously, this type of interchange would cause children to lose any desire to read!

The Difference Between Spelling and Sound

Examine the word "through." Although there are seven printed letters, or **graphemes**, in the word, there are only three speech sounds: "th," "r," and "oo." Now examine the word "phlegm." How many sounds (not letters) do you think are in this word? If you answered four, you are correct—"f," "l," "e," and "m." Obviously, letters do not always adequately represent the number of sounds in a word. Letters only tell us about spelling; they give no clues as to the actual pronunciation of a word. It is imprecise to talk about a sound that may be associated with a particular alphabet letter (or letters) because the letters may not be an accurate reflection of the sound they represent. For instance, the grapheme "s" represents a different sound in the word "size" than it does in the word "vision." What do you think is the sound associated with the letter "g" in the word "phlegm?"

EXERCISE 2.1

Say each of the following words out loud to determine the number of sounds that comprise each one. Write your answer in the blank.

Examples:

3	reed	4	frog	4	wince
4	lazy	3	smooth	3	cough
4	spilled	3	driven	1	oh
2	comb	2	why	5	raisin
3	thrill	3	judge	3	away

An alphabet that contains a separate letter for each individual sound in a language is called a **phonetic alphabet**. A phonetic alphabet maintains a one-to-one relationship between a sound and a particular letter. Our (Roman) alphabet is not phonetic because it contains only 26 alphabet letters to represent approximately 42 English speech sounds. In elementary school we all learned that the English vowels were "a, e, i, o, u, and sometimes y." In actuality, there are approximately 14 vowel sounds in our language, but we don't have 14 different letters to represent them.

Because the Roman alphabet contains fewer letters than the number of speech sounds in English, one alphabet letter often represents more than one speech sound. For instance, the grapheme "c," in the words "cent" and "car," represents two different sounds. Likewise, the grapheme "o" represents *six* different sounds in the words "cod," "bone," "women," "bough," "through," and "above." Sometimes the same sequence of letters represents different sounds in English. For instance, the letter sequence "ough" represents four different vowel sounds in the words "through," "bough," "cough," and "rough." (Note that the spelling "ough" also represents the inclusion of the consonant /f/ in the last two words.) These examples provide further evidence why it is inappropriate to discuss sounds in association with letters. After reading the previous information, how would you answer the question, What is the sound of the letter "o" or the letters "ough?"

Another way sound and spelling differ is that the same sound can be represented by more than one letter or sequence of letters. **Allographs** are different letter sequences or patterns that represent the same sound. The following groups of words contain allographs of a particular sound, represented by the underlined letters. You will see that the sound associated with some allographs is predictable, while the sound associated with others is not. Keep in mind that for each example, although the spelling is different, *the sounds they represent are the same*.

l<u>oo</u>p, thr<u>ough</u>, thr<u>ew</u>, fr<u>ui</u>t, can<u>oe</u>

m<u>ai</u>l, conv<u>ey</u>, h<u>a</u>te, st<u>ea</u>k

tr<u>i</u>te, tr<u>y</u>, tr<u>ied</u>, <u>ai</u>sle, h<u>eigh</u>t

<u>f</u>or, lau<u>gh</u>, <u>ph</u>oto, mu<u>ff</u>in

<u>sh</u>oe, <u>S</u>ean, cau<u>ti</u>on, pre<u>ci</u>ous, ti<u>ss</u>ue

<u>e</u>ked, v<u>i</u>sa, h<u>ee</u>d, m<u>ea</u>t

Note in some of the examples that *pairs* of letters often represent one sound because there are simply not enough single alphabet letters to represent all of the sounds of English. These pairs of letters are called **digraphs**. Digraphs may be the same two letters (as in "h<u>oo</u>t," "h<u>ee</u>d," or "ti<u>ss</u>ue") or two completely different letters (as in "<u>sh</u>oe," "st<u>ea</u>k," or "tr<u>ied</u>").

EXERCISE 2.2

Examine the underlined sounds (letter combinations) in the words in each row. Place an "X" in front of the one word that does not share an allograph with the others.

Examples:

____	r<u>ai</u>d	____	c<u>a</u>ke	____	h<u>ey</u>	X	b<u>a</u>ck
1.	X	<u>sh</u>oe	____	mea<u>s</u>ure	____	o<u>c</u>ean	____	suffi<u>c</u>ient
2.	____	<u>ch</u>ord	____	li<u>qu</u>or	____	bis<u>c</u>uit	X	ra<u>g</u>
3.	____	m<u>oo</u>n	____	thr<u>ough</u>	X	th<u>ough</u>	____	s<u>ui</u>t
4.	X	w<u>oo</u>d	____	d<u>o</u>ne	____	fl<u>oo</u>d	____	r<u>u</u>b
5.	____	<u>i</u>ce	____	wa<u>s</u>	____	pre<u>ss</u>	X	<u>s</u>ci<u>ss</u>ors

---

Another oddity of the spelling of words involves *silent letters*. Although the word "plumb" has five graphemes, the final letter has no connection to the pronunciation of the word. Consequently, "plumb" has only four speech sounds. These "silent" letters also can be found in the words "gnome," "psychosis," "rhombus," and "pneumonia."

Many oddly spelled English words, and those that contain silent letters, are often related to the origin of a word, and usually reflect a spelling common to the language from which it was borrowed. For example, words such as "pneumonia," "rhombus," and "cyst" are derived from the Greek language, helping explain their particular spellings. In addition, we borrow entire words from other languages, keeping their spelling intact. This only adds to our spelling irregularities. Examples of some words borrowed from other languages include:

quiche (French)	karaoke (Japanese)
kielbasa (Polish)	chutzpah (Yiddish)
sauerkraut (German)	taekwondo (Korean)
tequila (Spanish)	lasagna (Italian)

Morphemes

If our system of spelling is so irregular, how are we ever able to learn the complexities of the English language? How do we learn to read and write? Actually, our English spelling system is not as odd as it appears. In fact, only about 25 percent of the words in English have irregular spellings (Crystal, 1987). Unfortunately, many of the irregularly spelled words tend to be the ones used often in our language.

One key to the regularity of oddly spelled words can be found if we study the spelling patterns among words that share similar meaningful linguistic units, or morphemes. A **morpheme** is the smallest unit of language capable of carrying meaning. For instance, the word "book" is a morpheme. The word "book" carries meaning because it connotes an item that is composed of pages with print, binding, two covers, and so on. The word "chair" is also a morpheme; it conveys meaning.

Now consider the word "books." It contains two morphemes, the morpheme "book" and the plural morpheme, represented by -s. The -s ending indicates the plural form of the word, that is, more than one book. Since -s carries meaning, it is a morpheme. Other examples of morphemes include regular verb endings (such as -ed and -ing as in the words "walk*ed*" and "call*ing*"), prefixes (such as pre- and re- as in "prepaid" and "reread"), and suffixes (such as -tion in "constitution" and -ive as in "talkative"). Notice that syllables and morphemes are not the same thing. It is possible for a one-syllable word, such as "books" or "walked" to have more than one morpheme. Also, it is possible for words with more than one syllable to be comprised of only one morpheme (e.g., "celery" and "asparagus").

Take a moment to examine the following three pairs of words. Notice that each word pair shares the same morpheme. Say each pair aloud. What do you notice?

*music music*ian   *phlegm phlegm*atic   *press press*ure

Hopefully, you noted that although each pair shares the same morpheme, the pronunciation of the morphemes in each pair is different. English morphemes tend to be spelled the same even though the words that share them are pronounced in a different manner. English spelling may not appear to be so odd if one considers the spelling of the morphemes that form the roots of many irregularly spelled English words (MacKay, 1987).

Morphemes that can stand alone and still carry meaning, such as "book," "phlegm," "music," or "press," are called **free morphemes**. Morphemes (bold) such as **pre**(date), **re**(tread), (book)**s**, (music)**ian**, and (press)**ure** are called **bound morphemes** because they are bound to other words and carry no meaning when they stand alone.

EXERCISE 2.3

For each item below, think of another word that shares the same morpheme.

Example:

    create   creation

1. deduce   *deduction*
2. protect   *protection*
3. potent   _____
4. scrutiny   _____
5. labor   *laborer*

6. great   *greater*
7. honest   *honesty*
8. decent   *decently*
9. late   *later*
10. magnet   *magnetic*

EXERCISE 2.4

Indicate the number of morphemes in each of the following words.

Examples:

1 cucumber	2 reading	3 reworked	
1 caution	2 running	2 lived	3 relistened
2 warmly	1 finger	2 talker	1 kangaroo
2 prorated	2 clarinetist	2 sharply	2 swarming

Phonemes

Because it is difficult to use the Roman alphabet to represent speech sounds, the IPA has been adopted by linguists, phoneticians, and speech and hearing professionals for the purpose of speech transcription. The IPA was created for adoption by languages worldwide by the International Phonetic Association, formed in 1886. The IPA symbols are consistent from language to language. For example, the English word "sit" and the German word "mit" (meaning "with") both have the same vowel. Therefore, we would use the same vowel symbol to transcribe these words (/sɪt/ and /mɪt/, respectively). If you were familiar with all of the IPA symbols, you would be capable of transcribing languages other than English. Keep in mind that you would need to know the IPA symbols for speech sounds that are not part of the English language. A list of all the common IPA symbols used in English is located in Table 2.1. The complete IPA chart (revised to 2005) is located in Figure 2.1. Take some time to examine the IPA chart. There are several sections of the chart that need to be highlighted. The large area at the top, labeled CONSONANTS (PULMONIC), shows all the consonants of the world's languages that are produced with an airstream from the lungs. All English consonants are pulmonic consonants. Many of these symbols may appear foreign to you. Compare the IPA pulmonic consonants with the English consonant symbols given in Table 2.1. You will see that many of the

TABLE 2.1   The IPA Symbols for American English Phonemes.

	Symbol	Key Word
Vowels	/i/	key
	/ɪ/	win
	/e/	reb<u>a</u>te
	/ɛ/	red
	/æ/	had
	/u/	moon
	/ʊ/	wood
	/o/	<u>o</u>kay
	/ɔ/	law
	/ɑ/	cod
	/ə/ schwa	<u>a</u>bout
	/ʌ/ carrot	bud
	/ɚ/	butt<u>er</u>
	/ɝ/	bird
Diphthongs	/aʊ/	how
	/aɪ/	tie
	/ɔɪ/	boy
	/eɪ/	bake
	/oʊ/	rose
Consonants	/p/	pork
	/b/	bug
	/t/	to
	/d/	dog
	/k/	king
	/g/	go
	/m/	mad
	/n/	name
	/v/	vote
	/ŋ/	ri<u>ng</u>
	/f/	for
	/θ/	<u>th</u>ink
	/ð/	<u>th</u>em
	/s/	say
	/z/	zoo
	/ʃ/	<u>sh</u>ip
	/ʒ/	beige
	/h/	hen
	/tʃ/	<u>ch</u>ew
	/dʒ/	<u>j</u>oin
	/w/	wise
	/j/	<u>y</u>et
	/r/	row
	/l/	let

Handwritten annotations:

i   hi = key

I   KIT = kit

æ   sa<u>d</u>

ʊ

ɔ

ɑ cod

ɚ

burger ɝ

bɝgɚ

Bob = Bab
dog = dag
mean = min

THE INTERNATIONAL PHONETIC ALPHABET (revised to 2005)

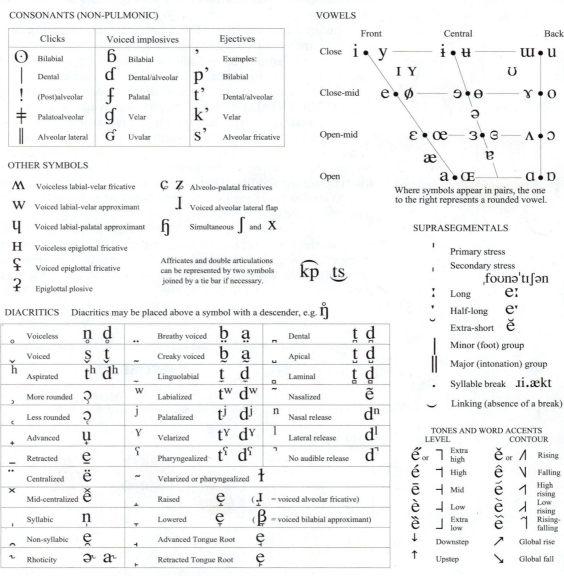

FIGURE 2.1 The International Phonetic Alphabet (revised to 2005). Reprinted with permission from The International Phonetic Association. Copyright 2005 by International Phonetic Association. www.langsci.ucl.ac.uk/ipa/

symbols in the IPA chart represent sounds not present in spoken English. However, some of the non-English symbols are used in transcription of disordered speech. This will be discussed in some detail in Chapter 8. Also, call your attention to the section of NON-PULMONIC CONSONANTS that are produced without the need for airflow from the lungs. Non-pulmonic consonants include the "clicks" often heard in some African languages.

A very important section of the IPA chart is labeled VOWELS. You will note that the vowels are placed in various locations around a four-sided figure. This *quadrilateral* is a schematic drawing of a speaker's mouth, or oral cavity. The placement of the vowel symbols within the quadrilateral is *roughly* based on where the tongue is located during production of the various vowels. As with the consonants, many of the IPA vowel symbols are representative of speech sounds not found in English.

The area marked DIACRITICS presents another array of specialized symbols that are used in conjunction with the IPA consonant and vowel symbols. **Diacritics** are employed to indicate an alternate way of producing a certain sound. The use of diacritical markings is explained in more detail in Chapter 8.

The last section of the IPA chart most important for our purposes is labeled SUPRASEGMENTALS. The suprasegmental symbols are used to indicate the stress, intonation pattern, and tempo of any particular utterance in a language.

As you look over the entire chart, you will notice that many of the unfamiliar symbols appear similar to the letters of the Roman alphabet. This was one of the guiding principles of the International Phonetic Association when creating the symbols for the IPA. That is, all symbols of the IPA were designed to blend in with the letters of the Roman alphabet (*Handbook of the International Phonetic Association,* 1999).

Initially, the IPA chart will be confusing to you. As you progress through this text, the IPA chart will become less confusing and more meaningful in your study of phonetics. Some good websites that will help you become acquainted with all of the sounds and symbols of the IPA can be found in the "Online Resources" at the end of the chapter.

EXERCISE 2.5

Examine the vowel symbols in Table 2.1. Which vowel symbol would be used to transcribe each vowel in the following words?

Example:

	beast	i

1.	lend	/ɛ/	4.	should	/ʊ/
2.	man	/æ/	5.	rude	/u/
3.	flick	/ɪ/	6.	week	/i/

EXERCISE 2.6

Examine the consonant symbols in Table 2.1. Which consonant symbol would be used to transcribe the *last* consonant in each of the following words? Hint: Listen to the last sound in each word as you say it aloud. Remember: Forget about spelling!

Examples:

        dog   <u> g </u>

        rich   <u> tʃ </u>

1.	ram	____		4.	sung	____
2.	laugh	____		5.	bath	____
3.	wish	____		6.	leave	____

EXERCISE 2.7

Which vowel or consonant IPA symbol would you use when transcribing the sounds represented by the digraphs (underlined) in the following words? Write your answer in the blank. (Consult Figure 2.1 and Table 2.1 to assist in completing this exercise.)

1.	<u>sh</u>oe	____		7.	mock<u>ed</u>	____
2.	<u>th</u>em	____		8.	wi<u>ng</u>	____
3.	<u>ch</u>ew	____		9.	exa<u>gg</u>erate	____
4.	g<u>ui</u>lt	____		10.	bis<u>cui</u>t	____
5.	w<u>oo</u>d	____		11.	vi<u>si</u>on	____
6.	rou<u>gh</u>	____		12.	lab<u>or</u>	____

Because the IPA is a phonetic alphabet, each symbol represents one specific speech sound, or **phoneme**. A phoneme is a speech sound that is capable of differentiating morphemes, and therefore is capable of distinguishing meaning. Note that a morpheme (such as "look") is composed of a string of individual phonemes. A change in a single phoneme always will change the identity and meaning of the morpheme. For example, by changing the initial phoneme from /l/ to /b/, the morpheme "look" becomes "book." Using our definition of phoneme, we can say that the phoneme /l/ (or the phoneme /b/) differentiates the two morphemes "look" and "book." By changing the final phoneme from /t/ to /b/ the morpheme "cat" is distinguished from the morpheme "cab." In these two examples, a change of only one phoneme results in the creation of two morphemes (words, in this case) with completely different meaning. Words that vary by only one phoneme (in the same word position) are called **minimal pairs** or **minimal contrasts**. "Look"/"book" and "cat"/"cab" are examples of minimal pairs because they vary by only one phoneme. In "look"/"book," the phoneme variation occurs at the beginning of the word, and in "cat"/"cab" the phonemes vary at the end of the word. Other examples of minimal pairs include "hear"/"beer," "through"/"brew," "clip"/"click," and "brine"/"bright." Notice that these words differ by only *one speech sound* even though spelling shows more than one letter change.

EXERCISE 2.8

For each word below, create a minimal pair by writing a word in the blank. The first five minimal pairs should reflect a change in the initial phoneme; the second five should involve a change in the final phoneme.

Examples: initial phoneme change   seal   <u>meal</u>

final phoneme change   card   <u>cart</u>

initial phoneme change

1. tame _____
2. late _____
3. call _____
4. could _____
5. boil _____

final phoneme change

6. heart _____
7. tone _____
8. web _____
9. cheap _____
10. rub _____

EXERCISE 2.9

Place an "X" next to the word pairs that are examples of minimal pairs.

_____ 1. kale, mail
_____ 2. blog, blot
_____ 3. smart, smarts
_____ 4. rinse, sins
_____ 5. bird, burned

_____ 6. find, fanned
_____ 7. daughter, slaughter
_____ 8. twitch, switch
_____ 9. rings, brings
_____ 10. limes, rhymes

Complete Assignment 2-1.

Allophones: Members of a Phoneme Family

Up to this point, the term *phoneme* has been discussed as a speech sound that can distinguish one morpheme from another. However, there is another way to define *phoneme*. We could also say that a phoneme is a family of sounds. Speech sounds are not always produced the same way in every word. For example the /l/ in the word "lip" is different from the /l/ in the word "bottle." You might say to yourself: How are they different? They are both /l/s. You need to consider how these /l/ sounds are produced in the mouth when saying these two words. In "lip," the /l/ is produced with the tongue toward the front of the mouth, and in the word "bottle" the /l/ is produced in the back of the mouth.

Say them to yourself and you will discover that this is indeed true. These are but two examples of the /l/ family of sounds.

Members of a phoneme family are actually variant pronunciations of a particular phoneme. These variant pronunciations are called **allophones**. The front (or light) /l/ and the back (or dark) /l/ are allophones or variant productions of the phoneme /l/. These two variants both can be found in the word "little" (the first /l/ is light; the second is dark). Try saying "little" by using the dark /l/ at the beginning of the word. Although the word may sound funny to you, it is still recognizable as the word "little." For this reason, the variants of /l/ are not individual phonemes. Saying the word "little" with either the front or back /l/ at the beginning of the word *does not change the identity or meaning of the original word*. That is, it does not result in the creation of a minimal pair.

EXERCISE 2.10

Try saying the /p/ sound in the word "keep" two different ways:

1. exploding (or releasing) the /p/

2. not exploding the /p/

(These are two allophones of the /p/ phoneme.)

Certain allophones must be produced a particular way due to the constraints of the other sounds in a word, that is, the *phonetic context*. For instance, the /k/ sound in the word "kid" is produced close to the front of the mouth because the vowel that follows it is a "front vowel," that is, a vowel produced toward the front of the mouth. On the other hand, the /k/ sound in "could" is produced farther back in the mouth because the vowel following /k/ is a "back vowel"—produced toward the back of the mouth. Say the two words, paying attention to the position of your lips and tongue as you pronounce them. Hopefully, you will see that there is a difference in the position of your speech organs. These two allophones of /k/ are *not* interchangeable due to the phonetic constraints of the vowel in each word. These allophones are said to be in **complementary distribution**. That is, these two allophones of /k/ are found in distinctly different phonetic environments and are not free to vary in terms of where in the mouth they may be produced.

Another example of complementary distribution involves production of /p/ in the words "pit" and "spit." In English, when /p/ is produced at the beginning of a word, a small puff of air occurs after its release. The puff of air is called *aspiration*. Say the word "pit" holding your hand in front of your mouth. You should be able to feel the puff of air escaping from your lips following the production of /p/. Whenever the phoneme /p/ follows the phoneme /s/, as in the word "spit," it will always be *unaspirated*. Say the word "spit" holding your hand in front of your mouth. You should feel less air than when you said the word "pit." Hold your hand in front of your mouth alternating the productions of these two words. You should be able to feel the variance in the airstream on your hand. These two allophones of /p/, aspirated and unaspirated, are in complementary distribution. In English, unaspirated phonemes never occur in the initial position of a word. However, unaspirated phonemes do occur at the beginning of words in many other languages including Vietnamese, Spanish, Mandarin Chinese, and Tagalog.

In contrast to the examples just given, some allophones are not linked to phonetic context and therefore can be exchanged for one another; they are free to vary. In Exercise 2.10 you were asked to say the word "keep" two different ways, either releasing the /p/ or not. In this case, it is up to the speaker to decide. The phonetic environment has no bearing on whether the /p/ will be exploded. In this case, the allophones of /p/ are said to be in **free variation**. Likewise, the final /t/ in the word "hit" may be released or unreleased, depending on the speaker's individual production of the word. These two variant productions (released or unreleased) are allophones of /t/ that are in free variation.

Syllables

In conversational speech, it is often difficult to determine where one phoneme ends and the next one begins. This is due to the fact that in connected speech, phonemes are not produced in a serial order, one after the other. Instead, phonemes are produced in an overlaid fashion due to overlapping movements of the articulators (speech organs) during speech production. Because there is considerable overlap in phonemes during the production of speech, many phoneticians and linguists suggest that the smallest unit of speech production is not the allophone or phoneme, but the **syllable**.

As you know, words are composed of one or more syllables. We all have a general idea of what a syllable is. If you were asked how many syllables were in the word "meatball," you would have little difficulty determining the correct answer—two. Even though you have a general idea of what a syllable is, in actuality it is quite difficult to answer the seemingly simple question, *What is a syllable?* The reason for this difficulty is that a syllable may be defined in more than one way. Also, phoneticians and linguists often do not agree on the actual definition of a syllable.

We will begin our definition by stating that a syllable is a basic building block of language that may be composed of either one vowel alone, or a vowel in combination with one or more consonants. This is the definition typically found in a dictionary or in a junior high school language arts textbook. However, for our purposes, this definition is not adequate. This definition is based on vowel and consonant letters, not vowel and consonant phonemes.

In most cases, it is easy to identify the number of syllables in a word. For instance, we would agree that the words "control," "intend," and "downtown" all have two syllables. Likewise, it is easy to determine that the words "contagious," "alphabet," and "tremendous" each have three syllables. However, it is not always so easy to determine the number of syllables in a word. Using our simple dictionary definition, the words "feel" and "pool" would be one-syllable words. That is, they each contain a vowel in combination with one or more consonant letters. Many individuals, however, pronounce these words as two syllables. On the other hand, some people pronounce these words as one syllable depending on their individual speaking style and dialect. The word "pool" is pronounced by many as "pull," as in "swimming pull." Likewise, some southern speakers pronounce the word "feel" as "fill," as in "I fill fine."

Another example involves the words "prism" and "chasm." According to the basic definition, these words would be considered one syllable because they contain only one vowel. However, most speakers would probably consider these words to consist of two syllables. One last example involves the pronunciation of words like "camera" or "chocolate." These words have three vowels, but can be pronounced as either two or three syllables, depending on whether the speaker pronounces the middle vowel (i.e., "camra" or "choclate"). Both pronunciations would be considered appropriate for either word.

Obviously, a better definition of "syllable" is necessary to help overcome these difficulties. One way to refine our definition might be to more fully describe a syllable's internal structure, using terms other than consonant and vowel. It is possible to divide English syllables into two components: **onset** and **rhyme**. The onset of a syllable consists of all the consonants that precede a vowel, as in the words "**spl**it," "**tr**ied," and "**f**ast" (onset is in bold letters). Note that the onset may consist of either a single consonant or a **consonant cluster** (two or three contiguous consonants in the same syllable).

In syllables with no initial consonant, there would be no onset. Examples of words with no onset would be "eat," "I," and the first syllable in the word "afraid." Note that the second syllable of "afraid" has an onset consisting of the consonants /f/ and /r/.

EXERCISE 2.11

Circle the syllables in the following one-syllable and two-syllable words containing an *onset*. (For the two-syllable words, circle *any* syllable with an onset.)

ouch	crab	hoe	oats	elm	your
react	cargo	beware	atone	courage	eating

The rhyme of a syllable is divided into two components, the **nucleus** and the **coda**. The nucleus is typically a vowel. The nuclei of the words "spl**i**t," "tr**i**ed," and "f**a**st" are indicated in bold letters. However, several *consonants* in English may be considered to be the nucleus of a syllable in certain instances. In the words "chasm" and "feel," the /m/ and /l/ phonemes would be considered to be the nucleus of the second syllable of each word (if "feel" is pronounced as a two-syllable word). In these words, the consonants /m/ and /l/ assume the role of the vowel in the second syllable. When consonants take on the role of vowels, they are called **syllabic consonants**.

The coda includes either single consonants or consonant clusters that follow the nucleus of a syllable, as in the words "spli**t**," "trie**d**," and "fas**t**." In some instances, the coda may in fact have no elements at all, as in the words "me," "shoe," "oh," and "pry." In these examples, remember to forget spelling and focus on the *sounds* in the words.

EXERCISE 2.12

Circle the letters that make up the *nucleus* in the following words. Some of the words have more than one nucleus.

shrine	scold	plea	produce	schism	away
elope	selfish	auto	biceps	flight	truce

EXERCISE 2.13

Circle the word(s) (or syllables) that have a *coda*.

through	spa	rough	bough	row	spray
lawful	funny	create	inverse	candy	reply

To further illustrate the nomenclature associated with syllables, the structure of the one-syllable words "scrub," "each," and "three" are detailed in "tree diagrams" (Figure 2.2). The onset, rhyme, nucleus, and coda of each word are labeled appropriately. The Greek letter sigma (σ) is used to indicate a syllable division. Note the null symbol (ɸ), which indicates the absence of the onset and coda in two of the examples. Diagrams of the two-syllable words "behave" and "prism" follow the diagrams of the one-syllable words (see Figure 2.3). Notice in Figure 2.3 that the consonant /m/ in "prism" forms the nucleus of the second syllable.

Syllables that end with a vowel phoneme (no coda) are called **open syllables**. Examples include "the" and both syllables of the word "maybe." Words that consist solely of a vowel nucleus, as in the words "I," "oh," and "a,"

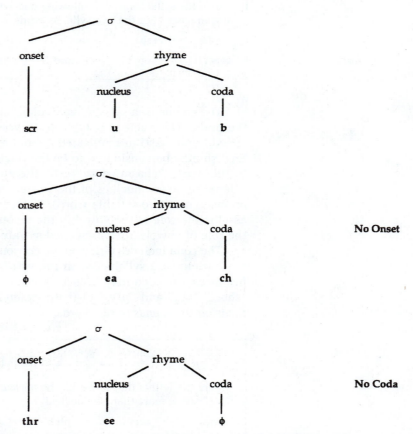

FIGURE 2.2 Syllable structure of the one-syllable words "scrub," "each," and "three."

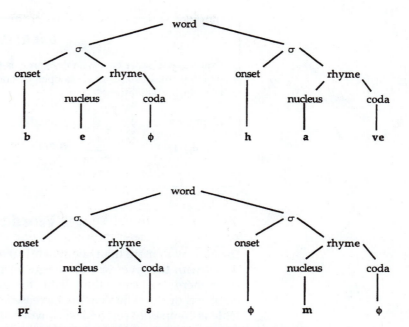

FIGURE 2.3 Syllable structure of the two-syllable words "behave" and "prism."

also are considered to be open syllables. Syllables with a coda—that is, those that end with a consonant phoneme—are called **closed syllables**. Examples of closed syllables are "had," "keg," and both syllables in the word "contain." When determining whether a syllable is open or closed, you need to pay attention to the phonemic specification of the syllable, not its spelling. More examples of open and closed syllables are given below.

Words with Open Syllables		*Words with Closed Syllables*	
One-Syllable	*Two-Syllable*	*One-Syllable*	*Two-Syllable*
he	allow	corn	captive
bow	daily	suave	chalice
may	belie	wish	dentist
rye	zebra	charge	English
through	hobo	slammed	invest

EXERCISE 2.14

Examine the following two-syllable words. Indicate whether the *first* syllable is open (O) or closed (C) by filling in the blank with the appropriate letter.

Examples: __O__ around   __C__ blistered

____ pliant   ____ comply   ____ coerced   ____ minutes

____ decree   ____ encase   ____ flatly   ____ preface

EXERCISE 2.15

Examine the same two-syllable words as those in the previous exercise. Indicate whether the *second* syllable is open (O) or closed (C) by filling in the blank with the appropriate letter.

Examples:	__C__	around	__C__	blistered		
____	pliant	____	comply	____	coerced	____ minutes
____	decree	____	encase	____	flatly	____ preface

Word Stress

In words with more than one syllable, there will be one syllable that will be produced with the greatest force or greatest muscular energy. The increased muscular energy will cause the syllable to stand apart from the others due to greater emphasis of the syllable. This increased emphasis in the production of one syllable is commonly referred to as **word stress** or **lexical stress**. The increase in muscular force or emphasis results in a syllable that is perceived by listeners as longer in duration, higher in pitch, and, to a lesser extent, louder (i.e., greater in intensity). The rise in pitch is particularly important in alerting listeners to the stressed syllable in a word (Lehiste, 1970). Phoneticians also refer to word stress, or lexical stress, as *word accent* (Calvert, 1986; Cruttenden, 2008).

Stress is not a trivial matter in learning and understanding spoken language. When we hear a word such as "confuse," we recognize it not only because of the particular phonemes that comprise it, but also because of the inherent stress pattern of the word. Try saying this word by changing the stress to the first syllable, that is, CONfuse. The word now sounds somewhat odd to you because the string of phonemes does not coincide with the new stress pattern. The unique combination of these individual phonemes and this particular stress pattern does not match any item stored in your mental dictionary. As language is developed, children (not just those learning English) must master not only the phonemes that make up individual words, but also their associated stress patterns. However, the stress patterns of different languages vary remarkably. One major reason why foreign speakers of English (or any second language) have difficulty with pronunciation is due to lack of knowledge of the stress patterns of the new language being learned. Second-language learners will often sound "foreign," that is, have an "accent," when using the stress pattern of their native language while speaking a second language.

In English, words that have more than one syllable will always have one particular syllable that will receive *primary stress* (i.e., the greatest emphasis). For example, the bisyllabic (two-syllable) word "SISter" has primary stress on the first syllable. The multisyllabic (more than two-syllable) word "courAgeous" has primary stress on the second syllable. Syllables in bisyllabic and multisyllabic words that do not receive primary stress may receive *secondary stress* or no stress, depending on the level of emphasis given to the individual syllable.

Word (lexical) stress is extremely important in learning the phonetic transcription of English because some of the IPA symbols indicate which syllable in a word receives primary stress. Although it is possible to learn how to mark levels of stress in multisyllabic words (i.e., primary versus secondary stress), for now we will focus primarily on indicating whether a syllable receives primary stress.

Some students will experience little difficulty in identifying the syllable with primary stress in bisyllabic and multisyllabic words. Unfortunately, for many this ability is extremely trying. Part of the reason for this difficulty is that although we know how to use stress correctly in *production of speech*, we are not accustomed to thinking about stress patterns in the *perception of speech*. As communicators, we simply are not used to listening to speech and identifying stressed syllables in words. Researchers have been successful in enumerating the rules that govern the location of primary stress in words (Chomsky & Halle, 1968; Cruttenden, 2008; Jones, 1967). However, the rules do have exceptions, and they are also difficult to remember. During transcription of speech, there is simply not enough time to think about the rules governing stress in words. For purposes of phonetic transcription, what is important is the ability to hear the location of primary stress in words, not the rules that govern how stress is assigned to syllables. Fortunately, the ability to identify (hear) the location of primary stress in words can be developed in time with much listening practice.

Examine the following bisyllabic words. Say them aloud. What do you notice about the stress patterns of these words? (**Hint:** They all have the *same* stress pattern.)

contain	aware	berserk	charade
inspect	reveal	suppose	detain

Hopefully, you determined that the *second* syllable of each of these words receives primary stress. Say the words again, paying careful attention to the increased pitch associated with the second syllable:

conTAIN	aWARE	berSERK	chaRADE
inSPECT	reVEAL	supPOSE	deTAIN

The IPA symbol used for indicating the primary stress of a word is a raised mark (ˈ) placed at the initiation of the stressed syllable. The words above would be marked in the following manner to indicate second-syllable stress:

conˈtain	aˈware	berˈserk	chaˈrade
inˈspect	reˈveal	supˈpose	deˈtain

Now, examine the following bisyllabic words. Each of these words contain *first* syllable primary stress:

ˈteacher	ˈcertain	ˈcareful	ˈpractice
ˈplural	ˈlarynx	ˈprimate	ˈcontact

EXERCISE 2.16

One word in each row does *not* have the same stress pattern as the others. Circle the word that does not have the same stress pattern.

1.	dandruff	shampoo	bottle	fragrance
2.	cologne	soufflé	surreal	careful
3.	always	never	okay	maybe
4.	Marie	Sarah	April	Lizzie
5.	intrude	instruct	invade	injure

Word stress, in addition to its role in pronunciation, also helps differentiate words that are spelled the same but vary in part of speech, or **word class** (i.e., whether a word is a noun, verb, adjective, adverb, etc.). For instance, the words "'contract" (noun) and "con'tract" (verb), although spelled the same, have different stress patterns. The noun form 'contract has stress placed on the first syllable, whereas the verb form con'tract has word stress on the second syllable. Note that the change in the stress pattern not only changes the meaning of the word, but also changes its pronunciation. Say these two words aloud. How do the two words differ in pronunciation? You probably noted that as stress changes, vowel pronunciation changes in one or both syllables. Other examples of two-syllable noun/verb pairs differing in word stress include:

Noun	*Verb*	*Noun*	*Verb*
'conflict	con'flict	'permit	per'mit
'record	re'cord	'subject	sub'ject
'digest	di'gest	'rebel	re'bel
'convert	con'vert	'conduct	con'duct

Note that in these word pairs, the noun form always receives first-syllable stress, and the verb form always receives second-syllable stress.

EXERCISE 2.17

Circle the words that can be spoken as both a noun *and* a verb by shifting the stress pattern between the first and second syllables.

propose	contest	protest	congress	research
project	consume	compress	reasoned	confines

CD #1
Track 1

Because identifying the primary stress in bisyllabic and multisyllabic words is a difficult chore, the following 12 word lists will provide you with some practice in listening for primary stress in words. These word lists (and accompanying exercises) are designed to make you focus on one particular stress pattern at a time. The lists begin with bisyllabic words and progress to multisyllabic words. As you examine each list, say the words aloud, focusing on the particular stress pattern being demonstrated. Listen to each list several times until you are comfortable with the stress pattern being demonstrated. If you experience any difficulty with Exercises 2.18, 2.19, and 2.20, review the word lists until you understand your errors.

CD #1
Track 2

List 1: Bisyllabic words; first-syllable stress (words beginning with "e")

edict	easy	eager	Easter
Egypt	ether	either	even
Ethan	eagle	eater	ego

Note: Keep in mind that words beginning with the letter "e" do not always have first-syllable stress. Examine the words in List 2.

CD #1
Track 3

List 2: Bisyllabic words; second-syllable stress (words beginning with "e")

eclipse	elapse	efface	effect
elate	elect	ellipse	elude
Elaine	emote	enough	erupt

CD #1
Track 4

List 3: Bisyllabic words; first-syllable stress (words beginning with "o")

over	ocean	omen	owner
Oprah	onus	oboe	ogre
okra	open	ozone	odor

Note: Keep in mind that words beginning with the letter "o" do not always have first-syllable stress. Examine the words in List 4.

CD #1
Track 5

List 4: Bisyllabic words; second-syllable stress (words beginning with "o")

overt	obey	oppress	olé
okay	oblique	obese	oblige

CD #1
Track 6

List 5: Bisyllabic words; first-syllable stress (words beginning with "in")

invoice	instant	inbred	insect
inner	inches	ingrate	infant
income	index	infield	inlay

Note: Keep in mind that words beginning with the letters "in" do not always have first-syllable stress. Examine the words in List 6.

CD #1
Track 7

List 6: Bisyllabic words; second-syllable stress (words beginning with "in")

inspire	instead	induce	inject
infect	inflict	indeed	inept
infer	inscribe	intrude	involve

CD #1
Track 8

List 7: Bisyllabic words; second-syllable stress (words beginning with "a")

around	abuse	abort	amass	avoid	abode
away	aware	arise	alike	afloat	avenge
abrupt	adorn	accost	atone	aloof	aghast
alas	akin	avow	adapt	afraid	anoint

Note: There are many words in English (such as those in List 7) that begin with the letter "a." The vowel phoneme associated with the sound at the beginning of these words is called *schwa*, represented with the IPA symbol /ə/. This unstressed vowel constitutes its own syllable in all of the words in List 7.

List 8: Bisyllabic words; first-syllable stress

engine	master	caring	lucky	staples	Harold
plastic	rowing	neither	happen	Dayton	careful
forest	whisper	quandary	listless	tantrum	nacho
siphon	solo	hidden	trophy	panda	Pittsburgh

Note: Most, but not all, two-syllable words in English have first-syllable primary stress. Examine List 9 for two-syllable words with second-syllable primary stress.

List 9: Bisyllabic words; second-syllable stress

remove	control	serene	carafe	pertain	repulse
arranged	remain	caffeine	repute	suppose	untrue
perspire	beside	react	Brazil	invoke	humane
manure	discrete	compress (verb)	admire	assist	beguile

List 10: Three-syllable words; first-syllable stress

realize	horrible	circulate	fidgety	element	hypnotize
hydrogen	insulin	character	mediate	critical	Michigan
premium	rivalry	sacrifice	tolerant	verbalize	readable
yesterday	xylophone	mystify	glorious	caraway	terrible

List 11: Three-syllable words; second-syllable stress

Missouri	insipid	metallic	Ohio	betrayal	inscription
confusion	diploma	abortion	courageous	erosion	contagious
awareness	preparing	computer	neurotic	palatial	morphemic
repulsive	reminded	semantics	charisma	aroma	transistor

List 12: Three-syllable words; third-syllable stress

interrupt	indiscreet	Illinois	prearrange	disrespect	contradict
minuet	intervene	buccaneer	decompose	interfere	masquerade
reprehend	obsolete	readjust	disinfect	reapply	connoisseur
reimburse	introduce	predispose	disenchant	represent	nondescript

Note: It is possible to pronounce most of the words in List 12 with stress on the *first* syllable, depending on your own speaking habit and dialect. In addition, the location of stress in a multisyllabic word may change, depending on the message the speaker wishes to convey.

CD #1
Track 14

EXERCISE 2.18

Circle the words that have *second*-syllable stress.

decoy	mirage	pastel	puzzle	regret	platoon
stipend	thesis	undo	reason	falter	Maureen
timid	planted	derail	virtue	restricts	peon
transcend	parade	circus	suspend	movie	shoulder
lucid	cajole	devoid	cassette	provide	merchant

CD #1
Track 15

EXERCISE 2.19

Circle the three-syllable words that have *first*-syllable stress.

pondering	edited	consequent	misery	calendar	ebony
plentiful	asterisk	pharyngeal	persona	distinctive	example
surrounded	December	caribou	underling	Barbados	lasagna
terrified	hydrangea	telephoned	contended	perfected	India
musical	skeletal	courageous	umbrella	Philistine	perusal

CD #1
Track 16

EXERCISE 2.20

Circle the three-syllable words that have *second*-syllable stress.

stupendous	pliable	creative	carefully	elevate	magical
corporal	answering	spectacle	presumption	placenta	bananas
plantation	clarinet	murderer	predisposed	decorum	horribly
heroic	violin	integer	discover	clavicle	majestic
daffodil	subscription	expertise	immoral	muscular	Hawaii

Complete Assignment 2-2.

Broad Versus Narrow Transcription

Throughout the book, we will be referring to different forms of phonetic transcription. Therefore, it is important to say a brief word regarding these different forms of transcription now. Transcription of speech, making no attempt at transcribing allophonic variation, is called **broad transcription** or **phonemic transcription**. Virgules (slash marks) always are used with phonemic transcription. An example of broad transcription would be transcribing the word "ball" as /bɑl/. The final /l/ is a *dark* /l/. However, broad transcription does not make that distinction since the intent of phonemic (broad) transcription is to capture on paper the transcription of phonemes, with no reference to allophonic variation.

Narrow transcription or **allophonic transcription**, on the other hand, relies on diacritics to show modifications in the production of a vowel or consonant phoneme during transcription. Allophonic transcription of the word "ball" with a velarized or *dark* /l/ would be [bɑɫ]. Notice that brackets, not virgules, are used with narrow transcription. Narrow transcription also would allow for differentiation between the released (exploded) /p/ and the unreleased /p/ in production of the words "keep" [kip] and [kip˺], respectively.

There are times when transcription of an *unknown* sound system may be necessary. Suppose you were asked to analyze the phonological system of someone who spoke a language with which you were not familiar. You would need to listen very carefully and would need to put down on paper every phonemic and allophonic detail associated with that person's speech production. Every detail would be important, because you would be interested in trying to understand the rules that explain how the speech sound system is structured. This type of transcription, where nothing is known about a particular speech sound system prior to analysis, is termed an **impressionistic transcription**, another form of narrow transcription. Impressionistic transcription also may be employed when working with a child who has a severe speech sound disorder affecting the rules associated with typical speech development. Brackets always are used when performing an impressionistic transcription.

EXERCISE 2.21

Match the terms that can be associated with *phonemic*, *allophonic*, or *impressionistic* transcription. There will be more than one correct answer for each term.

_____ phonemic

_____ allophonic

_____ impressionistic

1. broad transcription
2. narrow transcription
3. use of virgules
4. use of brackets

Review Exercises

A. How many phonemes are there in each of the following words? Circle the words that have the same number of phonemes as letters.

1. bread   4
2. coughs   4
3. throw   3
4. news   3

5. plot   4
6. stroke   5
7. fluid   4
8. spew   3

9. fat   3
10. tomb   2
11. walked   4
12. last   4

B. How many morphemes are there in the following words?

1. clueless   _2_   6. rewrite   _2_
2. tomato   _1_   7. winterized   _3_
3. pumpkin   _1_   8. edits   _2_
4. likable   _2_   9. thoughtlessness   _3_
5. cheddar   _1_   10. coexisting   _3_

C. Listed below are three columns of words. Decide if the words in columns 2 or 3 *end* in the same phoneme as the words in the first column. Circle the correct matches.

1. box	flack	(puss)
2. buzz	(dogs)	fits
3. flag	lounge	(league)
4. cooked	(pant)	nagged
5. throw	cow	(beau)
6. through	chow	(flew)
7. tomb	(limb)	bob
8. fleas	(wheeze)	mice
9. laugh	(giraffe)	bough
10. path	bathe	(cloth)

D. When the sounds in the words below are reversed, they make another word. What is the new word in each case, after reversing the sounds?

1. net   _ten_   6. main   _name_
2. sell   _less_   7. pin   _nip_
3. pots   _stop_   8. ban   _nab_
4. gnat   _tan_   9. tack   _cat_
5. need   _dean_   10. tune   _newt_

E. For the following set of items, circle the one that *begins* with a sound *different* from the other two.

1. church	(chef)	chop
2. see	cent	(cut)
3. (think)	this	these
4. knee	(came)	nut
5. phone	(please)	frost
6. (song)	sure	sheep
7. (gnaw)	geese	ghost
8. cup	choir	(chore)
9. gerbil	(goat)	George
10. (their)	thanks	thing

F. Give a minimal pair for each of the following words by changing the underlined phoneme.

1. s<u>p</u>it _slit_
2. h<u>a</u>nd _sand_
3. <u>p</u>ink _think_
4. <u>s</u>in _tin_
5. pai<u>l</u> _pain_
6. f<u>a</u>n _fin_
7. <u>th</u>ought _bought_
8. h<u>a</u>d _hid_
9. <u>t</u>ook _shook_
10. r<u>o</u>b _rib_

G. Circle the following pairs of words that are *minimal pairs*.

1. (maybe, baby)
2. (plaid, prod)
3. (looks, lacks)
4. mail, mailed
5. (prance, prince)
6. (bribe, tribe)
7. smart, dart
8. (shout, pout)
9. window, minnow
10. (lumpy, bumpy)

H. For the underlined syllables, indicate whether they are open (O) or closed (C).

1. mar<u>ble</u> _____
2. <u>pre</u>vious _____
3. pa<u>tron</u> _____
4. <u>tri</u>fle _____
5. <u>so</u>dium _____
6. <u>awe</u>some _____
7. mis<u>take</u> _____
8. <u>luck</u>y _____
9. <u>pro</u>fit _____
10. <u>sys</u>tem _____

I. Examine the following words. Indicate whether the *first* syllable has an *onset* and/or a *coda* by placing an "X" in the appropriate column.

	Onset		Coda	
Examples:	**Yes**	**No**	**Yes**	**No**
social	X	_____	_____	X
picture	X	_____	X	_____
1. mentions	_____	_____	_____	_____
2. icon	_____	_____	_____	_____
3. camper	_____	_____	_____	_____
4. instinct	_____	_____	_____	_____
5. able	_____	_____	_____	_____
6. lotion	_____	_____	_____	_____
7. charming	_____	_____	_____	_____
8. asterisk	_____	_____	_____	_____
9. Japan	_____	_____	_____	_____
10. aloof	_____	_____	_____	_____

J. Indicate the primary stress for each of the following two-syllable words. Write "1" if the first syllable has primary stress or "2" if the second syllable has primary stress.

CD #1
Track 17

_1_ 1. loser   _2_ 6. provoke   _1_ 11. plastic
_2_ 2. unsure   _1_ 7. stagnant   _2_ 12. divorce
_1_ 3. anxious   _2_ 8. beside   _1_ 13. western
_2_ 4. disturb   _2_ 9. germane   _1_ 14. language
_1_ 5. Grecian   _2_ 10. gourmet   _2_ 15. defer

K. Indicate the primary stress for each of the following three-syllable items. Write "1", "2," or "3" to indicate the syllable with primary stress.

CD #1
Track 18

_2_ 1. provincial   _1_ 6. hypocrite   _1_ 11. picturesque
_1_ 2. sorceress   _3_ 7. indisposed _1_ 12. relegate
_2_ 3. indigent   _1_ 8. uncertain   _2_ 13. foundation
_2_ 4. commander   _2_ 9. magenta   _2_ 14. contagious
_1_ 5. arabesque   _1_ 10. platypus   _1_ 15. constable

L. Indicate the primary stress for each of the following four-syllable words. Write "1," "2," or "3," or "4" to indicate the syllable with primary stress.

CD #1
Track 19

_3_ 1. problematic _1_ 6. correlation _1_ 11. protozoan
_1_ 2. mercenary   ___ 7. catamaran   _3_ 12. contradiction
_2_ 3. statistical _2_ 8. continuant   ___ 13. protoplasm
_1_ 4. ecosystem   _1_ 9. allegory   _3_ 14. Argentina
_2_ 5. gregarious   _2_ 10. carnivorous _2_ 15. obstructionist

Study Questions

1. What is a phonetic alphabet?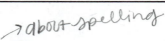
2. What is the difference between a *digraph* and an *allograph*?
3. Discuss three ways in which English spelling principles deviate from the ways words are pronounced.
4. Define the following terms:
   a. *morpheme*
   b. *phoneme*
   c. *grapheme*
5. Why are *allophones* not considered to be *phonemes*?
6. Contrast the terms *complementary distribution* and *free variation*.
7. What is the purpose of the IPA?
8. Why is the term *syllable* difficult to define?
9. Define the following terms: *onset, rhyme, coda, nucleus.*
10. What is the difference between an *open* and a *closed* syllable?
11. Why are the words "spread" and "bread" not *minimal pairs*?
12. What is the difference between *phonemic* (broad), *allophonic* (narrow), ~~and impressionistic transcription~~?

Online Resources

International Phonetics Association home page. (n.d.). Retrieved from
http://www.langsci.ucl.ac.uk/ipa/
(numerous resources including charts, sounds, and fonts)

SIL International. (2014). *IPA help*. Retrieved from
http://www.sil.org/computing/ipahelp/index.htm
(downloadable computer program for learning sounds of the IPA)

UCLA Phonetics Lab archive. (2009). Retrieved from
http://archive.phonetics.ucla.edu/
(provides information and audio recordings regarding the sounds of the world's languages)

UCLA Phonetics Lab data web page. (n.d.). Retrieved from
http://www.phonetics.ucla.edu/
(provides recorded samples of the sounds of the world's languages)

University of Victoria Department of Linguistics, Linguistics IPA Lab. (n.d.). *Public IPA chart*. Retrieved from
http://web.uvic.ca/ling/resources/ipa/charts/IPAlab/IPAlab.htm
(interactive IPA chart with pronunciations of all IPA symbols)

Anatomy and Physiology of the Speech Mechanism

Learning Objectives

After reading this chapter you will be able to:

1. Describe the role of the three major biological systems in production of speech: *respiratory, laryngeal,* and *supralaryngeal.*
2. Describe the role of the individual speech organs in the production of the English phonemes.

To fully understand the production of English phonemes, it is essential to have a basic understanding of the role of the speech organs. When you hear the term "speech organs," what comes to mind? Most likely, you think of the tongue, and perhaps the teeth and lips. If you already have taken an introductory course in speech-language pathology and audiology, you also may be familiar with the role of the alveolar ridge and the hard and soft palates. Speech production is, however, quite a complex process involving many other anatomical structures. For instance, the lungs are important in generating the breath stream for speech, and the larynx is important for generating voice. In this chapter we will explore the function of the various components of the speech mechanism and also discuss their role in respiration, phonation, and articulation. To understand these processes we will explore three major biological systems, namely the *respiratory, laryngeal,* and *supralaryngeal* systems, respectively.

The Respiratory System and Respiration

Generally, when we think of respiration, we think of breathing for vegetative, or for life, purposes. As a matter of fact, that *is* the primary role of the respiratory system. However, respiration is vital in the production of speech, because speech could not occur without a steady supply of air from the lungs. We tend to think primarily of the lungs when we think of respiration. The respiratory system involves not only the lungs but also the trachea, the rib cage, the thorax, the abdomen, the diaphragm, and other major muscle groups. Examine Figure 3.1, which displays the airway involved in respiration.

The process of speech production begins with the lungs. When a person begins to speak, a preparatory breath is taken (usually unconsciously) in order to have enough air to create an utterance (i.e., a word, phrase, or sentence).

diaphragm separates chest cavity from abdominal cavity

pleural membrane

as space in lungs↑, negative air pressure

air pressure in lungs = air pressure out

☒ As the diaphragm ☒ contracts,

air rushes out of lungs

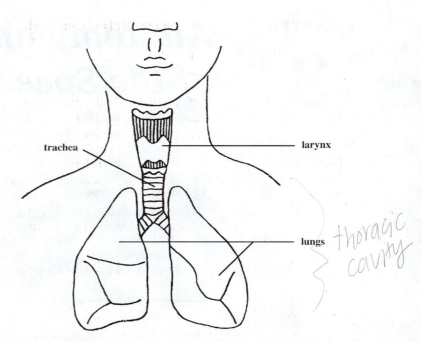

FIGURE 3.1   The anatomical relationship among the human larynx, trachea, and lungs.

This preparatory breath uses more air volume than is needed when sleeping, or when sitting quietly reading a book, or watching a DVD. More air volume is necessary in order to speak. Try speaking without taking a preparatory breath—you will run out of air very quickly. You probably have tried to speak when you are "out of breath"—your speech is choppy and characterized by gasps for air. Therefore, good breath support is essential during speech production. Singers also need good breath support to sustain their notes while performing so that they do not impair their vocal cords.

When sitting quietly, the period of time devoted to inhalation and exhalation is fairly equal. That is, inhalation and exhalation each comprise about 50 percent of one inhalation/exhalation cycle. When we breathe for speech, this 50–50 relationship drastically changes. For speech purposes, inhalation only takes up approximately 10 percent of the inhalation–exhalation cycle. The other 90 percent is devoted to exhalation (Borden, Harris, & Raphael, 1994). This is necessary to have enough breath support to sustain the airstream for speech.

During inhalation, the **thoracic cavity** (chest cavity) must expand in order to make room for the expansion of the lungs. This is accomplished, in part, by lowering the **diaphragm**. The diaphragm is a major muscle that separates the abdominal cavity from the thoracic cavity. The diaphragm contracts, thereby lowering, during inhalation. As the diaphragm lowers, the rib cage expands, enlarging the thoracic cavity and creating extra space for the inflating lungs. These actions are accomplished by several sets of muscles, most notably (but not limited to) the **external intercostal muscles**, located between the ribs. As the muscles of inhalation contract, the **sternum**, or breast bone, and the rib cage are also raised.

What causes the lungs to fill with air during inhalation? As the lungs expand, the air pressure in the lungs becomes less than the air pressure in the environment. This results in what is called a *negative pressure,* relative to atmospheric pressure, inside the lungs. That is, there is a drop in air pressure. To equalize the air pressure between the lungs and the environment, air rushes into the lungs.

During exhalation, the lungs deflate because they are composed of elastic tissue (not unlike letting the air out of a balloon). Simultaneously, the diaphragm begins to relax and rise, returning to its original position. Also, the rib cage becomes smaller as it lowers due to both the relaxation of the inhalation muscles and the contraction primarily of the **internal intercostal muscles** and the abdominal muscles. The internal intercostal muscles are located between the ribs, but are located *deep* to (beneath) the external intercostals. The end result is the expulsion of the airstream through the **trachea**, or windpipe. The trachea, which connects the lungs with the larynx, is a tube comprised of cartilaginous rings embedded in muscle tissue (see Figure 3.1).

The Laryngeal System and Phonation

The laryngeal system consists primarily of the **larynx**, or "voice box." The larynx is composed mainly of muscle and cartilages. It attaches *inferiorly* to (below) the trachea, and *superiorly* (above), by a broad curtain-like ligament, to a "floating" bone known as the **hyoid bone** (see Figures 3.2 and 3.3). This is the only bone in the human body that does not attach to another bone. The hyoid also has muscular attachments to the tongue and to the **mandible** (lower jaw).

Figure 3.2 displays the major structures of the larynx from the *anterior* (front) and *posterior* (rear) viewpoints. Located in the larynx are the **vocal folds**, or **vocal cords**. The vocal folds are elastic folds of tissue, primarily composed of muscle. They attach anteriorly to the **thyroid cartilage**. The thyroid cartilage is more sharply angled in males than in females, explaining why males have more prominent thyroid cartilages. The vocal folds attach posteriorly to

[Handwritten margin notes:]

hyoid → horseshoe shaped, at the base of tongue, anchor for the larynx

thyroid → largest, knotch on front (comes together at angle), superior & inferior horns, most anterior cartilage, function is to protect vocal folds

know location, structure, function

cricoid → at bottom of larynx and sits on top of trachea, wide band, post=large, ant=small, only completely ringed cart, class ring

arytenoid → connection to the vocal folds, only paired cart., sit on top posterior cricoid, function is to move vocal folds, open & close our airway

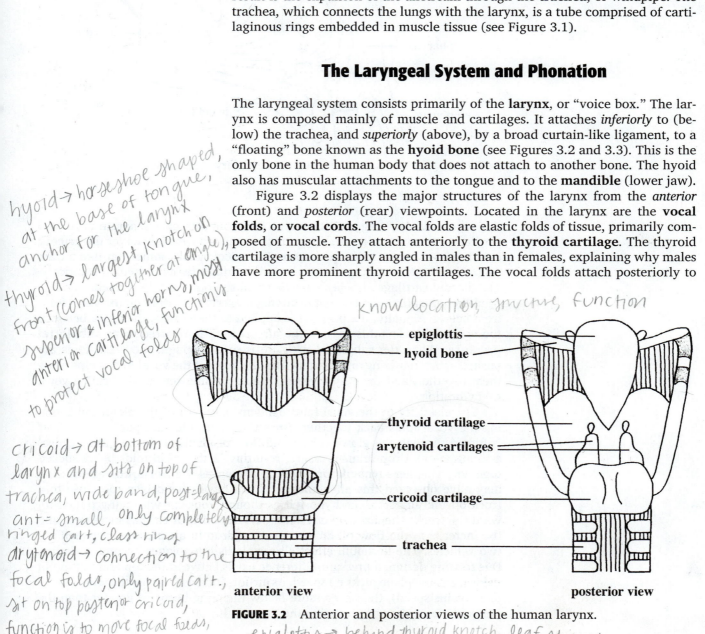

epiglottis
hyoid bone
thyroid cartilage
arytenoid cartilages
cricoid cartilage
trachea

anterior view   **posterior view**

FIGURE 3.2 Anterior and posterior views of the human larynx.

epiglottis → behind thyroid knotch, leaf shaped, function is to covers open airways during swallowing, protects airways

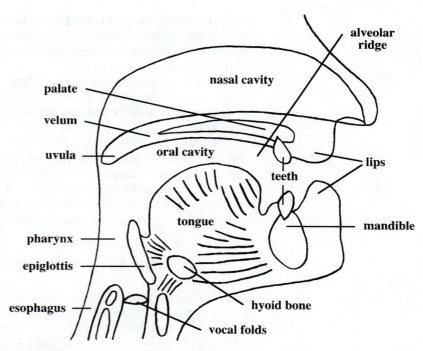

FIGURE 3.3   The vocal tract and related supralaryngeal structures.

the **arytenoid cartilages**. Each vocal fold connects to a separate arytenoid cartilage. The arytenoid cartilages attach to the superior portion of the **cricoid cartilage**, which encircles the larynx. The cricoid looks somewhat like a class ring, with the band facing anteriorly and the ring's features facing posteriorly. The thyroid cartilage attaches *laterally* to (at the sides of) the cricoid.

When the airstream enters the larynx, it exerts a pressure on the vocal folds from below. Actually, the pressure is applied to the **glottis**, the space between the vocal folds. For this reason, the air pressure is referred to as **subglottal pressure**. When the subglottal pressure is great enough, the vocal folds are pushed apart, releasing an air burst. The elasticity of the vocal folds helps bring them together, and the action repeats, thus creating the process called vocal fold vibration.

The elasticity of the vocal folds explains only part of the picture in bringing the vocal folds back together. Once the vocal folds are pushed apart, air is forced through the glottis. The rapid flow of air through the glottis causes a simultaneous drop in air pressure, resulting in the vocal folds being sucked together. This aerodynamic principle is known as the **Bernoulli effect**. You may have observed this phenomenon if you have ever driven too close to a truck on the interstate, and you felt as though your car was being pulled toward the truck. The airflow between the truck and your car has increased, and the increase in the flow of air has caused a drop in air pressure between the two vehicles. The Bernoulli effect also explains how planes become airborne. Due to wing design, a pressure difference exists between the top and bottom of the wing as the plane picks up speed. As airflow increases across the wing (as the plane gains speed), the air pressure below the wing becomes greater than the pressure above the wing, causing the plane to lift off.

The vibration of the vocal folds in creation of a vocal sound is called **phonation**. You can feel the vocal folds vibrating if you place your fingertips on your "Adam's apple" (the notch in the thyroid cartilage in the front of your neck) while sustaining, or prolonging, the phoneme /z/ ("zzzzzzz"). You should be able to feel the vocal fold vibration. The phoneme /z/ is called a **voiced** sound due to vocal fold vibration during its production. Some other examples of voiced phonemes include all of the vowels and several of the consonants— for example, /b/, /l/, /m/, /v/, and /g/.

Now place your fingers on your larynx while sustaining the phoneme /s/ ("sssssss"). The production of the phoneme /s/ does *not* involve phonation. Because the vocal folds do not vibrate, the phoneme /s/ is called a **voiceless** phoneme. Several English speech sounds are produced without participation of the vocal folds. Voiceless phonemes such as /s/ and /f/ are formed by forcing the airstream through a narrow constriction formed by the speech organs in the oral cavity, without participation of the vocal folds.

EXERCISE 3.1

Think of at least two other phonemes that are voiced and two others that are voiceless.

voiced _____   *voiceless* _____

During quiet breathing (when not speaking), the vocal folds remain apart— that is, in a state of **abduction**—to allow air to flow from the lungs through the glottis to the oral and nasal cavities. The vocal folds also remain apart during the production of voiceless sounds. However, when producing voiced phonemes, the vocal folds are in a state of **adduction**—they are brought together. The vocal folds then alternate during phonation between periods of abduction and adduction.

During phonation, the vocal folds open and close at the rate of approximately 125 times per second in the male larynx and approximately 215 times per second in the female larynx (Boone & McFarlane, 1994). This basic rate of vibration of the vocal folds is called the **fundamental frequency** of the voice. The fundamental frequency is responsible for the inherent voice pitch, or **habitual pitch**, of an individual. The pitch of the male voice is usually perceived to be lower than the pitch of the female voice due to the lower fundamental frequency. The pitch of the voice is largely dependent on the size (mass) of the individual larynx. Because the vocal fold tissue in the male larynx has greater mass than that of the female larynx, the male vocal folds vibrate more slowly. Hence, the male voice is perceived as being lower in pitch. Because children have smaller larynges than adults, their vocal pitch is the highest of all.

The fundamental frequency of the voice is not constant; voice pitch changes continually over time during speech production. When a word is given stress for emphasis (i.e., the *blue* car), the fundamental frequency rises. When someone asks a question, his or her voice pitch also rises, *doesn't it?* Singers change the fundamental frequency of their voices to sing a scale. Individuals who speak in a *monotone* ("one tone") rarely change the pitch of their voice. If you have ever had a professor who spoke in a monotone, you know how *monotonous* it was for the class. The pitch of the voice also conveys information regarding our moods, that is, whether we are happy, sad, excited, bored, or angry.

In addition to phonation, the larynx serves other important purposes. During a meal, the **epiglottis**, another cartilage of the larynx, diverts food away from the trachea and toward the esophagus to avoid food from "going down the wrong pipe" (see Figure 3.2). The larynx is also important in maintaining air pressure in the thoracic cavity during strenuous activities such as giving birth, lifting a heavy object, and elimination. During these activities, air is held in the lungs to provide extra muscular strength derived from the thorax. The vocal folds are held tightly together along their margins during these activities in order to stop the escape of air from the lungs. If you lift weights, you know the importance of good breath control to help you with your workout.

The Supralaryngeal System and Articulation

The supralaryngeal system refers to anatomical structures *above* the larynx. (The prefix "supra" means above.) These structures include the **pharynx**, or throat, the oral cavity, the nasal cavity, and the articulators (see Figure 3.3). Collectively, these structures comprise what is known as the **vocal tract**. The length of the vocal tract from larynx to lips is about 17 centimeters (cm); (almost 7 inches) in the average adult male and about 14 or 15 cm in the average adult female (Kent, 1997).

The pharynx directs airflow from the larynx to the oral and nasal cavities. It connects to the esophagus, which lies posteriorly to the larynx. The pharynx can be divided into three major sections. In ascending order from the larynx, they are (1) the *laryngopharynx,* the portion of the pharynx adjoining the larynx; (2) the *oropharynx,* adjacent to the posterior portion of the oral cavity; and (3) the *nasopharynx,* adjacent to the posterior portion of the nasal cavity.

The *nasal cavity* begins at the nostrils, or **nares**, and continues to the nasopharynx, posteriorly. Directly inferior to the nasal cavity (separated by the palate) is the oral cavity. The *oral cavity,* or mouth, begins at the lips and continues posteriorly to the oropharynx. The oral and nasal cavities join at the pharynx (see Figure 3.3).

During phonation (vocal fold vibration), air bursts or pulses escape from the glottis when subglottal pressure becomes sufficient to push the folds apart. These pulses are modulated by the opening and closing of the vocal folds. The air bursts collide with a column of air residing in the vocal tract. This collision sends acoustic vibrations at the speed of sound through the vocal tract to the lips (Daniloff, Schuckers, & Feth, 1980).

During production of voiceless phonemes, the vocal folds do not modulate the airstream because the vocal folds are abducted. Instead, acoustic vibrations are created when air, streaming from the lungs, is impeded by a constriction formed by the speech organs in the oral cavity. As the flow of air is forced through the constriction, a turbulent airstream is generated. The turbulence generates acoustic vibrations, which then travel toward the lips along with the airstream.

As the airstream from the lungs (and the accompanying acoustic vibrations) is directed to the oral and nasal cavities, the vibrations are modified by the speech organs to produce the individual phonemes of a language. This process is called **articulation**, which means "to join together." Articulation of speech, therefore, involves the joining together of the speech organs for the production of phonemes.

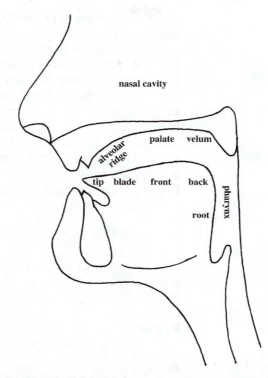

FIGURE 3.4 The landmarks of the tongue in relation to the other structures in the vocal tract.

The major articulators of the vocal tract are located in the oral cavity. It is these structures that are directly responsible for the production of speech sounds. A detailed description of these organs and their role in the production of speech follows. While reading the descriptions of the articulators in the next few paragraphs, you may find it helpful to refer to Figures 3.3 and 3.4.

The Lips

The purpose of the lips is to open and close in the production of several English speech sounds. The upper lip is supported by the **maxilla**, or upper jaw, and the lower lip is supported by the mandible. In production of English phonemes, the lower lip is more mobile because the mandible is quite active in speech production. The phonemes associated with the lips are called **labial** sounds. The labial sounds in English include /p, b, m, w, f, and v/. Because /p, b, m, and w/ are produced with both lips, they are called **bilabial** phonemes. Notice that the formation of the phoneme /w/ is slightly different from /p, b, and m/, the other three bilabial phonemes.

EXERCISE 3.2

Say the words "witch" and "bear" and pay attention to your lips in the formation of /w/ and /b/. What is the difference in the way the lips come together in the formation of these sounds?

The lips often become rounded during production of certain phonemes including /w/ and several of the vowels. In fact, all of the vowels in English can be classified in relation to whether the lips are rounded or not. The lips become *rounded* during production of the vowels in the words "loot," "could," "hurt," and "toad," whereas the lips are *unrounded* during production of the vowels in the words "then," "can," and "eat." More will be said of lip rounding in the next chapter.

EXERCISE 3.3

Say the following words aloud, paying particular attention to whether your lips become rounded or not. Place an "X" next to the words that involve lip rounding.

_____ choose	_____ way	_____ car
_____ lamb	_____ road	_____ look
_____ this	_____ heard	_____ mess

The Teeth

The role of the teeth in the production of speech is more important than one might imagine. The top front teeth, the upper **central incisors**, and the lower lip are used in combination to produce the phonemes /f/ and /v/ as in the words "fat" and "vat." Phonemes that involve the articulation of the lower lip and the teeth are called **labiodental** (lips and teeth). The upper and lower central incisors (with the assistance of the tongue) are important in production of the initial phonemes in the words "think" and "that." Phonemes that are produced by the tongue and the teeth are called **dental** or **interdental**. In addition to being directly involved in the production of several phonemes, the teeth (most notably the *molars*) also help guide the tongue in production of other speech sounds, such as the initial sounds in "top," "sit," "ship," and "zebra."

EXERCISE 3.4

The phonemes that begin the words "think" and "that" both have a "th" sound, yet they are considered to be two separate phonemes. What is the difference in their production?

The Alveolar Ridge

The **alveolar ridge** (or *gum ridge* of the maxilla) is the bony ridge containing the sockets of the teeth. It is located directly posterior to the upper central incisors. Say the word "team." The tip of your tongue touches the anterior alveolar ridge as you produce the initial /t/ phoneme. Other examples of **alveolar** phonemes include /d, l, n, s, and z/. Note that although the tongue does not directly contact the alveolar ridge during production of the phonemes /s and z/ (as in the words "sip" and "zip"), they are still considered alveolar because of the tongue's close proximity to the alveolar ridge during their production.

The Palate

The **hard palate** (or simply, **palate**) is the bony structure located just posterior to the alveolar ridge. You can feel the palate by sliding the tip of your tongue from the alveolar ridge toward the back of the mouth. The palate, often referred to as the roof of the mouth, separates the oral cavity from the nasal cavity. Individuals born with a *cleft palate* may have an incomplete closure of the hard (or soft) palate that allows air to escape from the oral cavity directly into the nasal cavity. Sounds produced in conjunction with the palate (and tongue) are called **palatal**. Examples of palatal sounds include the sounds at the beginning of the words "s̲hip" and "y̲ou."

The Velum

The **velum**, another name for the **soft palate**, is a muscular structure located directly posterior to the hard palate. (Some of you may be able to touch the soft palate with your tongue tip.) **Velar** sounds are those produced by articulation of the soft palate with the back of the tongue. Examples include the initial sounds in the words "kite" and "goat" and "ng" in the word "sing."

The **uvula** is the rounded, tablike, fleshy structure located at the posterior tip of the velum. Although the uvula is not used in production of speech sounds in English, there are *uvular* phonemes in other languages, such as French and Arabic. Uvular phonemes are produced by articulation of the uvula and the back of the tongue.

Because the velum is muscular, it is capable of movement. The velum acts as a switching mechanism that directs the flow of air coming from the lungs and larynx. When the velum is raised, it contacts the back wall of the pharynx, closing off the nasopharynx from the oropharynx. This process is called **velopharyngeal closure**. Closure of the velopharyngeal port prevents air from entering the nasal cavity. On the other hand, when the velum is lowered, air flows into both the oral and nasal cavities.

Phonemes produced with a raised (closed) velum are called **oral phonemes**; the airstream is directed solely into the oral cavity. Phonemes produced with the velum lowered are called **nasal phonemes** because the breath stream also flows into the nasal cavity during their production. In English, there are only three nasal phonemes: /m/, /n/, and /ŋ/. The symbol /ŋ/ represents "ng" as in the words "sing" and "hunger." All of the other phonemes in English are oral.

The Glottis

The *glottis* is the place of production for the English phoneme /h/ as in "heart." This phoneme is considered a **glottal** sound because it is produced when the airstream from the lungs is forced through the opening between the vocal folds. Because the vocal folds do not vibrate during the production of /h/, it is considered to be voiceless.

The Tongue

The tongue is the major articulator in the production of speech. It is composed of muscle and is a quite active and mobile structure. The tongue is supported by the mandible and the hyoid bone through muscular attachments. The tongue also has muscular attachments to several other structures, including the epiglottis, the palate, and the pharynx.

Sounds produced with the tongue are called **lingual** sounds. The tongue is the primary articulator for all of the English vowels. In addition, the tongue articulates with the lips, teeth, alveolar ridge, palate, and velum in production of the consonants. The **root** of the tongue arises from the anterior wall of the pharynx and is attached to the mandible (see Figure 3.4). As a result, tongue movement is very much related to movements of the lower jaw.

In addition to the root, the tongue has several other geographical landmarks (see Figure 3.4). These landmarks include the **apex** (*tip*) of the tongue and the **blade**, which lies immediately posterior to the tip. The **body** of the tongue is found just posterior to the blade. The body is comprised of two portions, the **front** and the **back**. The front of the tongue generally lies inferior to the hard palate, and the back lies inferior to the velum. The entire tongue body is sometimes referred to as the tongue **dorsum**. (The term *dorsum* also is used to refer specifically to just the back of the tongue.) The landmarks are useful in describing the portion of the tongue involved in production of the various English phonemes. For instance, /t/ is produced by placing the apex or blade of the tongue against the alveolar ridge, and /g/ is produced during articulation of the back of the tongue and the soft palate.

EXERCISE 3.5

Provide the name of the articulator referenced by each of the following adjectives.

1. velar _____
2. alveolar _____
3. lingual _____
4. labial _____
5. palatal _____
6. glottal _____
7. dental _____

The Vocal Tract and Resonance

Every phoneme in a language has a unique sound quality associated with it due to a unique vocal tract shape and accompanying vibratory pattern, or **resonance**. Resonance deals with the vibratory properties of *any* vibrating body (including the vocal tract, a guitar, a pane of glass, or a tuning fork). All objects have natural frequencies of vibration, or resonances. Consider blowing across the top of a bottle. When you blow across the opening, a particular tone is produced due to the inherent vibratory properties of the air mass in the bottle. Imagine adding some water to the bottle. Now what happens when you blow across the top? The tone that is produced will sound higher in pitch because the mass of air is less than before.

During the process of articulation, the tongue and other articulators constantly change their positions to produce different sounds as acoustic vibrations from the larynx (or from a vocal tract constriction) flow through the vocal tract on their way to the lips. As the articulators move from one position to the next, the natural frequencies of vibration (or resonances) of the vocal tract change accordingly. These resonance changes are the direct result of modifications in the air mass in the vocal tract brought about by the ever-changing shape of the tongue, pharynx, lips, and jaw during production of speech. (This process is similar to changing the water level in the bottle.)

Now, consider how the resonance of the vocal tract differs between an oral and a nasal sound. During production of an oral sound, only the oral and pharyngeal cavities resonate. During production of a nasal sound, the oral cavity is closed, the velum is lowered, and the acoustic vibrations entering the nasal cavity undergo resonance there as well. The addition of the nasal cavity in production of nasal phonemes dramatically alters the resonance of the vocal tract. Hence, the sound quality varies markedly when comparing oral and nasal phonemes.

Alterations in the resonance of the vocal tract are what allow you to recognize differences among the individual English phonemes. As a child, you learned that a particular sound quality is associated with the /r/ phoneme (for example) and that a totally different sound quality is associated with the /s/ phoneme. It is your ability to recognize these differences that allow you to perceive speech.

Although the term *quality* has been used freely in this discussion of resonance, it has not yet been defined. **Quality** is the perceptual character of a sound based on its acoustic resonance patterns. **Timbre** is a synonym often used for sound *quality*.

The size, shape, and composition of any vibrating body help determine its unique resonance characteristic (timbre). A middle "C" played on a piano has a different timbre than middle "C" on a clarinet even though both instruments produce the same note on the musical scale. The contrasting timbre allows you to recognize the difference in middle "C" played by these two instruments. Similarly, the vocal tract has a recognizable quality due to its own characteristic resonance and sounds nothing like the sounds produced from a pop bottle or a piano.

Review Exercises

A. Match each of the laryngeal cartilages at the right with its correct description.

   _B_   1. shaped like a class ring   a. epiglottis

   _C_   2. forms the Adam's apple   b. cricoid

   _D_   3. situated atop the cricoid   c. thyroid

   _A_   4. prevents food from entering the larynx   d. arytenoids

B. Fill in the blank with the appropriate answer.

1. The basic rate of vocal fold vibration is called ___frequency___.

2. The ___mandible___ is another name for the lower jaw.

3. a. The anatomical term *anterior* means ___front___.

   b. The anatomical term *inferior* means ___bottom___.

   c. The anatomical term *superior* means ___top___.

   d. The anatomical term *posterior* means ___back___.

4. The ___diaphragm___ is a major muscle that separates the chest cavity from the abdomen.

5. ___Sub glottal air pressure___ pressure is the air pressure *below* the vocal folds.

6. Inherent voice pitch is also known as _____ pitch.

7. The _____ is the portion of the tongue just posterior to the tip. The tip is also known as the _____.

8. The tongue dorsum is composed of the _____ and the _____.

9. Another name for sound quality is _____.

C. Match the anatomical term at the right to the structures referenced. The terms may be used more than once.

1. The pharynx is _____ to the esophagus.   a. anterior

2. The lips are _____ to the teeth.   b. posterior

3. The dorsum of the tongue is _____ to the tip.   c. superior

4. The uvula is _____ to the velum.   d. inferior

5. The nasal cavity is _____ to the oral cavity.

6. The tongue is _____ to the palate.

7. The larynx is _____ to the trachea.

8. The arytenoid cartilages are _____ to the thyroid cartilage.

9. The alveolar ridge is _____ to the hard palate.

10. The laryngopharynx is _____ to the oropharynx.

D. Circle T or F to indicate whether you think the statement is true or false.

T   F   1. The phoneme /s/ is an alveolar sound.

T   F   2. Vibration of the vocal folds is termed *articulation*.

T   F   3. The tongue is involved in production of *labiodental* phonemes.

T   F   4. The hyoid bone does not attach to any other bone.

T   F   5. The upper lip is supported by the *maxilla*.

T   F   6. When speaking, the period of time devoted to inhalation and exhalation is fairly equal.

T   F   7. The root of the tongue attaches to the mandible.

T   F   8. When the vocal folds are together, they are said to be *adducted*.

T   F   9. The oral and nasal cavities join at the larynx.

T   F   10. The diaphragm contracts and lowers during the process of inhalation.

E. Match the appropriate articulatory description at the right with the *initial phoneme* of each word. The descriptions may be used more than once.

1. window   a. dental

2. terrible   b. labial

3. them   c. palatal

4. laundry   d. alveolar

5. manage   e. velar

6. shocked

7. pollute

8. zebra

9. kerosene

10. think

Study Questions

1. Describe the process of inhalation and exhalation. Which anatomical structures are involved in these processes?
2. What is the *Bernoulli effect*? What is its importance in the production of speech?
3. Define the following terms:
    a. *glottis*
    b. *abduction/adduction*
    c. *hyoid bone*
    d. *uvula*
4. Which structures comprise the vocal tract?
5. What is the difference between a voiced and voiceless sound?
6. What is the *pharynx,* and what are its three major components?
7. What is the *larynx,* and what are its major cartilaginous components?
8. What is *phonation*? Which anatomical structures are involved in phonation?
9. What is *articulation*?
10. Identify and describe each of the geographical landmarks of the tongue.
11. What is the difference between an oral sound and a nasal sound?
12. Why does an adult male have a different habitual pitch than an adult female?

the length & mass of vocal folds — testosterone

Online Resources

University of Iowa. (2001–2013). fənɛtɪks: the sounds of spoken English. Retrieved from
http://www.uiowa.edu/~acadtech/phonetics/#
(schematic diagram of the articulators for speech; *follow the anatomy link* after selecting "American English" by clicking on the American flag at the top of the page)

Larynx—cartilages—3D anatomy tutorial. (2012). Retrieved from
http://www.youtube.com/watch?v = Z3S2dD9BrSY
(3D video of the laryngeal cartilages)

National Center for Voice and Speech. (2005). Tutorials. Retrieved from
http://www.ncvs.org/ncvs/tutorials/voiceprod/tutorial/index.html
(tutorials on a number of topics related to voice and speech); pay particular attention to the tutorials related to *laryngeal anatomy* (Chapter 1), *breathing* (Chapter 3), and *vocal fold oscillation* (Chapter 4)

UCLA Phonetics Lab demo page. (n.d.). Retrieved from
http://www.linguistics.ucla.edu/faciliti/demos/vocalfolds/vocalfolds.htm
(video of vocal fold vibration)

Vowels

Beginning with this chapter, the focus will be on phonetic transcription. This chapter will emphasize the vowel sounds, and Chapter 5 will introduce the consonants. In these two chapters, each phoneme of English will be identified in terms of the manner in which it is articulated. In addition, its phonetic symbol will be introduced in transcription practice.

As stated in Chapter 1, learning phonetics is much like learning a new language. In order for you to feel comfortable with the use of the IPA, ample opportunity will be given for practice. The importance of practice cannot be emphasized enough in the study of phonetic transcription. Therefore, in addition to the printed exercises in this text, you will also have the opportunity to transcribe speech while listening to the instructor and other speakers, either in class or with the optional audio CDs.

What Is a Vowel?

Vowels are phonemes that are produced without any appreciable constriction or blockage of air flow in the vocal tract. As you know, English has many more vowel sounds than those represented by the five Roman alphabet letters "a," "e," "i," "o," and "u." Table 4.1 lists all of the vowel phonemes in Standard American English along with the way in which they are classified.

The tongue is the primary articulator in the production of vowels. Because the tongue has muscular attachments to the mandible, changes in jaw position also are linked directly to vowel production. As the tongue changes position for production of the individual vowels, the size and shape of the pharynx also change correspondingly. The airstream passes through the oral cavity with virtually no obstruction by the tongue or other major articulators. If the tongue did create a constriction in the vocal tract, a consonant phoneme would be

TABLE 4.1 Standard American English Vowels (diphthongs and vowels only found in regional dialects are not included).

Vowel Phoneme	Key Word	Tongue Height	Tongue Advancement	Tense/ Lax	Lip Rounding
/i/	*key*	high	front	tense	unrounded
/ɪ/	*win*	high	front	lax	unrounded
/e/	*reb<u>a</u>te*	high-mid	front	tense	unrounded
/ɛ/	*red*	low-mid	front	lax	unrounded
/æ/	*had*	low	front	lax	unrounded
/u/	*moon*	high	back	tense	rounded
/ʊ/	*wood*	high	back	lax	rounded
/o/	<u>*o*</u>*kay*	high-mid	back	tense	rounded
/ɔ/	*law*	low-mid	back	tense	rounded
/ɑ/	*cod*	low	back	tense	unrounded
/ə/	<u>*a*</u>*bout*	mid	central	lax	unrounded
/ʌ/	*bud*	low-mid	back-central	lax	unrounded
/ɚ/	*butt<u>er</u>*	mid	central	lax	rounded
/ɝ/	*bird*	mid	central	tense	rounded

produced. How then are vowels produced if no obstruction occurs in the vocal tract? To answer this question, say the following five words aloud. Pay particular attention to the position of your tongue as you produce the vowel (the middle element) in each word.

b<u>ea</u>d, b<u>i</u>d, b<u>ay</u>ed, b<u>e</u>d, b<u>a</u>d

Now say the words again and leave off the consonant phonemes /b/ and /d/ so that you are saying only the vowel. Once again, pay attention to the position of the tongue. What did you observe? Hopefully, you noted that as you said these words in order, the position of your tongue continually lowered. Specifically, it was the body of the tongue that lowered during the production of these vowels. Also, you may have noted that your jaw lowered at the same time.

Vowel phonemes are categorized in relation to the position of the body of the tongue in the mouth during their production. Specifically, vowels are characterized by height and advancement of the tongue body. **Tongue height** refers to how high (or low) in the oral cavity the tongue is when producing a particular vowel. **Tongue advancement** relates to how far forward (or backward) in the mouth the tongue is when producing a particular vowel. All of the vowels in English can be described by using these two dimensions of tongue position in the oral cavity.

To better understand the idea of tongue height and advancement, it is convenient to think of the oral cavity as the space schematically represented in Figure 4.1. This figure is called the **vowel quadrilateral** due to its characteristic shape. All of the vowels in English are plotted on this two-dimensional figure to represent tongue advancement and height. Examination of Figure 4.1

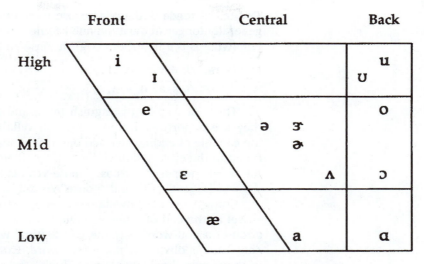

FIGURE 4.1 The vowel quadrilateral for American English vowels.

shows that tongue height can be divided into three dimensions: high, mid, and low. Tongue advancement also is divided into three dimensions: front, central, and back. It is these dimensions that will be discussed as each of the vowels are introduced in the following sections. Keep in mind that the vowel quadrilateral is only an approximation of tongue positions for the production of vowels.

A secondary characteristic of vowels involves lip rounding, that is, whether the lips are **rounded** or **unrounded** (retracted) in their production. For example, compare the vowel sounds in the following two words: "moon" and "mean." Notice that the first vowel is produced with the lips rounded, whereas the lips are unrounded in association with the second vowel. In English, most vowels produced in the back of the mouth are rounded; the front vowels are all unrounded. Other languages, such as German and French, have rounded front vowels. A summary of the rounded and unrounded vowels of English follows:

Unrounded: /i, ɪ, e, ɛ, æ, ɑ, ə, ʌ/

Rounded: /u, ʊ, o, ɔ, ɚ, ɝ/

**PRELIMINARY EXERCISE 1—
ROUNDED AND UNROUNDED VOWELS**

Using Table 4.1 as your guide, indicate whether the following one-syllable words have a rounded or an unrounded vowel (vowel graphemes are in **bold letters**). Write either R (rounded) or U (unrounded) in the blanks.

U 1. lean   R 6. throw
R 2. hook   R 7. back
R 3. road   U 8. then
U 4. mint   U 9. wait
R 5. chew   R 10. should

The terms **tense** and **lax** also are used to classify vowels. Tense vowels are generally longer in duration and require more muscular effort than lax vowels. Following is is a list of the English tense and lax vowels:

Tense: /i, e, u, o, ɔ, ɑ, ɝ/

Lax: /ɪ, ɛ, æ, ʊ, ə, ʌ, ɚ/

The best way to distinguish tense and lax vowels is to examine the way they are apportioned among English syllables when speaking. Tense vowels are capable of ending stressed open syllables. Examples of tense vowels can be found in the open syllables "he" /hi/ and "too" /tu/ and in the first syllable of the word "purpose" /pɝpəs/. Tense vowels also occur in closed syllables, as in the words "feet" /fit/ and "goose" /gus/.

Conversely, lax vowels never end a stressed open syllable. Placing a lax vowel at the end of a one-syllable word, for instance, would result in the creation of a non-word. Say the word "him" without the final /m/, for example, /hɪ/. This is obviously not a real word. Examples of lax vowels can be found in the words "had" /hæd/ and "look" /lʊk/ (closed syllables) and in the first syllable of the word "aloud" /əlaʊd/ (an *unstressed* open syllable).

PRELIMINARY EXERCISE 2—TENSE AND LAX VOWELS

Using Table 4.1 as your guide, indicate whether the following one-syllable words have a tense or a lax vowel (vowel graphemes are in **bold letters**). Write either T (tense) or L (lax) in the blanks.

_T_	1. seek	_L_	3. singe	_T_	5. hot	_L_	7. map
_L_	2. push	_L_	4. head	_T_	6. hoot	_T_	8. clerk

Every vowel in English has a unique description based on the combination of tongue height, tongue advancement, lip rounding, and whether the vowel is tense or lax. Because the oral structures (especially the tongue and pharynx) change during the production of each individual vowel, there is a corresponding change in resonance throughout the entire vocal tract. These changes in resonance not only give each separate vowel a unique acoustic characteristic or quality, they also provide acoustic cues to listeners so that each vowel can be recognized individually.

Most English vowels are **monophthongs** (one vowel sound) because they have one primary articulatory position in the vocal tract. Vowel sounds that have two distinct articulatory positions are called **diphthongs**. Each diphthong is an individual phoneme containing two vowels. Table 4.2 lists the English diphthongs.

During articulation of a diphthong, the tongue is placed in the appropriate position for production of the first element. The tongue then moves to the second element in a continuous gliding motion. The first element of a diphthong is referred to as the **onglide** portion, and the second element is referred to as the **offglide**. The tongue rises in the oral cavity when moving from the onglide to the offglide for all of the English diphthongs. Therefore, the offglide is always produced at a higher position in the oral cavity than the onglide (see Figure 4.2).

TABLE 4.2 The English Diphthongs.

Diphthong	Key Word
/aɪ/	*buy*
/aʊ/	*cow*
/ɔɪ/	*toy*
/eɪ/	*hate*
/oʊ/	*coat*

Note that all English offglides consist of only two vowels, either /ɪ/ (a front vowel) or /ʊ/ (a back vowel). Also, the onglide /a/, found in the diphthongs /aɪ/ and /aʊ/, exists only as a monophthong in some American regional dialects.

Because all English vowels are oral sounds, the velum is generally raised to prevent air from being directed into the nasal cavity during their production. In some instances, vowels may take on a nasal quality due to the phonemic environment of a word. This process is called **nasalization**. Generally, vowels tend to be nasalized when they precede or follow a nasal consonant. For example, the vowel /ɪ/ would be nasalized in articulation of the word "rim" [rɪ̃m]. (The *tilde* over the /ɪ/ indicates nasalization.) Because /m/ is a nasal consonant, the preceding vowel would become nasalized due to the fact that the velum remains lowered during production of the word. Say the word aloud and you will be able to observe the nasalization of the vowel. Nasalized vowels are typical of some dialects of English and, in some cases, also may be characteristic of a speech disorder. More will be said of vowel nasalization in Chapter 6.

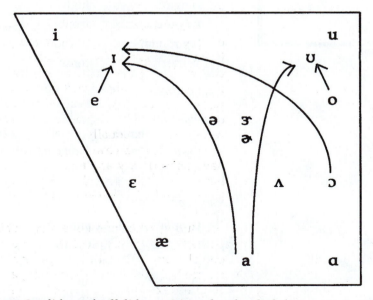

FIGURE 4.2 Onglide and offglide positions for the diphthongs /eɪ/, /oʊ/, /aɪ/, /ɔɪ/, and /aʊ/ (in reference to the traditional vowel quadrilateral).

Transcription of the English Vowels

In the following sections, the vowels of English will be introduced using the following format:

1. **Pronunciation Guide** for the phonemes being discussed
2. **Phonetic Symbol Name** of each phoneme (Pullum & Ladusaw, 1996)
3. **Description** of each vowel on four dimensions: tongue height, tongue advancement, lip rounding, and tense/lax
4. **Sample Words** containing the phoneme being discussed
5. **Allographs** commonly used to represent the phoneme in spelling
6. **Discussion** involving the production of the vowel, and examples of some dialectal variants
7. **Exercises**

The Front Vowels

Pronunciation Guide

/i/	as in "keep"	/kip/
/ɪ/	as in "hit"	/hɪt/
/e/	as in "rebate"	/ribet/
/eɪ/	as in "state"	/steɪt/ (allophone of /e/)
/ɛ/	as in "led"	/lɛd/
/æ/	as in "mat"	/mæt/

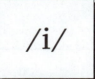

Lower-Case i

Description → "general phonetic description

Height:	high
Advancement:	front
Lip rounding:	unrounded
Tense/lax:	tense

Sample Words

fleet	we	eke	teacher
TV	eaves	creek	credence
Easter	yeast	reach	piece
seeks	edict	receipt	pilaf

Allographs

Grapheme	Example	Grapheme	Example
i	mosquito	ee	keel
e	she	ey	key
ei	seizure	ie	relieve
ea	reach	oe	amoeba

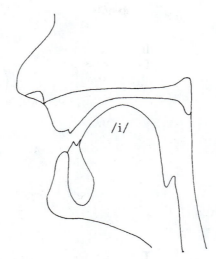

/i/

FIGURE 4.3 /i/ articulation.

Discussion The vowel /i/ is produced by raising the body of the tongue to a high front position in the oral cavity. During production of /i/ (as well as for the other front vowels), the tongue is raised in the vicinity of the hard palate (Figure 4.3). If you examine the vowel quadrilateral (Figure 4.1), you will see that the vowel /i/ is the highest and most fronted of all vowels. Because it represents an extreme point or corner of the vowel quadrilateral, it is referred to as one of the **point vowels**. The other point vowels in English include the front vowel /æ/ and the back vowels /u/ and /ɑ/. The lips are unrounded in production of /i/. In addition, /i/ is considered to be tense because it is capable of ending a one-syllable word (open monosyllable)—for example, "key" /ki/ and "pea" /pi/.

The mandible is raised during production of /i/ because the tongue is in a high position. In fact, the jaw is in a somewhat closed position. Also, the oropharynx enlarges during production of /i/ because the tongue body and root move superiorly and anteriorly away from the pharynx. As the tongue lowers in production of the front vowels (from /i/ to /æ/), the jaw lowers, and the size of the oropharynx decreases (as the tongue moves closer to the pharyngeal area). See Figure 4.4 for a comparison of the tongue, jaw, and pharyngeal positions for the two front vowels /i/ and /æ/.

> **Note:** In Exercise 4.1 and several others in this chapter, *consonant* IPA symbols are used. The IPA consonant symbols to be used are the same as their Roman alphabet counterparts. These consonant phoneme symbols are /b, d, f, g, h, k, l, m, n, p, r, s, t, v, w, and z/. For example: "ease" /iz/; "dean" /din/.

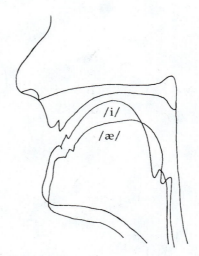

FIGURE 4.4   /i/ and /æ/ articulation.

EXERCISE 4.1 – THE VOWEL /i/

A.   Circle the words that contain the /i/ phoneme.

paper	train	(Cleveland)	(seaside)
(please)	picture	trip	trail
tribal	(machine)	labor	trees
settle	(screen)	Toledo	lip
nice	foreign	(Levi)	jeans

B.   Circle the phonetic transcriptions that represent English words.

(/ist/)	/flip/	(/min/)	(/hid/)
(/iv/)	/hig/	/lim/	(/wins/)
/rift/	/if/	(/trit/)	(/lik/)

C.   In the blanks, write each of the words using English orthography (i.e., use the Roman alphabet to write the words).

/lip/	*leap*	/it/	*eat*	/brizd/	*breezed*
/pip/	*peep*	/hip/	*heep*	/spik/	*speak*
/mit/	*meet*	/sip/	*seep*	/klin/	*clean*
/rid/	*read*	/did/	*deed*	/krist/	*creased*

D.   Place an "X" next to the pairs of words that share the same vowel sound.

_____	dream	drip	X	east	eaves
X	seek	wheel	_____	chief	vein
_____	same	land	_____	base	lease
X	creek	steam	X	need	pain
X	bean	heed	X	creed	cream

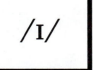

Small Capital *ɪ*

Description

Height:	high (lower than /i/)
Advancement:	front
Lip rounding:	unrounded
Tense/lax:	lax

Sample Words

flit	whittle	inside	dreary
business	king	sister	steer
listen	pistol	intend	prince
really	stink	choosy	kitty

Allographs

Grapheme	Example	Grapheme	Example
i	with, ring	e	England, pretty
y	gym	ea(r)	fear
ui	guilt	ee(r)	deer
u	business	i(r)	mirror
-y	baby	ei(r)	weird
ee	been	ie(r)	pierce
o	women	e(re)	here
ie	sieve		

Discussion   The body of the tongue is only slightly lower in production of /ɪ/ when compared to /i/ (compare Figures 4.3 and 4.5). This is why it is also classified as a high vowel. The jaw is in a fairly closed position during production of /ɪ/, and the lips are unrounded. One distinction between /ɪ/ and /i/ is that /ɪ/ is lax. Placing /ɪ/ in the final position of a monosyllable would result in a nonsense word, that is, /bɪ/ or /wɪ/. The phoneme /ɪ/ does occur in closed syllables such as in "listen" and "indent."

The vowel /ɪ/ has some peculiarities in phonetic transcription. In final, unstressed syllables that end in "y," in words like "cra**zy**," "gloo**my**," and "quanti**ty**," it has been debated by phoneticians and linguists as to whether the phoneme /i/ or /ɪ/ should be used in the transcription of the final sound (i.e., /kreɪzɪ/ or /kreɪzi/). In reality, what is heard by listeners is a phoneme that tends to be shorter in duration than the vowel /i/ found in stressed syllables (as in "heed"), but longer than /ɪ/ (as in "hid"). Also, the vowel in final, unstressed syllables tends to be retracted, that is, produced farther back in the oral cavity than the traditional place of articulation for /i/ (but not as low as /ɪ/) (Ball & Müller, 2005). Yavaş (2006) states that /i/ and /ɪ/ occur in *free variation* (see Chapter 2) in the final unstressed position of words for some speakers. In addition, Kretzschmar (2008), Ladefoged and Johnson (2011), and Yavaş (2006) suggest that the use of /i/ versus /ɪ/ in final, unstressed syllables may be associated with regional dialect. Although phoneticians and linguists differ in opinion as to which phoneme is the correct choice in transcribing the final sound in

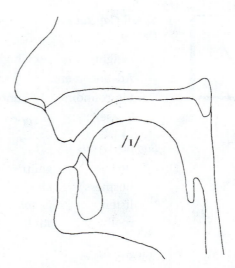

FIGURE 4.5   /ɪ/ articulation.

words like "crazy" or "gloomy," what is clear is that the correct sound can be thought of as an allophone of either /i/ or /ɪ/. Some sources (Singh & Singh, 2006; Shriberg & Kent, 2013) recommend the use of /ɪ/, while others (Ball & Müller, 2005; Kretzschmar, 2008; Ladefoged & Johnson, 2011) recommend the use of /i/ in transcription of this sound.

In this text, when transcribing the final "y" in final, unstressed syllables, the sound will be treated as an allophone of /ɪ/. Keep in mind that some individuals will treat this sound as an allophone of /i/ in this particular phonetic context. As pointed out in Chapter 1, the phonetic symbol you adopt in this context is not as important as your consistency and understanding of the underlying rationale for your selection of that symbol. Also remember that although we will be using the phonemic symbol /ɪ/ in this particular case, the symbol is representing an *allophone* of /ɪ/.

Another peculiarity with /ɪ/ involves words that contain the letter string "ing," such as in the words "running," "finger," and "ink." Their actual transcriptions are /rʌnɪŋ/, /fɪŋgɚ/, and /ɪŋk/. Notice the use of the phoneme /ɪ/ and not /i/ in these words. In this phonetic context, /ɪ/ is raised from its usual position (but not so high that it is produced as /i/). /ɪ/ also becomes nasalized due to the lowered velum associated with the nasal consonant "ng" /ŋ/ that follows. The raised and nasalized /ɪ/ in these words is actually an allophone of /ɪ/. Therefore, it is considered more accurate to use /ɪ/ instead of /i/ in this phonetic context.

Last, the vowel /ɪ/ is often found in combination with the consonant /r/ as in the words "hear" /hɪr/ and "ear" /ɪr/. In this case, /ɪ/ + /r/ become what is known as an **r-colored vowel** or **rhotic diphthong**. R-colored vowels possess an *auditory quality* known as **rhotacization**. Rhotacization simply means that the vowel is perceived as having an "r" quality or "r-coloring" associated with it.

The rhotic diphthong, /ɪr/, also may be transcribed as /ɪɚ/ or /ɪɚ͡/. The tie bar under the diphthong in the last example is used by some phoneticians and clinicians when transcribing the diphthong to signify the production of two speech sounds as one phoneme even though this is not an IPA convention.

This text will adopt the use of /ɪr/, as opposed to /ɪɚ/ or /ɪɚ/, when transcribing this phoneme. The rhotic diphthong /ɪr/ is only one of several found in English.

There are a few dialectal variants involving the phoneme /ɪ/. For instance, in the southeastern United States, some people pronounce the r-colored vowel /ɪr/ with /i/, as in "here" /hir/ or "ear" /ir/ (Hartman, 1985). /ɪ/ is also found to occur before /l/ in some southern pronunciations, as in "really" /rɪlɪ/ and "meal" /mɪl/. Both in African American English and in southern American dialect, words such as "many," "pen," and "cents" might be pronounced as /mɪnɪ/, /pɪn/, and /sɪnts/, respectively.

EXERCISE 4.2—THE VOWEL /ɪ/

A. Contrast the vowels in the following pairs of words (minimal pairs) by saying them aloud.

/i/	/ɪ/		/i/	/ɪ/
reed	rid		keel	kill
heed	hid		deal	dill
deep	dip		ceased	cyst
seat	sit		bean	been
sleek	slick		feet	fit

B. Circle the words that contain the /ɪ/ phoneme.

peace	friend	enthrall	bitter
mythical	silver	woman	tryst
click	ingest	build	fear
thread	pink	bowling	tried
pride	clear	sporty	synchronize

C. Circle the phonetic transcriptions that represent English words.

/vɪl/	/sɪst/	/fɪld/	/wɪns/
/izɪ/	/klip/	/spid/	/hik/
/hɪr/	/ɪl/	/sɪg/	/pɪgɪ/

D. In the blanks, write each of the words using English orthography.

/stip/	*steep*	/pɪk/	*pick*
/pliz/	*please*	/kɪst/	*kissed*
/mɪt/	*mit*	/bik/	*beak*
/dɪd/	*did*	/pɪp/	*pip*
/fɪr/	*fear*	/mɪstɪ/	*misty*
/rɪlɪ/	*really*	/ɪndid/	*indeed*

Continues

EXERCISE 4.2 (*cont.*)

E. Place an "X" next to the pairs of words that share the same vowel sound.

⨉ feel	teach	⨉ win	king
____ lip	thread	⨉ mint	inch
____ been	drink	⨉ deed	flea
____ vent	list	⨉ dish	ill
____ tied	pig	⨉ kick	mill

F. Indicate with an "X" the words that contain the r-colored vowel /ɪr/.

1. ____ flirt	5. ⨉ smeared	9. ____ stirred
2. ⨉ peerless	6. ____ worried	10. ____ stared
3. ____ bird	7. ⨉ steered	11. ⨉ earring
4. ____ shrill	8. ____ harder	12. ____ cursor

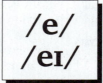

Lower-Case e
Description

Height:	high-mid
Advancement:	front
Lip rounding:	unrounded
Tense/lax:	tense

Sample Words   The following set of words all take /e/ in their transcriptions because the syllables that contain the vowel do not receive primary stress.

chaOtic	UNdulate
GYrate	layETTE
PHOnate	DECade
MANdate	ROtate

The following words all take the allophone /eɪ/ because the syllables are either stressed or at the end of a word.

aWAY (also ends the word)	conTAgious
touPEE (also ends the word)	STATed
creATE	BAby
TAble	BRAID

Allographs

Grapheme	Example	Grapheme	Example
ea	great	ei	veil
a..e	hate	ay	stray
au	gauge	ey	grey
ai	faint		

Discussion The /e/ vowel is produced with the body of the tongue slightly higher than the exact middle of the mouth, therefore it is referred to as a *high-mid vowel* (see Figure 4.6). /e/ also is unrounded. Like the vowel /i/, it is tense and can be found in the second syllable of the word "mandate." An allophone of /e/, written as /eɪ/, occurs in stressed syllables and at the ends of words (regardless of stress). This allophone of /e/ is actually a diphthong and occurs in these particular phonetic contexts as a result of vowel lengthening.

The diphthongal allophone consists of the onglide /e/ plus the offglide /ɪ/. In producing /eɪ/, the tongue and vocal tract assume the initial position for the /e/ vowel. The tongue then continues to glide to the high, front position for /ɪ/ (see Figure 4.2). As mentioned, the diphthongal form, /eɪ/, is usually produced in stressed syllables and at the end of words (regardless of stress) when the vowel is lengthened; the shorter monophthong /e/ generally occurs in unstressed syllables. Strictly speaking, phonemic (broad) transcription would dictate the use of /e/ when transcribing the diphthongal variant /eɪ/. However, many individuals prefer to indicate the use of the diphthong when it occurs, even though technically, use of the symbol /eɪ/ would result in an *allophonic* transcription. In this text, the diphthong /eɪ/ will be used in transcription when this particular allophone occurs in stressed syllables and at the ends of words (even though this breaks with the true definition of phonemic transcription). Check with your instructor to determine which method is preferred.

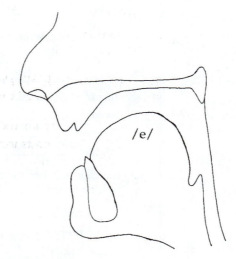

FIGURE 4.6 /e/ articulation.

The use of /eɪ/ may also vary with regional pronunciation. For example, some southern speakers in the United States use the diphthong /eɪ/ in words such as "fresh" /freɪʃ/ and "leg" /leɪg/.

EXERCISE 4.3–THE VOWEL /e/ – /eɪ/

A. Contrast the vowels in the following minimal pairs.

/eɪ/	/ɪ/		/eɪ/	/i/
grade	grid		tame	team
tape	tip		grain	green
drape	drip		trait	treat
take	tick		sale	seal
late	lit		Grace	grease
tale	till		wade	weed
faze	fizz		raid	reed

B. Circle the words that contain the /eɪ/ phoneme.

trail	rage	wheel	palatial
vice	razor	manage	green
transit	machine	whale	potato
lazy	bread	football	temperate
dale	tackle	daily	bright

C. Circle the phonetic transcriptions that represent English words.

/freɪd/	/deɪs/	/dɪnt/	/deɪlɪ/
/kreɪt/	/bɪz/	/spɪd/	/deɪm/
/neɪp/	/trɪps/	/treɪ/	/frɪl/
/pɪln/	/blid/	/feɪlm/	/streɪp/

D. In the blanks, write each of the words using English orthography.

/bleɪz/	blaze	/pleɪket/	playcate?
/pleɪd/	played	/rimeɪn/	remain
/beɪn/	bane	/ɪnmet/	inmate
/iveɪd/	evayed	/ribet/	rebae
/krɪmp/	crimp	/steɪnd/	stained
/rikt/	reeked	/deɪzɪ/	daisy

E. Indicate whether the syllable that contains /eɪ/ is either open or closed by writing O or C in the blank.

___ crayon	___ unmade
___ prepay	___ stay
___ baking	___ tailor
___ masonry	___ betrayed

Continues

EXERCISE 4.3 (*cont.*)

F.   Place an "X" next to the pairs of words that share the same vowel sound.

_____ braid	hid	__X__ state	rain
_____ feed	hate	_____ fist	flea
__X__ lane	aim	__X__ cringe	hid
__X__ fill	kissed	_____ deal	will
__X__ treat	sling	__X__ wheel	meat

G.   Indicate whether you should use /e/ or /eɪ/ when transcribing the following words.

_eɪ_ neighbor		_____ Crayola	
_eɪ_ crate		_____ basin	
_eɪ_ donate		_____ stay	
_eɪ_ hooray		_____ prostrate	
_____ saber		_____ incubate	

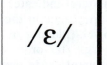

Epsilon
Description

Height:	low-mid
Advancement:	front
Lip rounding:	unrounded
Tense/lax:	lax

Sample Words

met	etch	bury	intend
steady	where	terror	tender
pretend	repent	heather	elephant
relish	stencil	marry	pleasures

Allographs

Grapheme	Example	Grapheme	Example
e	let	ai	said
ei	heifer	ai(r)	flair
ea	meant	ei(r)	their
a	many	ea(r)	bear
ie	friend	u(r)	bury
ue	guest	a(re)	bare
eo	Leonard	e(re)	where

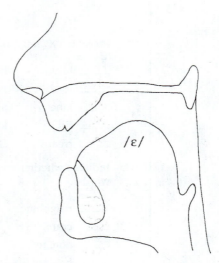

FIGURE 4.7   /ɛ/ articulation.

Discussion   The /ɛ/ vowel is commonly referred to as "epsilon," an IPA symbol borrowed from the Greek alphabet. It is categorized as a low-mid, front vowel (see Figure 4.7). Examination of the vowel quadrilateral indicates the tongue body is located midway between the mid and low positions in the mouth for its production. Epsilon is an unrounded and lax vowel. (Placing /ɛ/ at the end of a monosyllabic word creates a nonsense word, e.g., /tɛ/ or /wɛ/.) Epsilon becomes rhotacized when it occurs before the consonant /r/ in words such as "hair" /hɛr/ and "fair" /fɛr/. Therefore, /ɛr/ is another example of an r-colored vowel (rhotic diphthong). This phoneme is transcribed by some individuals as /ɛɚ/ or /ɛɚ/. In the northeastern and southeastern United States, /ɛr/ may be pronounced as /er/ as in "hair" /her/ and "fair" /fer/. Also, some speakers in the Great Lakes region substitute /ɛ/ for /ɪ/ in words such as "pillow" /pɛloʊ/ and "milk" /mɛlk/ (Hartman, 1985).

EXERCISE 4.4—THE VOWEL /ɛ/

A.   Contrast the vowels in the following minimal pairs by saying them aloud.

/ɛ/	/ɪ/		/ɛ/	/eɪ/
red	rid		wed	wade
dead	did		tread	trade
head	hid		shed	shade
etch	itch		met	mate
bell	bill		bread	braid
bear	beer		every	Avery
fair	fear		bell	bale

Continues

EXERCISE 4.4 (*cont.*)

B. Circle the words that contain the /ɛ/ phoneme.

pimple	trip	ensure	tryst
syrup	caring	women	contend
(pencil)	butter	build	pretzel
thing	thread	prepare	tried
jeep	pistol	unscented	remember

C. Circle the phonetic transcriptions that represent English words.

(/mɛrɪ/)   /hint/   /split/   (/istɛr/)

(/slɛpt/)   (/fɛr/)   /ɪrk/   (/meɪd/)

/sɪsɪ/   (/kleɪ/)   (/wɛl/)   (/krɪp/)

D. In the blanks, write each of the words using English orthography.

/reɪk/ _rake_   /stɛr/ _stare_

/fɪz/ _fiz_   /treɪl/ _trail_

/smɛl/ _smell_   /pritɛnd/ _pretend_

/sid/ _seed_   /hɛvɪ/ _heavy_

/kreɪn/ _crane_   /friz/ _freeze_

/breɪzd/ _braised_   /blɛst/ _blessed_

E. Place an "X" next to the pairs of words that share the same vowel sound.

___ fill	fear	_X_ step	edge
_X_ made	cage	___ bread	breathe
___ wind	best	___ flit	red
___ trade	peel	_X_ sill	kit
_X_ rid	sing	___ care	meant

F. Indicate whether the words below end with an open (O) or closed (C) syllable (write C or O in the blanks).

___ 1. trail   ___ 6. spree

___ 2. repay   ___ 7. arouse

___ 3. strike   ___ 8. rough

___ 4. plea   ___ 9. undo

___ 5. late   ___ 10. chow

G. Indicate with an "X" the words that contain the r-colored vowel /ɛr/.

_X_ 1. share   _X_ 6. careful

___ 2. early   _X_ 7. sparrow

_X_ 3. dearly   ___ 8. third

_X_ 4. compare   ___ 9. corridor

___ 5. fluoride   ___ 10. certain

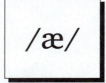

/æ/

Ash
Description

Height:	low
Advancement:	front
Lip rounding:	unrounded
Tense/lax:	lax

Sample Words

trash	jazz	smacked	language
thank	stand	asterisk	Capricorn
manage	batter	aster	blasphemy
Alabama	tamper	fantastic	trespass

Allographs

Grapheme	Example
a	back
a(ng)	hang
a(nk)	tank
au	laugh
ai	plaid

Discussion   The vowel /æ/, referred to as "ash," is the lowest of the five front vowels. (The vowel /a/, found in some eastern American dialects, is slightly lower.) It is also one of the four point vowels. In reference to the front vowels, the mandible and tongue are in their lowest position for /æ/ (see Figure 4.4). The size of the oropharynx is small for /æ/ because the tongue body is in an inferior and posterior position (see Figures 4.4 and 4.8). Like all of the other front vowels, /æ/ is unrounded. Also, /æ/ is lax; no monosyllables end with this sound. The one peculiarity of "ash" is its use in words in which it precedes the nasal /ŋ/, as in "rank" /ræŋk/ and "bang" /bæŋ/. You might be tempted to

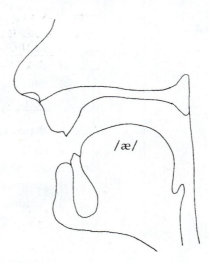

FIGURE 4.8   /æ/ articulation.

prance → præntʃ → præn†s intrusive /t/

use the vowel /eɪ/ in these words. Keep in mind that this vowel is an allophone of /æ/ in this particular context; its perception is affected by nasalization due to the nasal consonant that follows.

In the eastern and southern United States, speakers may use the vowel /æ/ in words such as "marry," "Harry," and "carry," that is, /mærɪ/, /hærɪ/, and /kærɪ/.

EXERCISE 4.5—THE VOWEL /æ/

A. Contrast the vowels in the following pairs of words by saying them aloud.

/ɛ/	/æ/	/eɪ/	/æ/
led	lad	bade	bad
tend	tanned	haze	has
den	Dan	shale	shall
Ben	ban	mate	mat
bed	bad	lane	language
Kent	can't	bane	bank
spend	spanned	Dane	dank

B. Circle the words that contain the /æ/ phoneme.

straddle	practice	lapse	revamp
pale	panther	repast	straight
Lester	pacific	pacify	farmer
baseball	hanged	chances	cards
jazz	pistol	tamed	bombastic

(circled: straddle, practice, lapse, revamp, panther, pacific, pacify, chances, baseball, jazz, bombastic)

C. Circle the phonetic transcriptions that represent English words.

/klæd/	/prid/	/strɪv/	/wæd/
/slæpt/	/bɪrd/	/bæz/	/trækt/
/web/	/steɪp/	/sprɪg/	/læzɪ/

(circled: /klæd/, /slæpt/, /bɪrd/, /trækt/, /sprɪg/)

D. In the blanks, write each of the words using English orthography.

/klæn/	clan	/spɪr/	spear
/sprɪnt/	sprint	/hɛrɪ/	hairy?
/rɛk/	wreck	/pækt/	packed
/teɪstɪ/	tasty	/dræg/	drag
/præns/	~~prance~~	/bɛrɪ/	berry
/læft/	laughed	/tinz/	teens

E. Place an "X" next to the pairs of words that share the same vowel sound.

____	badge	rage	____	hair	bend
____	seed	shade	____	lick	beer
____	cab	blonde	____	beak	bless
X	tray	whale	____	trap	bake
____	crank	shag	X	lapse	crag

Complete Assignment 4-1.

(handwritten margin notes: bʌs; ɛntsɚ; chickens—chickents; tʃɪkɪn†s)

The Back Vowels

Pronunciation Guide

/u/	as in "toot"	/tut/
/ʊ/	as in "look"	/lʊk/
/o/	as in "obese"	/obis/
/oʊ/	as in "vote"	/voʊt/ (allophone of /o/)
/ɔ/	as in "dawn"	/dɔn/
/ɑ/	as in "not"	/nɑt/

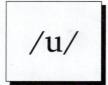

Lower-Case u
Description

Height:	high
Advancement:	back
Lip rounding:	rounded
Tense/lax:	tense

Sample Words

chew	ewe	uncouth	strewn
futile	truth	spew	loot
Truman	cruel	cucumber	tulip
clue	stupid	tuna	super

Allographs

Grapheme	Example	Grapheme	Example
u	Pluto	wo	two
ue	true	oe	shoe
u..e	tune	o	to
ui	suit	ew	stew
ou	through	ieu	lieu
oo	moon	eu	maneuver
o..e	move	ioux	Sioux

Discussion   If you compare the placement of /u/ with the placement of /i/ in the vowel quadrilateral, you will see that these two vowels are mirror images of one another, that is, they are the two highest vowels in English. Actually, all of the back vowels are approximate mirror images of their front vowel counterparts in terms of height. Because of the extremely high back tongue body position, /u/ is considered to be another point, or corner, vowel in English (see Figure 4.9). /u/ is a rounded vowel. As previously stated, although all of

ju = "you"

ju = beauty

u = booty

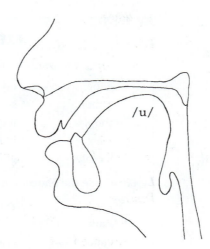

FIGURE 4.9 /u/ articulation.

the front vowels are unrounded, most of the English back vowels are rounded. The vowel /u/ is a tense vowel; it is found at the end of the one-syllable words "through," "you," and "true."

In raising the tongue to such a high position for /u/, the tongue root is forced to be somewhat advanced, widening the pharynx. As the tongue lowers in production of the back vowels from /u/ to /ɑ/, the pharynx narrows accordingly, due to the retreating movement of the tongue root, posteriorly. Figure 4.10 displays the different tongue, jaw, lip, and pharyngeal positions for /u/ and /ɑ/.

There is one peculiarity associated with the phoneme /u/ and its transcription. Notice that in words like "you," "few," and "music," /u/ is actually preceded by the consonant phoneme /j/ (/ju/, /fju/, and /mjuzɪk/). (The /j/ phoneme is the palatal "y" sound.) Without the /j/ phoneme, these words would sound like "oo," "foo," and "moosic." Some phonetics texts do treat the phoneme sequence /ju/ as a diphthong. In this text, however, we will treat /j/ + /u/ as separate monophthongs. As you examine the allographs of /u/ shown earlier, you will see several varied spellings for this phoneme.

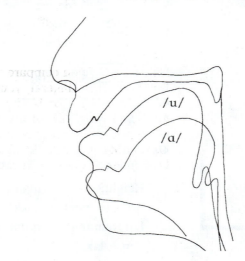

FIGURE 4.10 /u/ and /ɑ/ articulation.

EXERCISE 4.6—THE VOWEL /u/

A.   Circle the words that contain the /u/ phoneme.

(ghoul)   oboe   (crew)   plural

butter   stuck   (Lucifer)   must

should   luck   lusty   shook

(fuchsia)   look   molding   (stupor)

(loosely)   (glue)   blouse   choose

B.   Circle the phonetic transcriptions that represent English words.

/ust/   (/krud/)   /prus/   (/tul/)

/suv/   /tug/   /pus/   (/wund/)

(/pul/)   /rup/   (/lus/)   /slug/

C.   In the blanks, write each of the words using English orthography.

/spun/ *spoon*   /sup/ *soup*

/tun/ *tune*   /lud/ *lewd*

/rut/ *root*   /stru/ *strew*

/mud/ *mood*   /flu/ *flu*

/klu/ *clue*   /grum/ *groom*

/ruf/ *roof*   /snut/ *snoot*

D.   Indicate with an "X" the pairs of words that share the same vowel phoneme.

_____ 1. could   showed   _____ 6. brood   hood

__X__ 2. suit   loon   __X__ 7. stood   could

_____ 3. lute   book   _____ 8. hoops   poor

_____ 4. crew   scoot   __X__ 9. feud   moose

__X__ 5. push   foot   _____ 10. muse   cook

E.   Indicate with an "X" the words that have the phoneme sequence /j/ + /u/, as in "you."

_____ 1. oozing *uzing*   __X__ 6. fuming

__X__ 2. cute *k jut*   _____ 7. Pluto

__X__ 3. huge *h judʒ*   __X__ 8. useful

_____ 4. ruined   __X__ 9. viewing

_____ 5. sloop   _____ 10. spooky

/ʊ/

Upsilon
Description

Height:	high (lower than /u/)
Advancement:	back
Lip rounding:	rounded
Tense/lax:	lax

Sample Words

could	sugar	pushed	bull
should	would	cushion	lure*
hood	put	took	obscure*
wolf	full	stood	unsure*

*/ʊ/ in these words may be pronounced differently, depending on a speaker's dialect.

Allographs

Grapheme	Example
u	push
ou	could
u(r)	secure
oo	book
o	wolf

Discussion The vowel /ʊ/ (upsilon) is produced with the tongue body only slightly lower in the oral cavity than for /u/ (see Figure 4.11). Therefore, it also is termed high. Like /u/, the vowel /ʊ/ is rounded; unlike /u/, it is lax. You will never see open syllables ending with this phoneme, as in /bʊ/ or /tʊ/. Upsilon becomes rhotacized in combination with the consonant /r/, in formation of the r-colored vowel /ʊr/ (also transcribed as /ʊɚ/ or /ʊ͜ɚ/). The combination of /ʊ/ + /r/ may be used by some speakers in the pronunciation of the words "tour" /tʊr/ and "lure" /lʊr/. Others may pronounce these words as if they rhymed with "core," that is, /tɔr/ and /lɔr/ (see the vowel /ɔ/ on pages 79–80). Notice that there are many fewer allographs associated with /ʊ/ than for the vowel /u/.

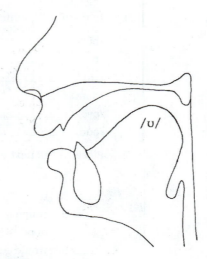

FIGURE 4.11 /ʊ/ articulation.

When the allograph "oo" is followed by /l/ (as in pool, cool, fool, and tool), the resulting pronunciation may be either /ʊ/ or /u/, depending on a speaker's dialect. Examine the following possible pronunciations of these words:

pool	/pʊl/	or	/pul/	*fool*	/fʊl/	or	/ful/
cool	/kʊl/	or	/kul/	*tool*	/tʊl/	or	/tul/

Some eastern speakers use the vowel /ʊ/ in words such as "room" /rʊm/ and "broom" /brʊm/.

EXERCISE 4.7—THE VOWEL /ʊ/

A.   Contrast the vowels in the following words.

/u/	/ʊ/	/u/	/ʊ/
who'd	hood	food	foot
cooed	could	shoed	should
Luke	look	stewed	stood

B.   Circle the words that contain the /ʊ/ phoneme.

hole	(wooden)	snooze	(stunned)
shut	(punched)	(luscious)	spook
(hood)	(couldn't)	(pulled)	(shook)
(flushed)	(mistook)	beauty	(person)
rudely	(cooker)	brood	(stood)

C.   Circle the phonetic transcriptions that represent English words.

/buk/	/stʊ/	(/rul/)	/sul/
/lʊv/	(/lum/)	(/rʊk/)	(/frut/)
(/trʊps/)	/stʊr/	(/buts/)	(/slʊg/)

D.   In the blanks, write each of the words using English orthography.

/pʊs/	puss	/tʊr/	tour?
/tru/	true	/hʊk/	hook
/stʊd/	stood	/lum/	loom
/dum/	doom	/fluk/	Fluke
/gru/	grew	/prun/	prune
/gʊd/	good	/krʊk/	crook

E.   Place an "X" next to the pairs of words that share the same vowel sound.

____ 1.	loot	foot	X 6.	what	look
X 2.	tune	mute	X 7.	nook	stood
X 3.	coupe	soon	____ 8.	rust	rook
____ 4.	flood	cute	X 9.	goof	cruise
____ 5.	would	soot	X 10.	mutt	look

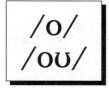

/o/
/oʊ/

Lower-Case o
Description

Height:	high-mid
Advancement:	back
Lip rounding:	rounded
Tense/lax:	tense

Sample Words The following words all take the allophone /o/ in their transcription because the syllables that contain the vowel are not stressed.

bo<u>D</u>Acious	RIb<u>o</u>flavin
Cr<u>o</u>Atian	fl<u>o</u>TILla
br<u>o</u>CADE	pr<u>o</u>HIBit
pt<u>o</u>MAINE	r<u>o</u>TAtion

The following words all take the allophone /oʊ/ because the syllables are either stressed (including monosyllables), or are at the end of a word.

cone	flow
bowl	whole
PR<u>O</u>bate	t<u>oa</u>d
ST<u>O</u>ic	SL<u>OW</u>er
BL<u>OA</u>Ted	reM<u>O</u>TE
beL<u>OW</u> (also end of word)	BELL<u>ow</u> (end of word)

Be sure to compare and contrast the words "below" and "bellow." The second syllable in "below" is stressed and the second syllable in "bellow" is not. However, both words are transcribed with /oʊ/ because this sound ends both words. In either case, the final phoneme is correspondingly lengthened.

Allographs

Grapheme	Example	Grapheme	Example
o	open	oe	foe
o..e	rose	oh	oh
oa	road	ou	soul
ow	bowl	eau	beau
ew	sew	au	cafe <u>au</u> lait

Discussion The body of the tongue is in the high-middle portion of the oral cavity during production of /o/ (see Figure 4.12). In many ways this phoneme is similar to the front allophones /e/ and /eɪ/. That is, the diphthong /oʊ/ occurs in stressed syllables and at the ends of words (regardless of stress), and the monophthong /o/ occurs in unstressed syllables. Therefore, /oʊ/ and /o/ are allophones of the same phoneme. The production of the diphthong begins with the tongue in position for the onglide /o/, in the mid-back portion of the mouth. The tongue then glides to a higher position for production of the offglide /ʊ/ (see Figure 4.2). *Phonemic* (broad) transcription would technically

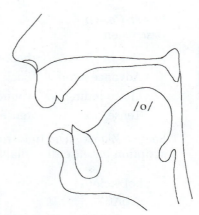

FIGURE 4.12 /o/ articulation.

dictate the use of /o/ when transcribing the allophone /oʊ/. In this text, however, the diphthong /oʊ/ will be used when transcribing this particular allophone when it occurs in stressed syllables and at the ends of words. Again, check with your instructor to determine which method is preferred.

EXERCISE 4.8—THE VOWEL /o/ – /oʊ/

A. Contrast the vowels in the following minimal pairs.

/oʊ/	/u/	/oʊ/	/ʊ/
grow	grew	coke	cook
slope	sloop	broke	brook
cope	coop	code	could
lobe	lube	hoed	hood
grope	group	showed	should
stowed	stewed	croak	crook

B. Circle the words that contain the /oʊ/ phoneme.

mope	aloof	root	toll
noose	slowed	pond	push
soda	lost	loaded	lasso
nosy	book	sugar	remote
dole	spoke	doily	wholly

C. Circle the phonetic transcriptions that represent English words.

/toʊ/	/boʊn/	/stup/	/prʊb/
/bʊt/	/floʊd/	/boʊd/	/krud/
/stub/	/stud/	/flʊk/	/woʊnt/

Continues

EXERCISE 4.8 (*cont.*)

D. In the blanks, write each of the words using English orthography.

/mould/ _mold_ /tupeɪ/ _tupay_
/kupt/ _cooped_ /bruzd/ _bruised_
/bounɪ/ _boney_ /bændeɪd/ _bandaid_
/ivouk/ _evoke_ /kʊkɪ/ _cookie_
/stoud/ _stode_ /kouɛd/ _coed_
/doupɪ/ _dopey_ /rizum/ _resume_

E. Indicate whether you should use /o/ or /ou/ when transcribing the following words.

_____ Romania   _____ snowman   _____ bowling
_____ corroded   _____ location   _____ though
_____ stolen   _____ jello   _____ notation
_____ magnolia   _____ coagulate _____ potential

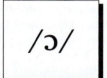

Open o
Description

Height: low-mid
Advancement: back
Lip rounding: rounded
Tense/lax: tense

Sample Words

prawn	thought	vault	wrong
awl	ought	autumn	haul
all	sought	off	gone
cord	frog	hoard	soar

Note: Some speakers (depending on dialect) may use the phoneme /ɑ/ in the production of some of these words.

Allographs

Grapheme	Example	Grapheme	Example
ou	wrought	o	log
au	laud	a	call
aw	lawn	oa	broad

Discussion The /ɔ/ vowel is often referred to as "open o." This rounded vowel is produced with the tongue slightly lower in the oral cavity than /o/, in the low-mid position (see Figure 4.13). In addition, it is a tense vowel, and it is

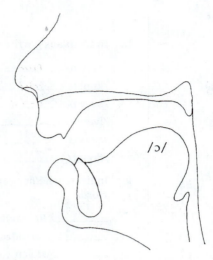

FIGURE 4.13   /ɔ/ articulation.

found in some individuals' pronunciations of the words "saw," "haul," "caught," and "awl." This vowel is difficult for many students to recognize since it is not produced by all speakers of American English; its use varies considerably with regional dialect. In many regions of the United States, the vowel has merged with /ɑ/ (discussed in the next section) so that both vowels are produced as /ɑ/. This topic will be discussed in greater detail in Chapter 9.

In words such as "corn," "bored," and "fort," it is the rhotacized, or r-colored vowel /ɔr/ (also transcribed as /ɔɚ/ or /ɔɝ/) that is used in their transcriptions—/kɔrn/, /bɔrd/, and /fɔrt/. Also, some individuals will pronounce the words "lure" and "tour" as /lɔr/ and /tɔr/, respectively. Others will use /ɔr/ in the production of the word "sure," that is, /ʃɔr/.

EXERCISE 4.9—THE VOWEL /ɔ/

A.   Circle the phonetic transcriptions that represent possible pronunciations of English words.

/bɔt/	/drʊm/	/stɔn/	/brɔn/ ⟵circled
/koʊt/	/grɔn/	/tɔk/ ⟵circled	/pʊl/
/lups/	/fɔrt/ ⟵circled	/flum/ ⟵circled	/ɔrn/

B.   In the blanks, write each of the words using English orthography.

/spɔrt/	sport	/sprɔl/	sprawl
/kʊd/	could	/stʊd/	stood
/proʊb/	probe	/frɔt/	fraught
/pruv/	prove	/kɔrps/	corpse
/stɔrd/	stored	/hʊkt/	hooked
/ɔfʊl/	awful	/doʊnet/	donate

Continues

EXERCISE 4.9 (*cont.*)

C. Indicate with an "X" the words that contain the r-colored vowel /ɔr/.

1. _____ farm   4. _____ storm   7. _____ lured
2. _____ third   5. _____ worm   8. _____ worth
3. _____ horrid   6. _____ thorn   9. _____ spar

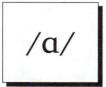

Script a
Description

Height:	low
Advancement:	back
Lip rounding:	unrounded
Tense/lax:	tense

Sample Words

rotten	ostrich	posse	cause
father	apart	latte	watch
bond	stop	car	problem
plod	bronze	Hans	smart

Note: Some speakers (depending on dialect) may use the phoneme /ɔ/ in production of some of these sample words.

Allographs

Grapheme	Example	Grapheme	Example
a	shawl	ea(r)	heart
o	rob	e(r)	sergeant
a(r)	mart		

Discussion   /ɑ/ is a point vowel due to the tongue's extremely low, back articulatory position in the oral cavity during its production (see Figure 4.14). It is the only unrounded back vowel in English. /ɑ/ is also tense. Due to dialectal variation in pronunciation, some individuals use this vowel instead of /ɔ/, especially in pronunciation of words such as "saw," "haul," "caught," and "awl." The /ɑ/ vowel is rhotacized when in combination with /r/ to form the r-colored vowel /ɑr/ (also transcribed as /ɑɚ/ or /ɑɚ/) as in the words "bark" /bɑrk/ and "art" /ɑrt/.

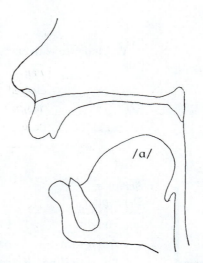

FIGURE 4.14   /ɑ/ articulation.

EXERCISE 4.10—THE VOWEL /ɑ/

A.   Contrast the vowels in the following words.

/oʊ/	/ɑ/ (or) /ɔ/ (depending on dialect)
boat	bought
bowl	ball
coat	caught
load	laud
sewed	sawed
loan	lawn

B.   Circle the phonetic transcriptions that represent possible pronunciations of English words.

/wond/	/tɔb/	(/harm/)	(/blab/)
/koʊd/	(/sɔt/)	/blad/	(/armɪ/)
(/frɔd/)	/pʊnt/	(/ad/)	(/kad/)

C.   In the blanks, write each of the words using English orthography.

/frast/	frost	/zɑr/	zhar
/lʊkt/	looked	/prund/	pruned
/bɔrd/	board	/blɔnd/	blonde
/kroʊm/	chrome	/ansɛt/	onset
/want/	want	/krɔdæd/	crawdad
/starvd/	starved	/ardvark/	ardvark

Continues

EXERCISE 4.10 (*cont.*)

D. Indicate with an "X" the words that contain the r-colored vowel /ɑr/.

1. ____ war	5. ____ starred	9. ____ poorly
2. ____ cleared	6. ____ dirt	10. ____ smarter
3. ____ quartz	7. ____ orchard	11. ____ carbon
4. ____ flare	8. ____ March	12. ____ spore

Complete Assignment 4-2.

The Central Vowels

Pronunciation Guide

/ə/	as in "<u>a</u>lone"	/əloʊn/	(unstressed)
/ʌ/	as in "but"	/bʌt/	(stressed)
/ɚ/	as in "p<u>er</u>haps"	/pɚhæps/	(unstressed)
/ɝ/	as in "heard"	/hɝd/	(stressed)

Schwa
Description

Height:	mid
Advancement:	central
Lip rounding:	unrounded
Tense/lax:	lax

Sample Words

<u>a</u>stound	p<u>a</u>rad<u>e</u>d	plantati<u>o</u>n	c<u>o</u>mmand
re<u>a</u>rrange	tang<u>e</u>nt	sp<u>u</u>moni	rel<u>e</u>v<u>a</u>nt
roast<u>e</u>d	s<u>a</u>lami	mount<u>ai</u>n	car<u>ou</u>sel
rans<u>o</u>m	ketch<u>u</u>p	tun<u>a</u>	<u>u</u>ndone

Note: /ə/ occurs in unstressed syllables in all of these words.

Allographs

Grapheme	Example	Grapheme	Example
u	<u>u</u>ntrue	ou	jeal<u>ou</u>s
o	c<u>o</u>logne	i	merr<u>i</u>ly
a	m<u>a</u>chine	oi	porp<u>oi</u>se
ai	vill<u>ai</u>n	e	happ<u>e</u>n
ia	parl<u>ia</u>ment	eo	surg<u>eo</u>n
io	nat<u>io</u>n		

Discussion   /ə/ is commonly known as "schwa." Schwa is produced with the tongue body in the most central portion of the mouth cavity. The entire vocal tract is in its most neutral configuration during production of /ə/. It is difficult to discuss this vowel without discussing another vowel concurrently, namely /ʌ/, referred to as *turned v* or "wedge." These vowels are used to represent allophones of the same sound, even though most phoneticians and clinicians treat them as two separate vowel phonemes. (There *is* actually a slight difference in their place of production in the oral cavity.) The basic distinction between these vowels is that schwa *occurs only in unstressed syllables* and turned v *occurs only in stressed syllables*. The distribution of these vowels is similar to /e/ and /eɪ/ and /o/ and /oʊ/, in reference to their occurrence in stressed and unstressed syllables:

Stressed	Unstressed
eɪ	e
oʊ	o
ʌ	ə

Schwa is unrounded because the lips do not protrude in its production. It is also a lax vowel.

EXERCISE 4.11 – THE VOWEL /ə/

A.   Circle the words that contain the /ə/ phoneme.

rowing	decision	control	untamed	laundry
lasagna	injure	glamour	opera	petunia
wooded	poorly	motion	puppy	cockroach
Laverne	ruled	holding	fuchsia	lotion

B.   Circle the phonetic transcriptions that represent English words.

/sətɪn/   /zəbrɑ/   /əbeɪt/   (/əluf/)

(/drɑmə/)   /ləpʊr/   (/bəlun/)   /rədæn/

(/səpoʊz/)   /rəpik/   (/brəzil/)   (/əndu/)

C.   In the blanks, write each of the words using English orthography.

/pinət/	peanut	/kənteɪn/	contain
/əkrɔs/	across	/lɛmən/	lemon
/vəlɔr/	valour	/bətɑn/	baton
/səport/	support	/əwɔrd/	award
/kɔfɪn/	coffin	/eɪprəl/	April
/plətun/	platoon	/kəsɛt/	caset

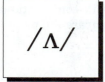

/ʌ/

Turned V
"Wedge"
Description

Height:	low-mid
Advancement:	back-central
Lip rounding:	unrounded
Tense/lax:	lax

Sample Words

r<u>u</u>b	b<u>u</u>tton	M<u>o</u>nday	m<u>u</u>stard
tr<u>ou</u>ble	l<u>u</u>ncheon	l<u>u</u>ckily	scr<u>u</u>mptious
fl<u>oo</u>d	und<u>o</u>ne	r<u>u</u>shing	p<u>u</u>blic
ab<u>u</u>ndance	st<u>u</u>mble	red<u>u</u>ndant	w<u>o</u>nderful

Note: /ʌ/ occurs in only the stressed syllables of these words.

Allographs

Grapheme	Example	Grapheme	Example
u	crumb	oe	does
o	done	ou	double
oo	flood		

Discussion   Turned v (sometimes referred to as "wedge") is found in monosyllabic words and stressed syllables. It is produced slightly lower and farther back in the oral cavity than /ə/ (see Figure 4.15). Like /ə/, /ʌ/ is unrounded and lax. Although /ʌ/ can occur in one-syllable words, it does not usually occur in open syllables in English. One exception might be in the production of the

'loˈtʃən

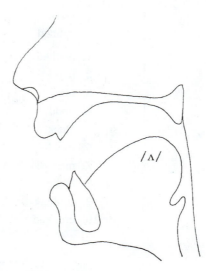

FIGURE 4.15   /ʌ/ articulation.

word "the," which usually does not receive stress in conversational English. Students often confuse /ʌ/ with the vowel /ʊ/. Compare the minimal pairs in Exercise 4.12A that contrast these two phonemes.

EXERCISE 4.12—THE VOWEL /ʌ/

A. Contrast the vowel /ʌ/ in the following minimal pairs.

/ʌ/	/ʊ/	/ʌ/	/u/	/ʌ/	/ɑ, ɔ/
cud	could	rub	rube	hut	hot
shuck	shook	done	dune	mum	mom
tuck	took	bust	boost	hug	hog
buck	book	dumb	doom	bust	bossed
stud	stood	rum	room	rub	rob
putt	put	spun	spoon	gun	gone
luck	look	glum	gloom	rubbed	robbed

B. Circle the words that contain the /ʌ/ phoneme.

awful	blunder	laundry	Hoover
custard	laborious	Sunday	lawyer
pushy	cushion	hundred	trumpet
cologne	abundant	plural	shouldn't
charades	mundane	wander	conducive

C. Examine the English words in the first column and the transcriptions in the second column. Place an "X" next to the transcription if it is wrong.

Examples:

	book	/bʊk/	_____
	subbed	/sʊbd/	X
1.	hooked	/hʌkt/	_____
2.	bond	/bʊnd/	_____
3.	bluff	/blʌf/	_____
4.	hood	/hud/	_____
5.	cluck	/klʌk/	_____
6.	rookie	/rʌkɪ/	_____
7.	mistook	/mɪstʊk/	_____
8.	lucky	/lʌkɪ/	_____
9.	rubbing	/rʊbɪŋ/	_____
10.	crooked	/krɔkəd/	_____

Continues

EXERCISE 4.12 (*cont.*)

D. Circle the phonetic transcriptions that represent English words.

/klʊstɪ/	/əpʊft/	/dʊkɪ/	/sʌntæn/
/rizən/	/krɑmd/	/pʊlɪ/	/vɪstʌ/
/mʌstɪ/	/əndʌn/	/plʌmət/	/plæzə/

E. In the blanks, write each of the words using English orthography.

/pɛrəs/	*Paris*	/robʌst/	*robust*
/hʌnɪ/	*honey*	/sʌdən/	*sudden*
/əlɑt/	*alot*	/kəbus/	*Kaboose*
/kənvɪns/	*convince*	/tʌndrə/	*tundra*
/gɑrdəd/	*guarded*	/kəlæps/	*collapse*
/flʌbd/	*flubbed*	/bəfun/	*bafoon*

F. Indicate whether /ʌ/ or /ə/ should be used in transcribing the following words by circling the appropriate symbol.

lumber	/ʌ/	/ə/	suspend	/ʌ/	/ə/
abort	/ʌ/	/ə/	suppose	/ʌ/	/ə/
shaken	/ʌ/	/ə/	induct	/ʌ/	/ə/
contain	/ʌ/	/ə/	serpent	/ʌ/	/ə/
thunder	/ʌ/	/ə/	rusty	/ʌ/	/ə/

G. Indicate with an "X" the following pairs of words that share the same vowel phoneme.

_____ 1. nuts	could		_____ 6. crook	fund
_____ 2. foot	stoop		_____ 7. blood	crust
_____ 3. done	rubbed		_____ 8. runs	floods
_____ 4. crumb	rust		_____ 9. loom	food
_____ 5. cook	should		_____ 10. rush	look

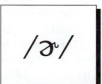

Right-Hook Schwa
"Schwar"
Description

Height:	mid
Advancement:	central
Lip rounding:	rounded
Tense/lax:	lax

Sample Words

pertain	luxury	chattering	percussion
surround	treasure	flirtatious	mattered
runner	under	countered	hibernation
ergonomic	ferocious	Saturday	harbor

Note: /ɚ/ occurs only in unstressed syllables in the sample words shown here.

Allographs

Grapheme	Example	Grapheme	Example
or	labor	er	winner
ar	lunar	ir	flirtatious
ur	urbane	yr	martyr

Discussion /ɚ/ is sometimes referred to as "schwar" because the phonetic symbol visually resembles schwa, but in addition possesses rhotacization (r-coloring). /ɚ/ is not easily defined by referring only to the four categories used previously to describe the other English vowels, that is, height, advancement, lip rounding, and tenseness. Production of /ɚ/ involves additional tongue movement and is formed by constricting the pharynx and increasing the space in the oral cavity in front of the tongue by either (1) raising the tongue tip and curling it posteriorly toward the alveolar ridge, or (2) lowering the tongue tip while bunching the tongue body in the region of the palate (*Handbook of the International Phonetic Association*, 1999; Ladefoged & Johnson, 2011; MacKay, 1987). In either case, the associated "r" quality is due to a constriction of the tongue in the epiglottal region of the pharynx (Ladefoged & Johnson, 2011).

The IPA chart (Figure 2.1) shows that schwar is missing from the vowel quadrilateral. At one time, the recommended IPA notation for this vowel was in the form of a rhotic diphthong, i.e., /əɹ/ or /ə˞/, indicating the rhotacization of the vowel (Pullum & Ladusaw, 1996). Currently, the IPA recommends the use of /ə/ plus /˞/, the diacritic for *rhoticity* (known as the "right-hook"), as the proper notation for transcribing this rhotacized mid-central vowel, i.e., /ə/ + /˞/ = /ɚ/. You will find the rhoticity diacritic /˞/ located in the IPA chart in the last row of the first column of the diacritics section (Figure 2.1). Interestingly, the *Handbook of the International Phonetic Association* (1999) also recommends the use of the rhoticity diacritic in transcribing other rhotic diphthongs (e.g., "far" /fɑ˞/ or "core" /kɔ˞/). Like schwa, /ɚ/ is produced only in unstressed syllables. Therefore, it is lax. One distinguishing feature of schwar is that it is produced with lip rounding. The degree of lip rounding varies from speaker to speaker. (Some phoneticians argue that this vowel is unrounded.)

Note: Words such as "ring" and "raisin" begin with the phoneme /r/, *not* with the phoneme /ɚ/. That is, /rɪŋ/ and /reɪzɪn/ *not* /ɚɪŋ/ and /ɚeɪzɪn/. Similarly, the words "unread" and "berate" should be transcribed as /ənrɛd/ and /bireɪt/, *not* /ənɚɛd/ and /biɚeɪt/.

EXERCISE 4.13 — THE VOWEL /ɚ/

A. Contrast the underlined sounds in the words below.

/ɚ/	/r/	/r/-colored vowels
slumb<u>er</u>	<u>d</u>ress	que<u>er</u>
p<u>er</u>use	<u>r</u>ibbon	me<u>re</u>
ov<u>er</u>	<u>cr</u>eam	sna<u>re</u>
stup<u>or</u>	th<u>r</u>ead	chai<u>r</u>
walk<u>er</u>	<u>fr</u>ost	sto<u>red</u>
must<u>ard</u>	a<u>r</u>ound	floo<u>r</u>

B. Circle the words that contain the /ɚ/ phoneme.

(clover) rebel barley dearly
fearless endear (perjure) fester
carbon torment harbor electric
tremor written poorly breezy
(laundered) (perhaps) torpedo (surprise)

C. Circle the phonetic transcriptions that represent English words.

(/kʌnvɚt/) /pəteɪn/ *pertayin* /pɚsɛnt/ (/lɛpəd/)
(/rɑbɚ/) /tɚoʊd/ (/drimɚ/) /fɚɚst/
(/sɚvɛs/) /ɚɛdɪ/ /ʌnfer/ (/hɪndɚ/)

D. In the blanks, write each of the words using English orthography.

/drɛsɚ/	dresser	/kəntɔrt/	contort
/kæmrə/	camera	/pɚanə/	perana
/rʌbɚ/	rubber	/pɚu/	purve
/mɑrbəl/	marble	/sɪmɚ/	simmer
/təreɪn/	turain	/kɛrosin/	kerosine
/flʌstɚd/	flustered	/əweɪtəd/	unweighted

/ɝ/

Right-Hook Reversed Epsilon
Description

Height:	mid
Advancement:	central
Lip rounding:	rounded
Tense/lax:	tense

Sample Words

c<u>ur</u>se	th<u>ir</u>d	Th<u>ur</u>sday	av<u>er</u>sion
det<u>er</u>	s<u>ur</u>geon	w<u>or</u>ry	rev<u>erse</u>
reh<u>ear</u>se	p<u>ur</u>ple	th<u>ir</u>sty	n<u>ur</u>sery
f<u>ur</u>nace	s<u>er</u>vice	p<u>er</u>colate	m<u>ur</u>der*

***Note:** The word "murder" would be transcribed as /mɝdɚ/.

Allographs

Grapheme	Example	Grapheme	Example
or	word	ir	shirt
ear	learn	ur	curt
er	perk	yr	Myrtle

Discussion   /ɝ/ occurs only in stressed syllables. It is produced in a manner similar to /ɚ/ with the lips rounded, although the degree of rounding varies among speakers (see Figure 4.16). (Like schwar, this vowel is considered unrounded by some phoneticians.) /ɝ/ is the only central vowel that is considered to be tense. It is found at the end of the one-syllable words "her," "stir," and "fur," and for some speakers "sure." Keep in mind that /ɝ/ occurs in only the stressed syllables of the sample words just provided.

We now can add /ɚ/ and /ɝ/ to the table of stressed and unstressed vowel allophones:

Stressed	Unstressed
eɪ	e
oʊ	o
ʌ	ə
ɝ	ɚ

Similar to the symbol for schwar /ɚ/, /ɝ/ is not located in the vowel quadrilateral. Instead the symbol is a combination of *reversed epsilon* /ɜ/ plus the right-hook diacritic /˞/, hence its name, "right-hook reversed epsilon." Reversed epsilon /ɜ/ is a non-rhotacized, mid-central vowel, part of the IPA chart, but not generally used by speakers of American English. However, in British English and in some American dialects, it is the vowel found in words such as "word" and "curtains" (i.e., /wɜd/ and /kɜtənz/). Try saying these two words without r-coloring when trying to produce reversed epsilon. The use of /ɜ/ in British English will be discussed in greater detail in Chapter 9.

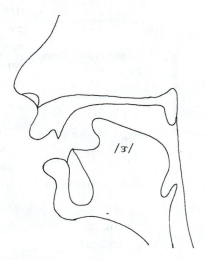

FIGURE 4.16   /ɝ/ articulation.

Right-hook reversed epsilon /ɝ/ is often confused with the rhotic diphthongs, previously introduced in this chapter. Especially confusing are /ɝ/
versus /ɪr/ and /ɛr/. Examine the following word combinations, paying close
attention to the distinction between /ɝ/ and the rhotic diphthongs. Each of the
words in the left column contain a different rhotic diphthong. All of the words
in the right column contain /ɝ/. Say each word pair (i.e., fear-fur; hair-her, etc.)
listening to the differences between the rhotic diphthongs and /ɝ/. Also, be sure
to look at Exercise 4.14A.

		/ɝ/				/ɝ/
/ɪr/	fear	___	fur	/ɪr/	beer	___ burr
/ɛr/	hair	___	her	/ɛr/	spare	___ spur
/ɑr/	star	___	stir	/ɑr/	shark	___ shirk
/ɔr/	court	___	curt	/ɔr/	ward	___ word
/ʊr/	tour	___	tur(n)	/ʊr/	lure	___ lear(n)

In some dialects of English, notably Southern and Eastern American English,
the central rhotic vowels /ɝ/ and /ɚ/ may undergo **derhotacization** (produced
without r-coloring), and pronounced as /ɜ/ and /ə/, respectively. The result is
the production of /ɜ/ in words that normally call for /ɝ/, and the production of
/ə/ in words that normally call for /ɚ/—"girl" /gɜl/ and "tiger" /taɪgə/. Derhotacization of vowels will be discussed in more detail in the section devoted to
regional dialects in Chapter 9.

EXERCISE 4.14—THE VOWEL /ɝ/

A. Contrast the vowel /ɝ/ with the rhotic diphthongs in the following minimal
contrasts.

/ɝ/	/ɑr/	/ɔr/	/ɪr/	/ɛr/
stir	star	store	steer	stare
purr	par	pore	peer	pair
fur	far	for	fear	fair
burr	bar	bore	beer	bare
myrrh	mar	more	mere	mare

B. Circle the words that contain the /ɝ/ phoneme.

forward	muster	warship	steered	morale
disturbed	pretend	wordy	distort	persistent
terrible	turban	January	conserve	choir
conversion	arid	stirrup	barren	fearless

Continues

EXERCISE 4.14 (*cont.*)

C.   Circle the phonetic transcriptions that represent English words.

/kʌstəd/   /lɝdɪ/   /kərɪr/ *career*   /vɝsəz/

/pɝsən/   /hɝdəd/   /fɝmɚ/   /dɝsənt/

/plædɚ/   /fɔrən/   /ɝbɔrt/   /kɝsɚ/

D.   In the blanks, write each of the words using English orthography.

/smɝkt/   smirked   /kənvɝt/   convert

/ovɝt/   overt   /wɪspɚ/   whisper

/kɛrət/   carrot   /bɝbən/   bourbon

/sʌbɚb/   suburb   /skwɝts/   squirts

/supɝb/   superb   /səhɛrə/   sahara

E.   Indicate whether /ɝ/ or /ɚ/ should be used in transcribing the following words by circling the appropriate symbol.

erasure	/ɝ/	(/ɚ/)	ermine	(/ɝ/)	/ɚ/
surprise	/ɝ/	(/ɚ/)	color	/ɝ/	(/ɚ/)
furnace	(/ɝ/)	/ɚ/	infer	(/ɝ/)	/ɚ/
curtail	/ɝ/	(/ɚ/)	terror	/ɝ/	(/ɚ/)
immerse	(/ɝ/)	/ɚ/	duster	/ɝ/	(/ɚ/)

F.   Indicate with an "X" the pairs of words that share the same vowel phoneme.

____ 1. herd	cheered	____ 6. hair	queer
____ 2. cord	word	_X_ 7. birch	lurk
____ 3. lured	stored	_X_ 8. hoard	lord
_X_ 4. ark	smart	____ 9. pear	heard
_X_ 5. fears	cheer	____ 10. term	peered

G.   For the following, indicate whether the word contains a rhotic diphthong or /ɝ/ (in any syllable) by placing the correct symbol in the blank.

Examples:

/ɪr/	cheer	/ɝ/	stir
_ɝ_ 1. mirth		____ 11. appearance	
____ 2. flared		____ 12. Carol	
____ 3. cirrus		____ 13. furtive	
____ 4. serenade		____ 14. larynx	
____ 5. Merlin		____ 15. experience	
____ 6. cherub		____ 16. disturbing	
____ 7. portion		____ 17. clearance	
____ 8. farming		____ 18. nervous	
____ 9. sparrow		____ 19. furious	
____ 10. nervous		____ 20. clairvoyant	

Complete Assignment 4-3.

More on Diphthongs

The diphthongs /eɪ/ and /oʊ/ were discussed earlier as allophones of /e/ and /o/, respectively. In English, there are three additional diphthong phonemes that do not exist in a monophthongal form. That is, they do not vary in relation to phonetic context. These three diphthongs are /aɪ/ as in "kite," /aʊ/ as in "loud," and /ɔɪ/ as in "void."

There is considerable variation in the symbols used to transcribe these three diphthongs. This is due to the fact that the exact articulation of these phonemes varies by dialect and by phonetic context. Similar to /eɪ/ and /oʊ/, these diphthongs should be thought of as having two distinctive articulations. That is, there is a gliding of the tongue from the first articulatory position (the onglide) to the second position (the offglide); the exact starting and ending position varies from speaker to speaker. As mentioned previously, the one commonality among all of the diphthongs (including /eɪ/ and /oʊ/) is the fact that the tongue always glides from a lower to a higher position in the oral cavity (see Figure 4.2). The symbols chosen for this text to represent the three diphthongs are the ones most often adopted by most phonetics texts. They also represent a fairly close approximation of the actual articulation of these sounds. Keep in mind that some people transcribe these diphthongs with a tie bar as in /a͡ɪ/, /ɔ͡ɪ/, and /a͡ʊ/.

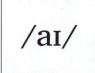

/aɪ/

Pronunciation Guide

/aɪ/	as in "buy"	/baɪ/
/aʊ/	as in "bough"	/baʊ/
/ɔɪ/	as in "boy"	/bɔɪ/

Sample Words

lye	ice
fiber	light
thyme	tie
buy	feisty

Allographs

Grapheme	Example	Grapheme	Example
i..e	write	uy	buy
i	sigh	ie	tried
ai	aisle	ei	height
ae	maestro	ey	eye
y	my	ay	aye

Discussion The tongue body begins in the low central or low back portion of the mouth (depending on dialect) in the production of the onglide /a/ and moves to the high front position for the offglide /ɪ/. The initial phoneme in this diphthong represents a vowel monophthong not commonly used by all speakers in the United States. It does exist in the speech patterns of individuals from Boston and other areas of the eastern United States in pronunciation of words such as "park" /pak/ or "car" /ka/.

Some speakers in the East and South produce this diphthong as the monophthong /a/ as in the words "might" /mat/ and "ice" /as/.

EXERCISE 4.15—THE DIPHTHONG /aɪ/

A.   Contrast the diphthong /aɪ/ in the following minimal pairs.

/aɪ/	/ɪ/	/eɪ/
kite	kit	Kate
height	hit	hate
sight	sit	sate
wind (verb)	wind (noun)	waned
lime	limb	lame
style	still	stale
tyke	tick	take

B.   Circle the words that contain the /aɪ/ phoneme.

power	spacious	machine	replaced
(slice)	delicious	Formica	traded
(contrite)	(spider)	maybe	(piped)
lever	(Cairo)	(cider)	(supplied)
(rivalry)	razor	piano	spigot

C.   Circle the phonetic transcriptions that represent English words.

/fraɪdɚ/   /braɪmɚ/   /taɪfraɪn/   (/rəvaɪz/)

/məbaɪ/   /naɪlɔn/   /prədaɪt/   (/traɪdɛnt/)

(/traɪd/)   (/laɪɚ/)   (/haɪəst/)   (/straɪpt/)

D.   In the blanks, write each of the words using English orthography.

/sɚpraɪz/	surprise	/klaɪmæks/	climax
/kəlaɪd/	collide	/preɪlin/	pralene
/treɪlɚ/	trailer	/baɪsɛps/	biceps
/praɪmet/	primate	/waɪɚd/	wired
/vaɪrəs/	virus	/taɪred/	tirade
/deɪlaɪt/	daylight	/daɪmənd/	diamond

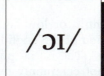

/ɔɪ/

Sample Words

toy	join	ah<u>oy</u>	flamb<u>oy</u>ant
expl<u>oi</u>t	b<u>oi</u>sterous	f<u>oi</u>ble	c<u>oi</u>ned

Allographs

Grapheme	Example
oy	soy
oi	foil

Discussion   The tongue body begins in the low-mid back position of the mouth (for /ɔ/) and glides to a high front position (for /ɪ/). When initiating this diphthong, the lips are rounded. As the tongue glides upward in the oral cavity toward the offglide portion, the lips become unrounded. In the South, some speakers will produce this diphthong as the monophthong /ɔ/, as in "oil" /ɔl/ and "soil" /sɔl/.

EXERCISE 4.16—THE DIPHTHONG /ɔɪ/

A. Contrast the diphthong /ɔɪ/ in the following minimal pairs.

/ɔɪ/	/aɪ/	/eɪ/
Boyd	bide	bade
soy	sigh	say
coil	Kyle	kale
hoist	heist	haste
loin	line	lane
boys	buys	bays
poise	pies	pays

B. Circle the words that contain the /ɔɪ/ phoneme.

repay	(hoisted)	(voiceless)	reward
(loiter)	crowded	fiery	tiled
straight	feisty	(coy)	(cloying)
crime	(broiler)	stoic	(destroy)
(goiter)	razor	(avoid)	supplied

C. Circle the phonetic transcriptions that represent English words.

(/kwaɪət/)	(/sprɔɪdɪn/)	/dɔɪəz/	/plɔɪdənt/
(/mɝdɚ/)	(/blaɪndlɪ/)	/ənstraɪt/	/taɪpsɛt/
(/pɔɪzən/)	(/vɔɪdəd/)	(/rikɔɪld/)	(/taɪwɑn/)

D. In the blanks, write each of the words using English orthography.

/ɔɪlɪ/	oily	/ændrɔɪd/	android
/maɪstroʊ/	miɑtro	/laɪvlɪ/	lively
/taɪfɔɪd/	taifoid	/ɪnvɔɪs/	invoice
/pɑrbɔɪl/	parboil	/ɔɪstɚ/	oyster
/haɪndsaɪt/	hindsight	/haɪɔɪd/	hyoid
/baɪaʊt/	buyout	/deɪlaɪt/	daylight

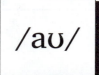

/aʊ/

Sample Words

loud	s<u>ou</u>r
clown	tr<u>ou</u>sers
ar<u>ou</u>nd	p<u>ow</u>der
fl<u>ó</u>wer	r<u>ou</u>sed

Allographs

Grapheme	Example
ou	house
ow	cow

Discussion   The tongue begins in the low back position of the mouth for the onglide /ɑ/ and glides upward to the high back position for the production of the offglide /ʊ/. When initiating this diphthong, the lips are unrounded. As the glide progresses toward the offglide, the lips become rounded.

EXERCISE 4.17—THE DIPHTHONG /aʊ/

A.   Contrast the diphthong /aʊ/ in the following minimal pairs.

/aʊ/	/oʊ/	/aɪ/	/ɔɪ/
bough	bow	buy	boy
sow	sew	sigh	soy
cowl	coal	Kyle	coil
row (quarrel)	row	rye	Roy
towel	toll	tile	toil
fowls	foals	files	foils

B.   Circle the words that contain the /aʊ/ phoneme.

toilet	(dowdy)	(frown)	(bounty)
(mousy)	(allowed)	loaded	probate
beauty	explode	soils	(proud)
(astound)	toil	(chowder)	crowbar
hello	toad	chastise	scrolled

C.   Circle the phonetic transcriptions that represent English words.

(/taɪəd/)	(/laʊzɪ/)	(/aɪvrɪ/)	/hoʊmbɔɪ/
/rɪbaʊ/	/blaʊkɚ/	(/rɔɪdɪ/)	/kaʊtaʊ/
/waʊntɪd/	/roʊgbɪ/	/paʊzɚ/	/aʊəlɪ/

D.   In the blanks, write each of the words using English orthography.

/bɔɪfrɛnd/	boyfriend	/roʊboʊt/	rowboat
/klɑndaɪk/	Klondike	/pɪspaɪp/	pigpipe
/daʊntaʊn/	downtown	/sɚaʊnd/	surround
/sloʊɚ/	slower	/doʊnʌt/	donut
/faʊndəd/	founded	/klaɪənt/	client
/vaɪzɚ/	viser	/braʊzɚ/	browser

Complete Assignment 4-4.

Review Exercises

A. Describe each of the following vowels by providing their tongue height, tongue advancement, lip rounding, and tense/lax characteristics. *general phonetic description*

	Height	Advancement	Rounded	Tense/Lax
i	high	front	no	tense
ʊ	high	back	*(marked)*	lax
ɝ	mid	central	*(marked)*	tense
ə	mid	central	*(marked)*	lax
o	mid	back	*(marked)*	tense
u	high	back	*(marked)*	tense
ɛ	mid	front	no	lax
ɚ	mid	central	*(marked)*	lax
ʌ	mid	central	*(marked)*	tense
e	mid	front	*(marked)*	tense
ɪ	high	front	no	lax
ɑ	low	back	*(marked)*	lax
ɔ	mid	back	*(marked)*	lax
æ	low	front	no	lax

(handwritten vowel chart in right margin with labels: lips, spread, rounded, front, central, back, closed, jaw, open, and vowel positions i, ɪ, e, ɛ, æ, ɝ, ʌ, ə, u, ʊ, o, ɔ, ɑ, high, mid, low)

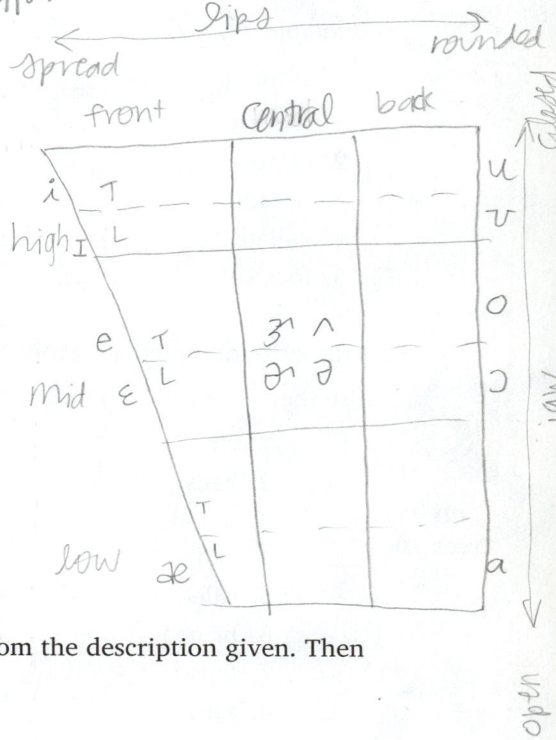

B. For the following items, fill in the blank with the appropriate vowels from the description given. Then write the word in English orthography.

Example:

	/mit/	high, front, tense vowel	meat
1.	/b_æ_d/	low, front	bad
2.	/s_ʌ_n/	low-mid, back-central	
3.	/sl_ɛ_pt/	low-mid, front	
4.	/s_u_p/	high, back, tense	soup
5.	/k_ɔ_rd/	low-mid, back	cord
6.	/f_ʊ_t/	high, back, lax	foot
7.	/f_ɪ_z/	high, front, lax	fiz
8.	/p_ɑ_rk/	low, back	park
9.	/w_ɝ_d/	mid-central, tense	word
10.	/kr_o_z/	high-mid, back	crows

(handwritten in right margin: aʊ, ɔɪ, aɪ, ju)

C. For each of the the following two-syllable words, indicate whether each vowel is tense (T) or lax (L).

Example:

	lasso	L	T
1.	Sunday	T	T
2.	bashful	L	L
3.	laundry	L	T

4.	confused	L	T
5.	fender	L	L
6.	concern	L	T

7. regroup   <u>T</u>   <u>T</u>   9. layette   <u>T</u>   <u>L</u>
8. obese   <u>I</u>   <u>T</u>   10. abrupt   <u>L</u>   <u>I</u>

D. For the following two-syllable words, indicate whether each vowel is rounded (R) or unrounded (U).

Example:

lasso   <u>U</u>   <u>R</u>

1. foolish   <u>R</u>   <u>U</u>   6. Pluto   <u>R</u>   <u>R</u>
2. curfew   <u>R</u>   <u>R</u>   7. person   <u>R</u>   <u>V</u>
3. decade   <u>V</u>   <u>U</u>   8. pursuit <u>R</u>   <u>R</u>
4. collate   <u>R</u>   <u>U</u>   9. rugby   <u>U</u>   <u>U</u>
5. football <u>R</u>   <u>R</u>   10. lower   <u>R</u>   <u>U</u>

E. Transcription Practice—Front Vowels

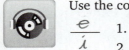

Use the correct IPA symbol(s) (i, ɪ, e, eɪ, ɛ, æ) for each of the front vowels in the following words.

<u>e</u> 1. straight   <u>ɛ</u> <u>i</u> 11. empty
<u>i</u> 2. bees   <u>e</u> <u>i</u> 12. rabies
CD #1 <u>ɛ</u> 3. bread   <u>I</u> <u>ɛ</u> 13. instead
Track 20 <u>ɛ</u> 4. can   <u>ɛ</u> <u>i</u> 14. stampede
<u>I</u> 5. filled   <u>e</u> <u>e</u> 15. vacate
<u>i</u> 6. bring   <u>i</u> <u>ɪ</u> 16. pleasing
<u>æ</u> 7. lapse   <u>ɛ</u> <u>I</u> 17. transit
<u>e</u> 8. sang   <u>i</u> <u>ɛ</u> 18. beer can
<u>ɛ</u> 9. fair   <u>I</u> <u>ɛ</u> 19. implant
<u>i</u> 10. mean   <u>ɛ</u> <u>ɪ</u> 20. barely

F. Transcription Practice—Back Vowels

Use the correct IPA symbol(s) (u, ʊ, o, oʊ, ɔ, ɑ) for each of the back vowels in the following words.

<u>o</u> 1. moat   <u>ɑ</u> <u>ʊ</u> 11. awful
<u>ʊ</u> 2. push   <u>ɔ</u> <u>ɑ</u> 12. Clorox
CD #1 <u>ɑ</u> 3. laud   <u>o</u> <u>o</u> 13. loco
Track 21 <u>ɑ</u> 4. locks   <u>o</u> <u>o</u> 14. oboe
<u>u</u> 5. crude   <u>ɑ</u> <u>o</u> 15. taco
<u>o</u> 6. chose   <u>ɑ</u> <u>ɑ</u> 16. monarch
<u>ɑ</u> 7. raw   <u>ɑ</u> <u>ɔ</u> 17. popcorn
<u>ʊ</u> 8. lure   <u>u</u> <u>ʊ</u> 18. truthful
<u>ɔ</u> 9. sword   <u>ɑ</u> <u>u</u> 19. costume
<u>ɑ</u> 10. card   <u>u</u> <u>ɑ</u> 20. crouton

G. Transcription Practice—Central Vowels

CD #1
ack 22

Use the correct IPA symbol(s) (ə, ʌ, ɚ, ɝ) for each of the central vowels in the following words.

ɝ	ə	1. certain	ɝ	ə	11. purpose
ʌ	ə	2. rusted	ʌ	ə	12. sudden
ɚ	ɝ	3. perturb	ʌ	ɚ	13. luster
ə	ɝ	4. assert	ɝ	ə	14. purchase
ʌ	ɚ	5. upper	ɝ	ɚ	15. sherbet
ɝ	ɚ	6. merger	ʌ	ɚ	16. mother
ʌ	ɚ	7. clutter	ə	ɝ	17. converge
ɝ	ə	8. verbal	ɝ	ɚ	18. herder
ə	ɝ	9. traverse	ɝ	ə	19. worded
ɝ	ɚ	10. learner	ʌ	ɚ	20. mustard

H. Diphthong Practice

Some of the following words have the wrong diphthong/vowel symbol in their transcriptions. If there is an error, write the correct symbol in the blank.

1. word	/wɝd/		16. maestro	/maɪstroʊ/	
2. lard	/lɔrd/	lard	17. flour	/floʊɚ/	flaʊɚ
3. carp	/kɝp/	karp	18. pouring	/pɔrɪŋ/	pɔrɪŋ
4. war	/wɑr/	wɔr	19. liar	/laɪɚ/	
5. mere	/mɪr/	mir	20. appear	/əpɛr/	əpɪr
6. wide	/weɪd/	waɪd	21. tighter	/taɪtɝ/	taɪtɚ
7. curd	/kʊrd/	kɝd	22. parrot	/pɝət/	pɛrət
8. stay	/steɪ/		23. corner	/kɔrnɚ/	
9. pray	/praɪ/	pre	24. oyster	/ɔɪstɛr/	ɔɪstɚ
10. crow	/kraʊ/	kro	25. squarely	/skwɛrlɪ/	skwɛrlɪ
11. coin	/kɔɪn/		26. silence	/sɪləns/	saɪləns
12. pride	/praɪd/		27. smarter	/smɔrtɚ/	smartɚ
13. firm	/fɪrm/	fɝm	28. avoid	/əvaɪd/	əvɔɪd
14. tour	/tʊr/		29. prowess	/proəs/	praʊɛs
15. fair	/fɛr/		30. license	/leɪsəns/	laɪsəns

I. Using /ɝ/ and the rhotic diphthongs listed below, create as many meaningful English words as possible for each of the following items.

/ɪr, ʊr, ɔr, ɑr, ɛr, ɝ/

Example:

b ____ beer, boor, bore, bar, bear, burr

1. p ____ peer, poor, pore, par, pear, purr
2. r ____ rear, roar, rare
3. d ____ t door, dare
4. w ____ d weed, wood, would, wear, were
5. k ____ d keyed, cooed, core, care

J. Using the vowels listed below, create as many meaningful English words as possible for each of the following items.

/i, ɪ, eɪ, ɛ, æ, u, ʊ, oʊ, ɔ, ɑ, ɝ, ʌ/

Example:

	z	ease, is, as, ooze, owes, awes, Oz
1.	___ d	add, owed, odd
2.	___ n	in, an, own, on, earn, urn
3. l	___ st	lean, loon, loan, learn
4. sk	___ n	skin, skan, scone
5. st	___ d	steed, stayed, stead, stood, stirred, stud
6. b	___ rd	beard, beared, bored, board, bird, barred
7. t	___ nt	tent, tint, taint, taunt
8. s	___ t	seat, sit, set, sat, rut, sought,
9. r	___ t	rate, rat, root, rot, rut, wrote
10. r	___ bd	ribbed, robed, robbed, rubbed
11. sp	___ t	spit, spat, spot, spirt
12. w	___ d	weed, wed, wood, wad, word

K. Write each of the following transcribed words in English orthography.

1. /kʌstəmz/   customs
2. /əbaʊnd/   abound
3. /twɔrd/   toward
4. /slɛndɚ/   slender
5. /kɛrfri/   carefree
6. /veɪkənt/   vacant
7. /bʌntəd/   bunted
8. /klaʊdɪ/   cloudy
9. /steɪplɚ/   stapler
10. /kəntɔrt/   contort
11. /saɪrənz/   sirens
12. /klɔɪstɚd/   cloistered
13. /ohaɪoʊ/   Ohio
14. /reɪdɪoʊ/   radio
15. /kɚoʊsɪv/   corrosive
16. /plətɑnək/   platonic
17. /rɛzənet/   resonate
18. /daɪgrɛs/   digress
19. /saɪfənd/   siphoned
20. /ɑrkənsɔ/   Arkansas
21. /wʌndɚfʊl/   wonderful

22. /kæləndɚ/   _calendar_
23. /rimɔrsfʊl/   _remorseful_
24. /stupɛndəs/   _stupendous_
25. /læksətɪv/   _laxative_
26. /sɪnsɪrlɪ/   _sincerely_
27. /kɑləndɚ/   _callender_
28. /rezənɛts/   _raisenettes_
29. /bɛrəton/   _baritone_
30. /disɛmbɚ/   _December_
31. /mɛksɪkou/   _Mexico_
32. /kwægmaɪɚ/   _Quagmier?_
33. /ɔrdəlɪ/   _orderly_
34. /hɝbəsaɪd/   _herbicide_
35. /rəpʌlsɪv/   _repulsive_
36. /kɛrəktɚ/   _character_
37. /sæsəfræs/   _sasafras_
38. /zaɪləfon/   _xylophone_
39. /kwɔrtɚbæk/   _quarterback_
40. /ɛmbɛrəst/   _embarassed_

L. Transcription Practice—Front, Back, and Central Vowels

Use the correct IPA symbol(s) for each of the vowels in the following words.

ɛ	ɪ	1. epic		i	ɨ	21. inkling
æ	ɚ	2. faster		ɛ	e	22. Fairbanks
ʌ	ɚ	3. wonder		ɑ	u	23. car pool
ɑ	ɛ	4. octet		ə	i	24. machine
ʊ	ɛ	5. woolen		æ	ɪ	25. Athens
i	o	6. depot		ɑ	ə	26. autumn
ɔ	ɚ	7. soldier		i	ə	27. rebus
ɪ	i	8. itchy		ɔ	ɛ	28. torment
ɝ	ɪ	9. worship		ʌ	ɚ	29. utter
æ	ɪ	10. palace		ʌ	ə	30. bushel
ɛ	ɨ	11. barely		ɔ	ə	31. corner
e	ə	12. nation		ɑ	i	32. quandary
i	ə	13. genius		æ	ɚ	33. aster
ʌ	ɚ	14. cupboard		o	u	34. phone booth
ɑ	u	15. cartoon		ʌ	ɛ	35. turban
æ	ɨ	16. nasty		i	e	36. key case
i	ɛ	17. fearless		ɔ	ɚ	37. boarder
ʌ	ɚ	18. number		ɛ	ɨ	38. blaring
e	ə	19. sanction		e	ə	39. strangle
o	ə	20. ocean		ɑ	ə	40. awesome

M. Transcribe the vowels in the following words.

CD #1
Track 24

ɔɪ	ɚ	1.	broiler
aʊ	æ	2.	mousetrap
ɔ	a	3.	boardwalk
o	ʊ	4.	closure
aɪ	a	5.	nylons
ɛ	ɔɪ	6.	steroid
a	ə	7.	starstruck
ɛ	i	8.	regime
æ	ə	9.	bashful
ɝ	ɚ	10.	perjure
i	ɛ	11.	spearmint
aɪ	ə	12.	lightbulb
ə	ɔɪ	13.	destroy
e	ɛ	14.	banquet
aɪ	ɔ	15.	eyesore

ɛ	ɚ	16.	gender
aɪ	ə	17.	China
a	ɪ	18.	jaundiced
ʌ	ɔɪ	19.	turquoise
ɪ	ɔɪ	20.	invoice
aɪ	ɛ	21.	financed
ɝ	ɛ	22.	merchant
o	e	23.	proclaim
o	e	24.	probate
ʊ	aɪ	25.	July
a	ɪ	26.	martian
ju	ɚ	27.	future
a	ɛ	28.	prospect
a	ə	29.	product
o	u	30.	tofu

Study Questions

1. What is the vowel quadrilateral and what is its importance in the study of phonetics?
2. Which vowels in English are tense? Which ones are lax? How does your understanding of syllables help in understanding the use of tense and lax vowels in English?
3. How are vowels produced in the vocal tract?
4. Which vowels in English are rounded? Which ones are unrounded?
5. What is a point vowel? List the English point vowels.
6. Why isn't the final sound in the word "lucky" transcribed with /i/?
7. Define the terms *onglide* and *offglide*.
8. Which vowels in English are affected by syllable stress?
9. What is the difference between a monophthong and a diphthong?
10. What is the relationship between tongue movement and pharyngeal shape during vowel production?

Online Resources

University of Iowa. (2001–2013). fənɛtɪks: the sounds of spoken English. Retrieved from
    http://www.uiowa.edu/~acadtech/phonetics/#
    (video and animation of English, German, and Spanish vowel/diphthong production)
University of Victoria Department of Linguistics, Linguistics IPA Lab. (n.d.). *Public IPA chart.* Retrieved from
    http://web.uvic.ca/ling/resources/ipa/charts/IPAlab/IPAlab.htm
    (interactive IPA chart with pronunciations of all IPA vowel symbols)

Consonants

What Is a Consonant?

Although this seems like a simple question, unfortunately the answer is not so simple. The term **consonant** can be defined in several ways. It is possible to define consonants in terms of the letters used to represent them or by the way they are formed by the articulators. Consonants also can be defined in terms of their particular role in the structure of syllables, or by their acoustic and physical properties. To best answer the question *What is a consonant?* we need to consider all of these issues.

We already know that there are many more consonant letters in the Roman alphabet than vowels. Likewise, there are more consonant than vowel phonemes. In Chapter 4, we learned that there are approximately 14 vowel phonemes in American English plus 5 diphthongs. In this chapter, 24 consonant phonemes will be introduced. As you are aware, the IPA symbols for the consonants are well represented by the letters of the Roman alphabet. There are only a few new symbols to learn in order to transcribe English consonants. In this respect, consonant transcription is easier to learn than vowel transcription. In addition to the 24 consonant phonemes, some of the more common allophonic variations of some of the consonants will be introduced.

Consonants Versus Vowels

In terms of production, vowels and consonants vary considerably. Unlike vowels, consonants are not produced solely by changes in tongue and lip positioning. Consonants are produced by vocal tract constrictions that modify the breath stream coming from the larynx. Consonant production generally involves the coming together of two articulators to modify the flow of air as it passes through the oral and/or nasal cavities. The tongue, the primary articulator in production of consonants, makes contact with other articulators to form most of the English consonants. In addition, there are several consonants that do not utilize the tongue in their production, for example, /h/, /b/, and /f/.

Another way in which vowels and consonants vary is in relation to where the sound generator (or sound source) is located during their production. The sound source for all of the vowels is at the level of the vocal folds. Thus, for vowel production, the breath stream coming from the larynx is voiced (vocal folds vibrating) creating resonance throughout the entire vocal tract. As you recall, changes in lip and tongue position cause alterations in the resonant frequencies of the vocal tract, giving each vowel its characteristic timbre. Similar to the vowels, the **sonorant consonants**, or simply *sonorants,* are produced with resonance occurring throughout the entire vocal tract. This is why the sonorants are also sometimes referred to as **resonant consonants**. The sonorant consonants include the nasals, the liquids, and the glides, all of which are voiced. The sonorants are produced with little constriction in the vocal tract and with little turbulence in the airstream as it passes through the oral cavity. Refer to Table 5.1 for a classification of all the English consonants.

The sound source for several consonants, however, is not in the larynx. For some consonants, the primary sound source is the noise (or turbulence) created at the point of constriction in the oral cavity, formed by the articulators, as air flows through the supralaryngeal system. Consonants produced in this manner are called **obstruents** (because the airflow is obstructed during their articulation). Obstruents are sometimes referred to as **non-resonant consonants**. Obstruents include the stop, fricative, and affricate consonants. In the production of obstruents, resonance does not occur throughout the entire vocal tract, as it does for the vowels and the sonorants. Instead, resonance occurs primarily in the portion of the vocal tract anterior to the constriction formed by the articulators. For voiceless obstruent sounds, such as /s, f, t, and k/, the sound source is solely at the point of constriction in the vocal tract. However, for voiced obstruents, such as /z, v, d, and g/, the vibrating vocal folds do provide a second sound source, creating a modulation of the breath stream coming from the lungs.

TABLE 5.1   The Classification of English Consonant Phonemes.

	Bilabial		Labiodental		Interdental		Alveolar		Palatal		Velar		Glottal
	vl	v	vl	v	vl	v	vl	v	vl	v	vl	v	vl
Obstruents													
Stops (Plosives)	p	b					t	d			k	g	ʔ
Fricatives			f	v	θ	ð	s	z	ʃ	ʒ			h
Affricates									tʃ	dʒ			
Sonorants													
Nasals		m						n				ŋ	
Approximants													
Glides		w								j		w	
Liquids								l		r			

vl = voiceless; v = voiced.

Whereas vowels can stand alone and create a meaningful utterance—for example, "oh," "a," and "I"—consonants do not have the ability to stand alone. Consonants are generally found at the beginning and/or the end of syllables. As such, they are often classified as to their position in relation to the vowel in each syllable. Consonants that occur before a vowel in any syllable are referred to as **prevocalic** and those that occur after a vowel are referred to as **postvocalic**. Consonants located between two vowels are termed **intervocalic**. See Table 5.2 for some examples of prevocalic, postvocalic, and intervocalic consonants.

TABLE 5.2 Examples of Prevocalic, Postvocalic, and Intervocalic Consonants (consonant graphemes and IPA symbols are underlined).

Prevocalic		Postvocalic		Intervocalic	
tee	/ti/	eat	/it/	easy	/izɪ/
hoe	/hoʊ/	move	/muv/	anew	/ənu/
cow	/kaʊ/	group	/grup/	okay	/okeɪ/
see	/si/	ran	/ræn/	array	/əreɪ/
ray	/reɪ/	eyes	/aɪz/	upper	/ʌpɚ/

PRELIMINARY EXERCISE 1—PREVOCALIC, INTERVOCALIC, AND POSTVOCALIC CONSONANTS

Match the appropriate term to each of the words below to indicate whether the underlined IPA symbol is in the prevocalic, intervocalic, or postvocalic position.

a. prevocalic   b. intervocalic   c. postvocalic

_____ 1. seem   /sim/   _____ 6. oily   /ɔɪlɪ/

_____ 2. trade   /treɪd/   _____ 7. hotdog   /hatdɑg/

_____ 3. away   /əweɪ/   _____ 8. hasten   /heɪsən/

_____ 4. cruise /kruz/   _____ 9. open   /oʊpən/

_____ 5. oaf   /oʊf/   _____ 10. football /fʊtbɑl/

As you learned in Chapter 2, vowels generally serve as the center or nucleus of a syllable. Vowels are considered to be the nucleus of a syllable because they are of greater intensity than consonants and are, therefore, the prominent aspect of a syllable. Because vowels can form the nucleus of a syllable, they are said to be **syllabic**. We will see later that in some instances a few consonants may become syllabic in some phonetic contexts. Consequently, they have the special ability to become the nucleus of a syllable as well.

Manner, Place, and Voicing

One last way in which consonants and vowels differ is the way in which consonant articulation is classified. Vowels are usually classified in terms of lip and tongue position. Consonants, on the other hand, are classified according to three different phonemic dimensions: *manner of production*, *place of articulation*, and *voicing*.

Manner of production refers to *the way in which the airstream is modified* as it passes through the vocal tract. For instance, stops are produced when the articulators completely impede the airstream passing through the vocal tract. Fricatives, on the other hand, are produced by forcing air through a narrow channel formed by the articulators in the oral cavity. Stop and fricative consonants belong to separate manners of production. In addition to stops and fricatives, the other English manners of production include affricates, nasals, glides, and liquids. Examine Table 5.1 in order to see the distribution of the English consonants among the various manners of production.

PRELIMINARY EXERCISE 2—MANNER OF PRODUCTION

Referring to Table 5.1, match each of the following consonants to their manner of production.

F 1. /r/   a. stop
A 2. /d/   b. fricative
E 3. /w/   c. affricate
B 4. /f/   d. nasal
D 5. /n/   e. glide
C 6. /tʃ/   f. liquid

To define **place of articulation** we must answer this question: *Where* in the vocal tract is the constriction located during the production of a particular consonant? In other words, to determine place of articulation, we need to know which speech organs are active in production of that consonant. From Chapter 3, you should be familiar with the various adjectives that refer to specific articulators located in the vocal tract. It is these adjectives that are used to refer to place of articulation. For example, if both lips are used to produce a phoneme, the place of production is *bilabial*. Likewise, if a phoneme is created by placing the tongue against the alveolar ridge, the place of articulation is considered to be *lingua-alveolar* or simply *alveolar*. (It is redundant to say lingua-alveolar because it is understood that the primary articulator is the tongue.) Table 5.3 reviews the various places of articulation most common to spoken English.

TABLE 5.3 Most Common Places of Articulation in English.

Place of Articulation	Articulators Involved
Bilabial	upper and lower lips
Labiodental	lower lip and upper central incisors
Dental	tongue apex (or blade) and teeth
Alveolar	tongue apex (or blade) and alveolar ridge
Palatal	blade of tongue and hard palate
Velar	back of tongue and velum
Glottal	vocal folds
Lingual	tongue

The last dimension used in classifying consonants is **voicing**. Voicing refers to whether the vocal folds are vibrating during the production of a particular consonant. Several phonemes in English share the same manner of production and place of articulation, yet differ only in the voicing dimension (/s/ and /z/, for example). Phonemes that differ only in voicing are called **cognates**. Other examples of voiceless/voiced cognates include /k/ and /g/, /f/ and /v/, and /p/ and /b/. Word pairs differing only in the voicing of one phoneme are minimal pairs—"bit"/"pit" and "tuck"/"duck."

PRELIMINARY EXERCISE 3—VOICED/VOICELESS COGNATES

Place an "X" by each word pair having initial consonants that are voiced/voiceless cognates. You may need to refer to Table 5.1 for assistance.

_____	1. me, we		_____	6. shoot, suit
_____	2. seal, zeal		_____	7. flame, blame
_____	3. plan, clan		_____	8. dram, tram
_____	4. lice, rice		_____	9. yes, chess
_____	5. grain, crane		_____	10. vender, fender

Transcription of the English Consonants

In the following sections, the consonants of English will be introduced using the following format:

1. **Pronunciation Guide** for each consonant within each manner class, along with a detailed explanation of each manner.
2. **Phonetic Symbol Name** of each phoneme (Pullum & Ladusaw, 1996).
3. **Description** of each consonant on three dimensions: voicing, place of articulation, and manner. Voiced/voiceless cognates will be introduced together.
4. **Sample Words** and **Minimal Pairs** containing the phoneme(s) being discussed.
5. **Allographs** commonly used to represent the phoneme in spelling.
6. **Discussion** involving the production of each consonant.
7. **Practice Exercises** for the entire manner class—exercises will *not* be given for each separate phoneme, as with the vowels.

The Stop Consonants (Plosives)

Pronunciation Guide

/p/	as in "pan"	/pæn/		/b/	as in "ban"	/bæn/
/t/	as in "tune"	/tun/		/d/	as in "dune"	/dun/
/k/	as in "could"	/kʊd/		/g/	as in "good"	/gʊd/
/ɾ/	as in "better"	/bɛɾɚ/				
/ʔ/	as in "kitten"	/kɪʔn̩/				

Stop consonants, or **plosives**, are produced by *completely* obstructing the airstream once it enters the oral cavity. This is why stops are part of the class of consonants termed obstruents. The obstruction in the vocal tract is more occluding for this manner of articulation than for any of the others. Stop production is marked not only by a closure in the oral cavity, but also by a closure of the velopharyngeal port. That is, the velum is raised to prevent the breath stream from entering the nasal cavity. The English stop consonants are produced by forming a closure in the oral cavity at one of three places of articulation: bilabial (both lips coming together), alveolar (the tip or blade of the tongue contacting the alveolar ridge), or velar (the back of the tongue contacting the velum).

The articulatory process in stop consonant production is very rapid. In fact, of all the phonemes in English, stops are among the shortest in duration. Although it is possible to prolong the production of a vowel (iiiiiiiii), it is not possible to prolong the production of a stop consonant.

During the period of closure, **intraoral pressure** (air pressure within the oral cavity) increases due to the fact that the impeded airstream cannot escape the oral cavity. Once the constriction is released, the intraoral air pressure is relieved, resulting in the expulsion of an audible noise burst from the oral cavity (hence the name *plosive*). The burst of air is referred to as noise, since the airflow becomes turbulent when the stop is released.

One last thing to consider relating to the production of plosives is their sound source. Stops may have one or two sound sources, depending on whether they are voiced or not. In English there are three voiceless stops (/p, t, k/) and three voiced stops (/b, d, g/). The primary sound source for voiceless stop consonants is considered to be at the point of constriction in the vocal tract, formed by the articulators. More specifically, the source of sound is the turbulent airflow generated when the intraoral pressure is released. For this reason, the sound source for voiceless stops is considered to be a noise source. For voiced stops, the vocal folds vibrate in conjunction with the release of the stop in the oral cavity. Therefore, voiced stops have two separate sound sources: (1) the noise source produced at the constriction in the vocal tract, and (2) the vocal tone produced by the vibrating vocal folds.

Each stop consonant has a characteristic vocal tract shape due to the position of the articulators that form the stop constriction. Therefore, there is a separate, characteristic vocal tract resonance for the labial, alveolar, and velar places of production. Vocal fold vibration causes modifications in the vocal tract resonance during production of the voiced stops. The differences in the resonance of the larynx, pharynx, and oral cavity during production of the various stop consonants provide listeners the auditory cues necessary to distinguish their place of articulation.

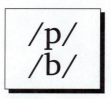

Lowercase p
Lowercase b

Description

/p/   voiceless, bilabial stop
/b/   voiced, bilabial stop

Sample Words

/p/	/b/
played	breeze
appear	rube
spite	stubborn
leapt	rubbed
ripped	club
stripe	abrade

Minimal Pairs

/p/	/b/	/p/	/b/
pet	bet	ape	Abe
punt	bunt	rip	rib
patch	batch	rope	robe
prim	brim	lap	lab
packed	backed	staple	stable
plead	bleed	ample	amble

Allographs

	/p/		/b/
Grapheme	**Example**	**Grapheme**	**Example**
p	pig	b	bear
pp	apple	bb	blubber

Discussion   The airstream is impeded as both lips are brought together during production of the stops /p/ and /b/. Therefore, these two phonemes are classified as bilabial (see Figure 5.1). The jaws are in an almost closed position so that the lips can come together. The velopharyngeal port remains closed so that air does not flow into the nasal cavity. Upon release, the burst of air for

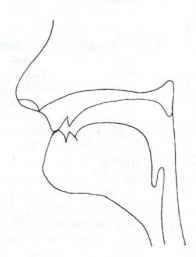

FIGURE 5.1   Bilabial articulation.

/p/ is more powerful than for /b/ because the amount of intraoral pressure is greater for voiceless phonemes. During production of /p/ or /b/, the tongue's position is determined by the following vowel. The use of the /p/ and /b/ phonemes in transcription is fairly straightforward (see the sample words just listed).

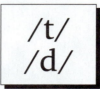

Lowercase t
Lowercase d

Description

/t/   voiceless, alveolar stop
/d/   voiced, alveolar stop

Sample Words

/t/	/d/
taste	dunce
stick	address
attack	pedestal
sate	door
tempest	edict
walk<u>ed</u>	mail<u>ed</u>

Minimal Pairs

/t/	/d/	/t/	/d/
talk	dock	pat	pad
to	do	trot	trod
touch	Dutch	state	stayed (staid)
troll	droll	straight	strayed
taffy	daffy	trait	trade
tram	dram	post	posed

Allographs

/t/		/d/	
Grapheme	**Example**	**Grapheme**	**Example**
t	toe	d	doe
ed	look<u>ed</u>	ed	wad<u>ed</u>

Discussion   To produce the alveolar stops /t/ and /d/, the apex, or blade, of the tongue makes contact with the alveolar ridge, impeding oral airflow (see Figure 5.2). The sides of the tongue are placed against the upper molars so that air does not escape from the sides of the tongue. In essence, a small airtight cavity is formed by the tongue and teeth so that an increase in intraoral pressure may occur.

The air burst associated with the release of the voiceless /t/ is greater than for the voiced /d/, due to greater intraoral pressure for the voiceless cognate. In certain phonetic contexts, the velopharyngeal port may open during release of /t/ or /d/, allowing release of air through the nasal cavity instead of through the oral cavity. In the words "ridden" and "sudden," for instance, the tongue may remain in contact with the alveolar ridge during the release of the consonant; the stop would then be released through the nasal cavity instead of

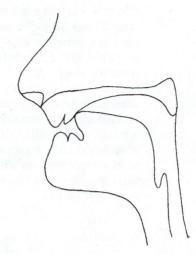

FIGURE 5.2   Alveolar articulation.

through the oral cavity. This maneuver is accomplished by lowering the velum. The release of air through the nasal cavity is called **nasal plosion** for obvious reasons. Nasal plosion can be indicated in narrow transcription by using a raised "n" following the phoneme in question (e.g., "sudden" [sʌdⁿn̩]).

One other consideration regarding /t/ and /d/ is their use in transcribing the morpheme "-ed," used to represent the past tense ending in words. Notice that the words "bagged" /bægd/ and "reaped" /ript/ each end with a different phoneme. In the first case, "ed" is represented by /d/ and in the second case with /t/. Now, examine the following words and see if you can determine a pattern as to the use of /t/ and /d/ in representing the morpheme "-ed."

Example	*Final Phoneme*	*Example*	*Final Phoneme*
crowed	/d/	taped	/t/
teamed	/d/	hiked	/t/
hogged	/d/	lacked	/t/
carded (carted)	/d/	docked	/t/

Perhaps you noticed that if the phoneme preceding the "-ed" morpheme is voiced, the final phoneme also will be voiced, that is, /d/. Notice that a final /d/ also will be used if a tap precedes "-ed," as in the words "carded"/"carted" (see the following discussion). Conversely, if the phoneme preceding "-ed" is voiceless, then the voiceless /t/ will represent the morpheme "-ed." Reexamine the previous words to make sure you understand this concept.

Allophones of /t/ and /d/

Alveolar Tap | /ɾ/ |

Sample Words
whittle   battle   coddle
Toto   cutie   ladder/latter

Glottal Stop | /ʔ/ |

Sample Words
button   mountain   hat
fatten   Latin   atlas

Alveolar Tap   An allophone of /t/ and /d/ often occurs in casual speech in words like "latter"/"ladder" and "Plato"/"play dough." Say these word pairs aloud to yourself and you will not see a difference in their production. For example, the pronunciation of the word "latter" is not truly a /t/, as in the pronunciation /lætɚ/, nor is it truly a /d/, as in /lædɚ/; the pronunciation is somewhere between the two. In this context, the (alveolar) **tap** /ɾ/ is the allophone used to represent the combination of /t/ and /d/ as in /læɾɚ/ or /pleɪɾoʊ/. Tap articulation involves a very rapid movement of the tongue tip against the alveolar ridge, creating a very brief stop consonant. The motion associated with a tapped stop consonant is more rapid than the "traditional" stop articulation of /t/ or /d/. The tap generally occurs in words with an intervocalic "t" or "d" digraph, in which the first syllable receives stress. Some examples include:

| better | stutter | matted | battle |
| madder | huddle | coddle | riddle |

The tap also is used in transcription when an intervocalic /t/ closes a stressed syllable. Examine the following words by saying them aloud:

| fated | flirted | static | data |

Notice that the /t/ becomes partially voiced, due to the voiced environment provided by the vowels preceding and following the consonant. Use of the tap in this instance is more accurate in transcription than using /t/ or /d/.

Glottal Stop   Another allophone of /t/, the **glottal stop** /ʔ/ appears quite often in American English. It generally occurs in syllable-final position. This stop is most readily noted in British English in the phrase, "Li'l bi' of tea" (Little bit of tea). The vocal folds are the articulators that both impede and release the flow of air in the production of this speech sound. Because the vocal folds do not vibrate during the production of the glottal stop, it is considered to be voiceless.

In American English, the glottal stop is found in some speakers' productions of words such as "kitten," "mountain," and "Dayton," where /t/ or /nt/ is followed by the /n/ phoneme. In saying these words, the /t/ is not released through the oral cavity. Instead, the release occurs at the level of the vocal folds. The reason for this is the tongue tip stays in place for both the /t/ and the following /n/ phonemes because they share the same (alveolar) place of articulation. Phonemes that share the same place of articulation are said to be **homorganic**. The transcription of the words "kitten," "mountain," and "Dayton" would be /kɪʔn̩/ , /maʊnʔn̩/ , and /deɪʔn̩/, respectively.

Notice the use of the symbol /n̩/ in the transcription of the words /kɪʔn̩/, /maʊnʔn̩/, and /deɪʔn̩/ above. The /n̩/ represents an entire syllable, that is, both the consonant and the vowel, because there is no fully articulated vowel in these words. In this context, /n̩/ has become a syllabic consonant. (Remember that vowels are considered to be syllabic because they are the nucleus of a syllable.) The syllabic marking indicates that /n̩/ has become the nucleus of the syllable and therefore also represents the vowel in the syllable.

Syllabic consonants (or simply syllabics) result most often when adjacent homorganic consonants occur in either the same word or in separate words in connected speech. Syllabics also can be found in conversational speech as in "cat 'n dog" /kæʔn̩dɑg/ and "sittin'" /sɪʔn̩ (note the use of the glottal stop here). We will return to the topic of syllabics in the sections focusing on nasals and liquids later in the chapter.

The glottal stop also occurs between vowels in individual words such as "Hawaii" /həwaɪʔɪ/, and in connected speech between vowels in adjacent words, as in "she eats" /ʃiʔits/ and "Hi Ilene" /haɪʔaɪlin/. Depending on dialect, some speakers replace syllable-final /t/ with a glottal stop. When this occurs, it almost sounds as though the speaker has deleted the /t/. Examples include "hat" /hæʔ/, "litmus" /lɪʔməs/, "Atlanta" /æʔlænə/, and "beatnik" /biʔnɪk/. In cases of disordered speech, it is important to listen carefully in order to determine if syllable-final /t/ is being deleted or if a glottal stop is being substituted.

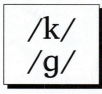

Lowercase k
Lowercase g

Description

/k/   voiceless, velar stop
/g/   voiced, velar stop

Sample Words

/k/	/g/
cotton	gold
wreck	rugged
opaque	Ghandi
queue	lager
squirts	aggressive

Minimal Pairs

/k/	/g/	/k/	/g/
crow	grow	luck	lug
cane	gain	back	bag
cut	gut	broke	brogue
cram	gram	shack	shag
kill	gill	pluck	plug
kale	gale	lacked	lagged

Allographs

	/k/		/g/
Grapheme	*Example*	*Grapheme*	*Example*
k	like	g	gone
ck	rock	gg	leggings
c	cat	gh	ghost
cc	occult	gu	guard
ch	chord		
cq	acquit		
cu	biscuit		
qu	liquor		

Discussion   The constriction in the oral cavity for production of /k/ and /g/ is considered to be velar because the stop is formed between the back of the tongue and the anterior portion of the velum (see Figure 5.3). As you would

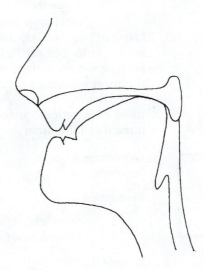

FIGURE 5.3 Velar articulation.

expect, there is greater intraoral pressure for the voiceless /k/ than for the voiced /g/. The release for both /k/ and /g/ is through the oral cavity. It is interesting to note the many allographs of the phoneme /k/. Of all the stop consonants, /k/ has the most variant spellings.

In some phonetic contexts, the back of the tongue may move slightly forward to articulate with the posterior portion of the palate during production of /k/ or /g/. To demonstrate, let us compare the production of the phoneme /k/ in two different phonetic contexts, that is, in the words "coop" and "keep." To produce the /k/ in /kup/, the back of the tongue would be close to the anterior portion of the velum because, in this context, it is followed by the back vowel /u/. To produce the /k/ in "keep," the tongue would be pulled forward, closer to the posterior portion of the palate, because /k/ is followed by the front vowel /i/. In anticipation of the forward place of articulation for /i/, the /k/ is produced more forward than normal. Keep in mind that a phoneme's identity often is altered by the other phonemes that precede or follow it.

EXERCISE 5.1—THE STOP CONSONANTS

A. Place an "X" by the words with a stop consonant in their transcriptions.

_____ 1. wish	_____ 6. runs	_____ 11. church	_____ 16. think
_____ 2. spring	_____ 7. whisper	_____ 12. tomb	_____ 17. rummage
_____ 3. loom	_____ 8. question	_____ 13. logical	_____ 18. realm
_____ 4. brush	_____ 9. system	_____ 14. jeans	_____ 19. guess
_____ 5. window	_____ 10. phase	_____ 15. Stephen	_____ 20. fox

Continues

EXERCISE 5.1 (*cont.*)

B. For each item, select the word(s) that have the specified criterion *in their transcriptions.* (There may be more than one correct response for each question.)

man   about   perky   could   plaque   green

Example:

Contains a bilabial sound   man, about, perky, plaque

1. Contains a high front vowel   *green*
2. Contains a voiceless alveolar stop   *about*
3. Contains no stops   *man, green*
4. Contains a velar stop   *perky, green*
5. Contains a central vowel   *about, perky*
6. Ends with a voiceless sound   *about, plaque*
7. Begins with a voiced sound   *man, could, plaque*
8. Contains a back vowel and a voiced stop   _____
9. Begins with a voiceless sound   _____
10. Contains a front vowel and a voiceless stop   _____

C. Indicate which of the following words have either a tap (T) or a glottal stop (G) in their transcriptions. Indicate which it would be by writing T or G in the blank.

____ 1. table   ____ 6. uncle   ____ 11. pushin'   ____ 16. talkin'
____ 2. better   ____ 7. written   ____ 12. splatter   ____ 17. bitten
____ 3. errand   ____ 8. beaten   ____ 13. rotted   ____ 18. wedded
____ 4. listen   ____ 9. walked   ____ 14. sweatin'   ____ 19. rotten
____ 5. quittin'   ____ 10. Lincoln   ____ 15. bottle   ____ 20. fodder

D. The words below all end with the "-ed" morpheme. Indicate in the blank whether the final phoneme should be transcribed as /t/ or /d/.

____ 1. wished   ____ 6. danced   ____ 11. sailed   ____ 16. crabbed
____ 2. loaded   ____ 7. wrapped   ____ 12. leased   ____ 17. placed
____ 3. endorsed   ____ 8. hanged   ____ 13. reached   ____ 18. meshed
____ 4. endangered   ____ 9. hoped   ____ 14. toted   ____ 19. burned
____ 5. robbed   ____ 10. traded   ____ 15. wrecked   ____ 20. carved

E. Circle the real English words given below.

1. /kipət/   5. /pɝkt/   9. /pɝpət/   13. /tʊkɪ/
2. /təkɪd/   6. /pækət/   10. /pɪkɪ/   14. /gækət/
3. /ədɛbt/   7. /tɛpɪd/   11. /ətæk/   15. /dɛrbɪ/
4. /paʊrɚ/   8. /taɪrɚ/   12. /tɔrkot/   16. /pipʔd/

Continues

EXERCISE 5.1 (*cont.*)

F. In the blanks, write each of the words using English orthography.

1. /pɑɾɚɪ/ _____   7. /gʌpɪ/ _____
2. /pʌkəd/ _____   8. /pækɪŋ/ _____
3. /pəteɪɾoʊ/ _____   9. /daɪpəd/ _____
4. /dɑktɚ/ _____   10. /peɪpɚbɔɪ/ _____
5. /tɑrgət/ _____   11. /dækɚɪ/ _____
6. /pʌpət/ _____   12. /daɪɹətəd/ _____

G. For each item below, correct any vowel, diphthong, or stop consonant transcription errors by marking out the incorrect IPA symbol and placing the correct symbol above it. If no error is present, indicate by circling "no error."

Examples:

a. cap   /kæp/   (no error)

                             ɪ
b. tick   /tɛ̶k/   no error

1. direct   /dɚɛkt/   no error
2. tighter   /taɪɾɚ/   no error
3. goaded   /goʊded/   no error
4. corker   /kɔrkɚ/   no error
5. Carter   /cɑrɾɚ/   no error
6. partake   /pɔrteɪk/   no error
7. repeat   /repit/   no error
8. poet   /poʊət/   no error
9. oboe   /oʊboʊ/   no error
10. paper   /pɑpɚ/   no error

H. Word Analysis
Read the phonetic descriptions of the following words. Then write the appropriate IPA symbols and the English orthography on the two lines.

Example:

voiceless alveolar stop + low front lax   /tæg/
vowel + voiced velar stop   tag

1. voiceless velar stop + high front lax   _____
    vowel + voiced alveolar stop   _____

2. high front tense vowel + voiced velar   _____
    stop + mid-central lax rounded vowel   _____

3. voiceless alveolar stop + low-mid front   _____
    vowel + voiceless bilabial stop + high   _____
    front lax vowel + voiced alveolar stop

Continues

EXERCISE 5.1 (*cont.*)

4. mid-central unrounded lax vowel +
   voiced bilabial stop + low-mid back-
   central unrounded lax vowel +
   voiceless alveolar stop
   _____

   _____

5. voiced alveolar stop + low back tense
   vowel + voiceless velar stop +
   voiceless alveolar stop
   _____

   _____

6. voiced velar stop + low-mid back tense
   vowel + voiced alveolar stop + high
   front lax vowel
   _____

   _____

I. Written Transcription Practice
   Transcribe the following words. Remember to enclose your transcriptions with virgules.

1. cape	_____	21. bigger	_____
2. pared	_____	22. beaker	_____
3. dog	_____	23. tuba	_____
4. tied	_____	24. cabby	_____
5. kept	_____	25. peered	_____
6. debt	_____	26. backed	_____
7. bake	_____	27. perky	_____
8. pour	_____	28. geared	_____
9. bored	_____	29. dagger	_____
10. pork	_____	30. giddy	_____
11. peat	_____	31. carpet	_____
12. taupe	_____	32. doctor	_____
13. took	_____	33. ticket	_____
14. putt	_____	34. decked	_____
15. coat	_____	35. tired	_____
16. apart	_____	36. bagboy	_____
17. guarded	_____	37. debate	_____
18. boater	_____	38. torrid	_____
19. Bobby	_____	39. parrot	_____
20. barter	_____	40. dirty	_____

Complete Assignment 5-1.

The Nasal Consonants

Pronunciation Guide

/m/	as in "man"	/mæn/
/n/	as in "new"	/nu/
/ŋ/	as in "ring"	/rɪŋ/

The three nasal consonants /m, n, and ŋ/ are produced in a manner similar to the stop consonants. That is, the airstream is completely obstructed in the oral cavity during their production. Also, the obstruction occurs at the same three places of articulation as the stops, that is, bilabial, alveolar, and velar (see Figures 5.2, 5.3, and 5.4). However, this is where the similarity ends. Nasal consonants are sonorants, not obstruents. Nasal consonants are produced with the velum lowered so that the airstream and acoustic vibrations continually flow into the nasal cavity. The obstruction at the lips, alveolar ridge, or velum is maintained during the production of the nasal consonants as it is for stops. Therefore, there is no release of intraoral pressure from the oral cavity. The articulators simply block the flow of air out of the oral cavity so that the airstream may continually flow through the nasal cavity and out through the nares. If you sustain the production of /m/, and place your index finger under your nose (as if you were trying to stifle a sneeze), you can feel a lightly escaping airstream.

Another difference between stop and nasal consonants is the fact that all nasal consonants are voiced; they have no voiceless counterparts in English. Like vowels, the sound source for nasals is the vibration of the vocal folds. Recall that in some instances, nasal phonemes may become syllabic. In the word "written" /rɪʔn̩/, the syllabic /n̩/ marks both the consonant and the vowel in the second syllable.

Lowercase m

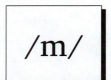

Description

/m/   voiced, bilabial nasal

Sample Words

/m/

mark	cramp
slam	dimpled
mend	alarming
maybe	amounted
drama	stomach
grump	mother

Minimal Pairs

/m/	/p/	/b/
mark	park	bark
roamed	roped	robed
messed	pest	best
crams	craps	crabs
sum	sup	sub
slam	slap	slab

Allographs

Grapheme	Example
m	cram
mm	hammer

Discussion   During production of /m/, the velum is lowered so that the airstream enters the nasal cavity. The lips are brought together in order to halt the airstream coming from the larynx (similar to the constriction for the phoneme /b/). Because /m/ is voiced, the vocal folds vibrate during its production. The oral resonating cavity for /m/ is the largest of the three nasals; it includes the entire oral cavity, extending from the lips to the oropharynx. The tongue is poised in position for the vowel following production of /m/. Figure 5.4 shows the articulation of the bilabial nasal /m/. Compare this figure with the articulation of a bilabial stop, as shown in Figure 5.1. Note the differing position of the velum in these two figures: It is lowered in Figure 5.4, and it is raised in Figure 5.1.

In some instances, /m/ may become syllabic in conversational speech, depending on the phonetic environment. For example, the word "happen" becomes /hæpm̩/, and the phrase "wrap them up" becomes "wrap 'em up" /ræpm̩əp/. Note the occurrence of syllabic /m/ in these examples due to the homorganic /p/ preceding the bilabial /m/.

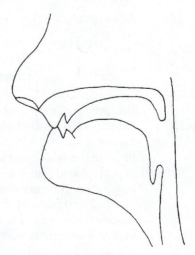

FIGURE 5.4   Bilabial nasal articulation.

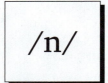

Lowercase n

Description

/n/ voiced, alveolar nasal

Sample Words

/n/	
note	runner
nail	Andover
Nile	nervous
loaned	answered
tunes	astound
snowball	mannerism

Minimal Pairs

/n/	/m/	/n/	/m/
nail	mail (male)	nine	mine
note	mote (moat)	Nate	mate
loan	loam	cunning	coming
grin	grim	warned	warmed
noon	moon	sunning	summing
roan	roam	dinner	dimmer

Allographs

Grapheme	**Example**
n	nice
nn	dinner

Discussion   The phoneme /n/ is produced in a manner similar to /m/, except for its place of articulation. /n/ is an alveolar consonant, similar to /t/ (see Figure 5.2). The tongue tip (or blade) contacts the alveolar ridge in order to impede the flow of air coming from the larynx. Because the place of articulation is posterior to that for /m/, the oral cavity is slightly smaller, causing a different resonance to be created in the vocal tract.

Transcription of this sound is fairly straightforward. However, when /n/ occurs at the end of a word, and the preceding consonant is an alveolar (homorganic) *obstruent,* such as /d, t, s, or ʔ/, the /n/ often becomes the nucleus of the syllable (syllabic). Some examples follow with the homorganic consonant allograph underlined.

ri<u>dd</u>en	/rɪdn̩/	go<u>tt</u>en	/gɑʔn̩/
rea<u>s</u>on	/rizn̩/	cho<u>s</u>en	/tʃouzn̩/
le<u>ss</u>on	/lɛsn̩/	ea<u>t</u>en	/iʔn̩/

Note that for the word "ridden," the stop /d/ may be released through the nasal cavity as the velum is lowered in production of /n/ (nasal plosion).

Examine the following words. Although the preceding consonant (underlined) is not homorganic, many individuals still use the syllabic /n̩/ in transcription because the vowel between the consonants is almost nonexistent.

ri<u>bb</u>on	/rɪbn̩/
ha<u>pp</u>en	/hæpn̩/ (or /hæpm̩/)
mu<u>ff</u>in	/mʌfn̩/

One last word about the use, or actually nonuse, of /n/. Keep in mind that in words containing the letter string "-ing," the phoneme /ŋ/ is used, not /n/ (see the following section on /ŋ/).

Eng

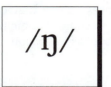

Description

/ŋ/ voiced, velar nasal

Sample Words

/ŋ/

ring	clank	stinky
wrangler	ankle	lingo
being	dangle	wrinkle
finger	larynx	wrangler

Allographs

Grapheme	Example
ng	sing
nk	link

Discussion   /ŋ/ is produced similarly to the other two nasal consonants in terms of voicing and velar opening. However, for /ŋ/, the point of constricted airflow in the oral cavity is the most posterior, between the back of the tongue and the anterior portion of the velum (or sometimes the posterior portion of the hard palate, in a manner similar to /k/ and /g/; see Figure 5.3). The oral resonating cavity for /ŋ/ is the shortest of all (when compared to /m/ and /n/) given that the constriction in the vocal tract is adjacent to the pharynx.

/ŋ/ never begins a word in English; it is found only in the intervocalic or postvocalic positions of a word. In relation to transcription, /ŋ/ poses some interesting dilemmas for beginning transcribers. Note the use of /ŋ/ with the following letter strings:

Letter String	Sample Word	Transcription
ink	kink	/kɪŋk/
ank	lanky	/læŋkɪ/
ynx	lynx	/lɪŋks/
inx	sphinx	/sfɪŋks/

It would not be possible to say these words using /n/ instead of /ŋ/ (try it for yourself). In some words, such as "English" and "finger," /ŋ/ is always followed by the voiced, velar stop /g/ in its pronunciation. However, there are other words in English, such as "longing" and "stinger," in which the production of /g/ is variable. Contrast the following two sets of words:

Word	Transcription		Word		Transcription	
linger	/lɪŋgɚ/		hanger	/hæŋgɚ/	or	/hæŋɚ/
ingot	/ɪŋgət/		singer	/sɪŋgɚ/	or	/sɪŋɚ/
anger	/æŋgɚ/		clanging	/klæŋgɪŋ/	or	/klæŋɪŋ/

Note that all of the words in the first set always have /g/ in their transcriptions, whereas the words in the second set may be pronounced with or without the /g/, depending on individual speaker differences and/or dialect; they are in free variation. Similar to /m/ and /n/, /ŋ/ may become syllabic when it follows a homorganic velar obstruent such as /k/ or /g/ as in "bacon" /beɪkŋ/ or "wagon" /wægŋ/.

EXERCISE 5.2—THE NASAL CONSONANTS

A. Place an "X" by the words with a nasal phoneme in their transcription.

X 1. ring	X 6. jasmine	X 11. moan	X 16. ripen
X 2. bomb	___ 7. crease	X 12. spanking	X 17. unfair
___ 3. pet	X 8. inside	___ 13. possible	X 18. monkey
___ 4. stop	___ 9. trait	X 14. trench	___ 19. lure
X 5. tomb	X 10. loaner	X 15. lung	___ 20. failure

B. Indicate with an "X" the words that have /ŋ/ in their transcription.

X 1. angle	___ 8. singe	X 15. banging
___ 2. angel	___ 9. ginger	___ 16. manx
X 3. brink	___ 10. danger	___ 17. ingest
X 4. mango	X 11. blinker	X 18. singer
___ 5. Angie	X 12. hanger	X 19. hunger
X 6. single	X 13. ringing	X 20. jangle
___ 7. conjure	X 14. mingle	___ 21. congeal

C. Circle the words in B that could have /ŋ/ followed by /g/ in their transcriptions. (Some words may be pronounced differently due to speaker dialect.)

reference top of page (discussion in class on Thurs.)

D. Place an "X" next to the words that have /g/ in their transcriptions.

___ 1. hinge	___ 7. ring	X 13. tango
X 2. bangle	X 8. drank	___ 14. flange
___ 3. wings	___ 9. onyx	___ 15. engine
X 4. single	X 10. tingle	X 16. English
___ 5. wrong	___ 11. bungee	___ 17. tongue
X 6. mangle	X 12. kangaroo	___ 18. dangerous

Continues

EXERCISE 5.2 (*cont.*)

E. Place an "X" next to the words that have /ŋ/ in their transcriptions.

_____ 1. pharynx	X 7. engine	X 13. ginger
X 2. England	_____ 8. flank	_____ 14. blanket
X 3. bungee	_____ 9. tingle	_____ 15. tongue
_____ 4. length	X 10. lunge	X 16. danger
_____ 5. lungs	_____ 11. strength	X 17. vengeance
_____ 6. jungle	_____ 12. tango	X 18. ranges

F. For each item, select the word(s) that have the specified criterion *in their transcriptions*. (There may be more than one correct response for each question.)

good	mutton	curving	bank
napped	taken	carton	code

1. Contains an initial labial sound   _____

2. Contains a voiced initial sound   _____

3. Ends with a stop   _____

4. Contains a central vowel   _____

5. Ends with a voiceless sound   _____

6. Contains a velar nasal   _____

7. Contains a syllabic consonant   _____

8. Contains no nasals   _____

9. Contains a low front vowel and a labial consonant   _____

10. Contains a velar consonant and a back vowel   _____

G. Circle the words that represent real English words.

1. (/kæmp/)	5. /tɪŋgə/	9. /dænk/
2. (/neɪm/)	6. /nɪŋgɪd/	10. (/bʌmpɪ/)
3. /mɛlɪ/	7. (/kræŋkɪ/)	11. (/pɪntoʊ/)
4. /pɪnt/	8. (/kɔrn/)	12. /pɑrmɔɪ/

H. In the blanks, write each of the words using English orthography.

1. /næb/	nab	7. /kændɪ/	candy
2. /kɑnd/	conned	8. /əpɔɪnt/	appoint
3. /əmæs/	amass	9. /kʊkɪŋ/	cooking
4. /æŋgɚ/	anger	10. /tumɚ/	tumor
5. /mɔrnɪŋ/	morning	11. /taɪʔn̩/	tighten
6. /bɛndɪŋ/	bending	12. /maɪndəd/	minded

Continues

EXERCISE 5.2 (*cont.*)

I. For each item below, correct any vowel, diphthong, nasal, or stop consonant transcription errors by marking out the incorrect IPA symbol and placing the correct symbol above it. If no error is present, indicate by circling "no error."

1.	camper	/kæmpɚ/	(no error)
2.	adorn	/ədɔrn/	(no error)
3.	duffer	/dəfɝ/	(no error) dʌfɚ
4.	bunting	/bʌntɪŋ/	(no error)
5.	bingo	/bɪŋoʊ/	no error ˈbɪŋo
6.	pecking	/pɛckɪŋ/	no error pɛkɪŋ
7.	Dayton	/deɪʔən/	(no error) deʔən
8.	batter	/bædɝ/	no error bæɾɚ
9.	baking	/bakɪŋ/	no error bekɪŋ
10.	doorknob	/dɔrknɑb/	no error dɔrnɑb

✗ Word Analysis
Read the phonetic descriptions of the following words. Then write the appropriate IPA symbols and the English orthography on the two lines.

1. voiceless velar stop + low front vowel + alveolar nasal + voiced alveolar stop

    _____
    _____

2. voiced bilabial nasal + low-mid, back-central vowel + alveolar nasal + high front lax vowel

    _____
    _____

3. mid-central lax unrounded vowel + voiceless alveolar stop + high-mid front vowel + alveolar nasal

    _____
    _____

4. voiceless velar stop + low back vowel + velar nasal + voiced velar stop + high-mid back vowel

    _____
    _____

5. voiced bilabial stop + mid-central tense rounded vowel + voiceless bilabial stop + voiceless alveolar stop

    _____
    _____

K. Transcription Practice
Transcribe the following words, using the IPA.

1.	mink	mɪŋk	8.	gnome	nom
2.	pert	pɝt	9.	monk	mʌŋk
3.	tan	tɛn	10.	coin	kɔɪn
4.	king	kɪŋ	11.	earn	ɝn
5.	done	dʌn	12.	newt	nut
6.	knead	nɪd	13.	town	taʊn
7.	bang	bɛŋ	14.	mood	mud

Continues

EXERCISE 5.2 (*cont.*)

15. knight	naɪt	28. bongo	ˈbaŋgo
16. dumb	dʌm	29. madam	ˈmaedəm
17. could	cʊd	30. gander	ˈgɛndɚ
18. torn	tɔrn	31. omit	oˈmɪt
19. tongue	tʌŋ	32. negate	nəˈget
20. gone	gɑn	33. tunic	ˈtunɪk
21. under	ˈʌndɚ	34. donkey	ˈdɑŋki
22. tankard	ˈtɛŋkɚd	35. command	kəˈmɛnd
23. peanut	ˈpinət	36. mirror	ˈmiɚɚ
24. dandy	ˈdɛndi	37. countin'	ˈkaʊntɪn
25. partake	parˈtek	38. daring	ˈdɛrɪŋ
26. Monday	ˈmʌnde	39. empire	ˈɛmpaɪr
27. nomad	ˈnomaed	40. coward	ˈkaʊɚd

Complete Assignment 5-2.

The Fricative Consonants

Pronunciation Guide

/f/	as in "form"	/fɔrm/	/v/	as in "van"	/væn/
/θ/	as in "thick"	/θɪk/	/ð/	as in "them"	/ðɛm/
/s/	as in "sip"	/sɪp/	/z/	as in "zoo"	/zu/
/ʃ/	as in "shell"	/ʃɛl/	/ʒ/	as in "rouge"	/ruʒ/
/h/	as in "ham"	/hæm/			

Fricatives are produced by forcing the breath stream (whether voiced or voiceless) through a narrow channel, or constriction, in the vocal tract. The articulators do not close completely during fricative production as they do in stop consonant production. They simply converge to form a slit to create the channel necessary for production of each fricative phoneme. There are five different places of articulation (points of constriction) in the vocal tract used for production of the nine English fricatives. These include the linguadental, labiodental, alveolar, palatal, and glottal places of articulation. Fricatives have voiced/voiceless cognate phonemes at each place of articulation. The only exception is the glottal fricative /h/, which is most often voiceless in English. Unlike stops and nasals, there are no bilabial or velar fricatives in English. However, these phonemes do exist in other languages. For instance, bilabial fricatives occur in Spanish and in Ewe, a West African language, and velar fricatives exist in German and Hebrew. Interestingly, bilabial and velar fricatives are sometimes produced by English-speaking adults and children as a result of a speech sound disorder.

Because the airstream from the lungs is being forced through a narrow channel, a turbulent, frictional noise is generated at the point of constriction. Fricatives, like stops, are considered to be obstruents, because their production involves an obstruction of the airstream in the vocal tract.

Voiceless fricatives, like voiceless stop consonants, are produced without the benefit of the vibrating vocal folds as the sound source. Therefore, the breath stream from the lungs must be forceful enough to create an audible turbulence at the point of constriction in the vocal tract. Similar to voiced stops, voiced fricatives have a second sound source—the vibrating vocal folds. In order to maintain voicing during their production, voiced fricatives have less airflow through the constriction in the oral cavity when compared to voiceless fricatives. Therefore, voiced fricatives are less intense than the voiceless fricatives; they are perceived as being softer than voiceless fricatives.

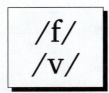

Lowercase f
Lowercase v

Description

/f/	voiceless, labiodental fricative
/v/	voiced, labiodental fricative

Sample Words

/f/	/v/
free	veal
foam	love
phobia	calves
coffer	vane
rough	over
turf	vase

Minimal Pairs

/f/	/v/
fail	veil
fend	vend
fan	van
leaf	leave
first	versed
proof	prove

Allographs

	/f/		/v/
Grapheme	**Example**	**Grapheme**	**Example**
f	fix	v	vote
ff	muffin	f	of
gh	rough	ph	Stephen
ph	phone		

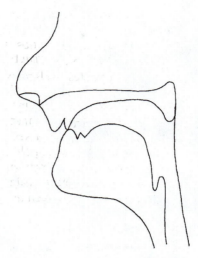

FIGURE 5.5 Labiodental articulation.

Discussion The point of constriction for /f/ and /v/ is formed by bringing the lower lip close to the edges of the upper central incisors (see Figure 5.5). The lower jaw must be raised near the upper jaw to accomplish this maneuver. The breath stream is forced through the narrow constriction formed by the lower lip and upper teeth.

The labiodental fricatives are quite easy to transcribe. The only allographs associated with /f/ that may cause trouble at first are "ph" and "gh." /v/ is generally used with words containing the letter "v" except in the rare case of "f" and "ph" (see the allographs just listed for examples).

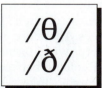

Theta
Eth

Description

/θ/	voiceless, interdental fricative
/ð/	voiced, interdental fricative

Sample Words

/θ/	/ð/	/θ/	/ð/
thermal	though	bath	bathe
thought	lathe	breath	breathe
froth	feather	thigh	thy
with	wither	ether	either

Note: "Either" and "ether" are minimal pairs, as are "thigh" and "thy."

Allographs

	/θ/		/ð/
Grapheme	*Example*	*Grapheme*	*Example*
th	thistle	th	although

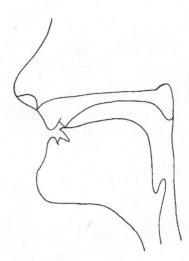

FIGURE 5.6   Interdental articulation.

Discussion   The interdental fricatives are named "theta" /θ/ (voiceless) and "eth" /ð/ (voiced). These phonemes are produced by forcing the breath stream through a constriction formed by the apex (or blade) of the tongue and the lower edge of the upper central incisors. The tongue is placed between the teeth for this articulation, hence the label *interdental*. Simultaneously, the sides of the tongue contact the upper molars to help direct the voiced or voiceless breath stream toward the constriction (see Figure 5.6).

A second way in which these phonemes may be produced is by forming a constriction between the apex of the tongue and the posterior portion of the upper central incisors. This particular articulation of these phonemes would be termed appropriately *dental,* as opposed to interdental.

/θ/ and /ð/ are both represented, in spelling, by the digraph "th." This is the only spelling representation of these two phonemes. Therefore, it is confusing at first for students learning how to transcribe words with /θ/ and /ð/. You may need to practice listening for the difference in voicing between the two phonemes since the spelling is the same for both sounds. Take a look at the *sample words* on the previous page. Practice saying them aloud while listening to the voicing differences of the two phonemes.

/s/
/z/

Lowercase s
Lowercase z

Description

/s/	voiceless, alveolar fricative
/z/	voiced, alveolar fricative

Sample Words

/s/	/z/	/s/	/z/
sew	zenith	lesson	xylophone
centaur	azalea	cease	pays
assert	fuzzy	awesome	Aztec

Minimal Pairs

/s/	/z/	/s/	/z/
seal	zeal	brace	braise
lacy	lazy	spice	spies
sip	zip	seek	Zeke
close	close	sue	zoo
loose	lose	noose	news
race	raise	purse	purrs

Allographs

/s/		/z/	
Grapheme	**Example**	**Grapheme**	**Example**
s	sink	z	zone
ss	press	zz	fizz
sc	science	s	was
c	ice	ss	scissors
		x	Xanadu

Discussion   The constriction for the alveolar fricatives is formed in one of two ways, depending on the individual speaker. The first involves the articulation of either the tongue apex or blade and the alveolar ridge. The tongue is raised so that it only approximates the ridge; the tongue does not make direct contact. At the same time, the tongue forms a tapering groove along its central or midline portion as the back of the tongue contacts the upper molars.

The second method for producing the alveolar fricatives is by placing the tip of the tongue behind the lower central incisors while the front of the tongue is raised to approximate the alveolar ridge. The tongue is still grooved along its central portion, and the sides of the tongue make contact with the upper molars. For both articulations, the channel formed by the tongue and teeth helps to direct the airstream anteriorly through the closely held upper and lower teeth.

In terms of transcription, the biggest problem for students is learning the correct use of /s/ and /z/ to represent the plural "-s" morpheme in words. Examine the following word pairs. Is the final phoneme transcribed as /s/ or /z/?

taps	seats	walks	chicks
tabs	seeds	runs	hogs

Whenever the final consonant of a word is voiceless, its plural marker will be transcribed as the voiceless phoneme /s/. The words "taps," "seats," "walks," and "chicks" all have a voiceless phoneme immediately preceding the plural morpheme /s/. The remaining words, which all have a voiced phoneme prior to the plural marker, are transcribed with /z/. Whenever the plural form of a word is "es" as in "babies" or "ladies," the plural phoneme is also represented by /z/ because it follows a (voiced) vowel. (The singular form of these words "baby" and "lady" ends with the vowel /ɪ/.) This voicing rule should seem familiar to you because similar practice is involved in using the phonemes /t/ and /d/ to indicate the "-ed" morpheme.

The phoneme /z/ is used by some speakers in pronunciation of words that are normally transcribed with an /s/. Examples include:

resource → /rizɔrs/   greasy → /grizɪ/   absurd → /æbzɝd/

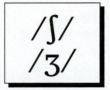

Esh
Yogh

Description

| /ʃ/ | voiceless, palatal (postalveolar) fricative |
| /ʒ/ | voiced, palatal (postalveolar) fricative |

Sample Words

/ʃ/	/ʒ/
shook	fusion
sure	casual
mansion	profusion
machine	measure
cashier	regime
pressure	television
national	seizure
omniscient	erosion

Allographs

/ʃ/		/ʒ/	
Grapheme	*Example*	*Grapheme*	*Example*
sh	shape	z	azure
ss	pressure	g	garage
sci	conscience	s	measure
ce	ocean	si	vision
ch	machine	zi	brazier
ci	social		
s	sugar		
si	pension		

Discussion   These two fricatives are created when the breath stream is forced through a constriction formed in a manner quite similar to the alveolar fricatives. The tongue has a groove along its central portion (although it is broader), and the sides of the tongue contact the upper molars. The airstream is directed anteriorly toward the front teeth. The more open constriction for /ʒ/ and /ʃ/ is formed by the closely held tongue blade and the hard palate. This articulation is posterior to the constriction formed for the alveolar fricatives /s/ and /z/. Therefore, /ʃ/ and /ʒ/ are considered by many phoneticians and linguists to have a **palatoalveolar** or **postalveolar** articulation (see Figure 5.7). (The IPA chart lists these phonemes as *postalveolar*.) Unlike /s/ and /z/, the lips are rounded in production of /ʃ/ and /ʒ/.

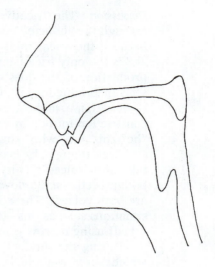

FIGURE 5.7   Palatal articulation.

The transcription of the phonemes /ʃ/ and /ʒ/ is a bit tricky at first. Students will often confuse them with the two affricates /tʃ/ as in "cheap" and /dʒ/as in "jam." Compare the following words:

sheep   /ʃip/   —   cheap /tʃip/
shoe   /ʃu/   —   chew /tʃu/
leisure /lɛʒɚ/   —   ledger /lɛdʒɚ/

Hopefully, you hear the difference in the pronunciation of these words. An explanation of the affricate manner of production will follow this section.

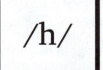

Lowercase h

Description

/h/   voiceless, glottal fricative

Sample Words

        /h/

hook	whose
helium	behave
hairy	ahead
Harold	unhook

Allographs

        /h/

Grapheme	Example
h	hit
wh	who

Discussion   The fricative /h/ is created when the breath stream is forced through the abducted vocal folds (the glottis). /h/ is considered to be voiceless because the vocal folds are not vibrating during its production. In English, /h/ is the only fricative without a voiced cognate. Unlike the other fricatives, production of /h/ does not involve a true constriction in the vocal tract as is seen in production of /f/ or /ʒ/, for example. When /h/ precedes the high vowels /i, ɪ, u, and ʊ/, the friction noise is created entirely, or nearly so, at the constriction formed by the tongue and palate, not at the glottis. Say the words "he" /hi/ and "who" /hu/ and you will see that this is so.

Even though /h/ is considered voiceless, in some phonetic contexts it may take on a voiced quality. For instance, in the word "ahead" /əhɛd/, a vowel both precedes and follows /h/, causing it to become voiced (because the vowels are both voiced). There is an IPA symbol for voiced /h/ that could be used in situations such as this—/əɦɛd/ (see Figure 2.1). It also could be transcribed as [əɦɛd] using narrow transcription.

During the production of /h/, the articulators will take on the shape of whichever vowel follows. For example, compare the shape and position of your lips for the words "hoop" and "heap." You will immediately notice that your lips are rounded—even before you produce the /h/ phoneme—in the word "hoop." Similarly, your lips are unrounded before the production of /h/ in "heap." The transcription of /h/ should pose few problems for students because the only allographs of /h/ are "h" and "wh."

EXERCISE 5.3—THE FRICATIVE CONSONANTS

A.   Place an "X" by the words with a fricative phoneme in their transcription.

X 1. push	X 6. brazen	___ 11. Montana	___ 16. hombre
X 2. thesis	X 7. cares	X 12. pleasure	X 17. leaks
___ 3. loom	___ 8. burlap	X 13. leather	X 18. worthy
X 4. happy	X 9. croissant	___ 14. marrow	___ 19. crouton
X 5. caution	X 10. vender	X 15. other	X 20. rajah

B.   Indicate which of the following words have /ʃ/ or /ʒ/ in their transcription. Write the correct phoneme next to the word. (Hint: Watch out for /tʃ/ and /dʒ/!)

___ 1. mishap	___ 8. badge	ʃ 15. Sean
ʒ 2. usually	ʒ 9. lesion	ʃ 16. passion
ʒ 3. decision	ʃ 10. lotion	ʃ 17. ricochet
___ 4. cheese	ʒ 11. corsage	___ 18. college
___ 5. largest	___ 12. changed	ʒ 19. allusion
___ 6. reason	ʃ 13. friction	___ 20. inject
ʃ 7. election	___ 14. juice	ʒ 21. Persia

C.   For the following words, indicate whether the "th" sound is voiced (/ð/) or voiceless (/θ/) by placing the correct IPA symbol in the blank.

ð 1. smoothly	ð 3. other	θ 5. moth
θ 2. method	ð 4. those	ð 6. gather

Continues

EXERCISE 5.3 (*cont.*)

θ	7. wrath	θ	13. thimble	θ	19. withstand
ð	8. writhe	θ	14. booth	ð	20. wither
ð	9. lathe	θ	15. oath	θ	21. author
θ	10. thought	ð	16. scathing	ð	22. smother
ð	11. clothes	ð	17. another	ð	23. bothers
ð	12. weather	θ	18. anything	θ	24. atheist

D. For each item, create real words (or proper names) by placing one of the nine fricatives in the blank. Write your answers in the blank at the right of each item. More than one answer is possible for each item.

/f, v, θ, ð, s, z, ʃ, ʒ, h/

Example:

/__u/   /s/, /z/, /ʃ/, /h/

(The words created are "sue," "zoo," "shoe," and "who.")

1. /mu__/   /v/, /s/, /z/
2. /wɪ__/   /θ/, /ð/, /z/, /ʃ/
3. /ʌ__ɚ/   /ð/, /ʃ/
4. /lɛ__ɚ/   /v/, /ð/, /s/ /ʒ/
5. /__ɛrɪ/   /f/, /v/, /ʃ/, /h/
6. /ru__/   /f/, /θ/, /z/, /ʒ/
7. /__aɪ/   /θ/, /s/, /ʃ/, /h/
8. /__ɪr/   /f/, /v/, /s/, /ʃ/, /h/

E. For each item, select each word from the list that has the specified criterion in its transcription. More than one answer is possible for each item.

them   beige   hug   wreath   tape   cash   soon   vend

1. Begins with a voiceless fricative   them
2. Begins with a voiced obstruent   _____
3. Ends with a voiceless obstruent   _____
4. Contains a front vowel and a
   voiceless fricative   _____
5. Contains an alveolar sound   _____
6. Contains all voiced phonemes   _____
7. Contains a stop and a fricative   beige
8. Contains a nasal and a fricative   them, soon
9. Contains a fricative and a central
   vowel   hug
10. Contains no fricatives   tape

ðɛm
beʒ
hʌg
riθ
tep
kæʃ
sun
vɛnd

Continues

EXERCISE 5.3 (*cont.*)

F. Indicate whether the following words should be transcribed with a final /s/ or a final /z/.

/z/ 1. babes   /z/ 7. bananas   /z/ 13. dramas
/s/ 2. chafes   /s/ 8. drinks   /s/ 14. croaks
/z/ 3. cars   /z/ 9. passes   /s/ 15. meats
/s/ 4. books   /z/ 10. throws   /z/ 16. affairs
/s/ 5. carpets   /z/ 11. loaves   /s/ 17. loafs
/z/ 6. pushes   /s/ 12. roasts   /z/ 18. birds

G. Circle the words that represent real English words.

1. (/ʃʊk/)   5. (/vɛrɪ/)   9. /pɜ˞s/   13. (/feɪvɚ/)
2. /ʒɪŋ/   6. /ðaɪ/   10. (/ʃɑrk/)   14. (/kreɪzd/)
3. /zɔrt/   7. /θrʊ/   11. /ɪrðu/   15. /bɪʒɚ/
4. (/θɜ˞d/)   8. /vɔɪnz/   12. /ʃæku/   16. /hoʊðɚ/

H. In the blanks, write each of the words using English orthography.

1. /eɪʒən/   Asian
2. /vɔrtɛks/   vortex
3. /vɑrnɪʃ/   varnish
4. /bɑðɚ/   bother
5. /spɛrd/   spared
6. /θæŋks/   thanks
7. /hɪrseɪ/   heresy
8. /ɜ˞bən/   urban
9. /sɜ˞vəst/   serviced
10. /ʌðɚz/   others
11. /froʊzn̩/   frozen
12. /ʃɪvɚd/   shivered
13. /fæʔn̩/   _____
14. /hɔrɚ/   _____
15. /gəziboʊ/   gazibo
16. /bɜ˞θdeɪz/   birthdays

I. For each item below, correct any vowel or consonant transcription errors by marking out the incorrect IPA symbol and placing the correct symbol above it. If no error is present, indicate by circling "no error."

#	word	transcription		correction
1.	bijou	/biʃu/	no error	biʒu
2.	neither	/niθɚ/	no error	niðɚ
3.	verify	/vɛrifaɪ/	no error	vɛrɪfaɪ
4.	hosed	/hosd/	(no error)	hoʒd
5.	Hoosier	/huʒɚ/	(no error)	
6.	panther	/pændɚ/	no error	pænθɚ
7.	assure	/əʃur/	(no) error	
8.	favored	/fevɚd/	(no error)	
9.	shining	/shaɪnɪng/	no error	ʃaɪnɪŋ
10.	earthy	/ɛrθi/	no error	ɜ˞θi
11.	amnesia	/æmniʒə/	(no error)	
12.	unthinking	/ʌnθɪnkɪŋ/	(no error)	ʌnˈθɪnkɪŋ

Continues

EXERCISE 5.3 (*cont.*)

J. Transcription Practice
Transcribe the following words using the IPA.

1.	Garth	/gɑrθ/	21.	thunder	/ˈθʌndɚ/
2.	fence	/fɛns/	22.	heather	/ˈhɛðɚ/
3.	sure	/ʃʊr/	23.	satin	/ˈsætɪn/
4.	dozed	/dozd/	24.	sheepish	/ˈʃɪpɪʃ/
5.	soared	/sɔrd/	25.	surrounds	/səˈraʊndz/
6.	hives	/hɑɪvz/	26.	Horton	/ˈhɔrtən/
7.	shout	/ʃaʊt/	27.	thirty	/ˈθɜ˞ti/
8.	thorns	/θɔrnz/	28.	vision	/ˈvɪʒən/
9.	those	/ðoz/	29.	pharynx	/ˈfɛrɪnks/
10.	haste	/hest/	30.	third base	/θɪrd bes/
11.	perhaps	/pɚˈhæps/	31.	goiter	/ˈgɔɪtɚ/
12.	shorter	/ˈʃɔrtɚ/	32.	terror	/ˈtɛrɚ/
13.	perused	/pɚˈuzd/	33.	thousand	/ˈθaʊsɛnd/
14.	unversed	/ənˈvɜ˞st/	34.	contour	/ˈkantɔr/
15.	mother	/ˈmʌðɚ/	35.	shortcake	/ˈʃɔrtkek/
16.	consumed	/kənˈsumd/	36.	varied	/ˈvɛrɪd/
17.	mirage	/mɚˈaʒ/	37.	defies	/dɪˈfɑɪz/
18.	potions	/ˈpoʃənz/	38.	discussed	/dɪsˈkʌst/
19.	overt	/oˈvɜ˞t/	39.	shorthand	/ˈʃɔrthɛnd/
20.	Tarzan	/ˈtarzɛn/	40.	muttered	/ˈmʌtɚd/

Complete Assignment 5-3.

The Affricate Consonants

Pronunciation Guide

/tʃ/   as in "chair"   /tʃɛr/
/dʒ/   as in "jar"   /dʒɑr/

The **affricate** manner of production involves a combination of the stop and fricative manners. For this reason, affricates are obstruents. Both English affricates are considered to have a palatal place of articulation. During production of the two affricates, the articulation begins as an alveolar stop. The tongue tip contacts the posterior alveolar ridge; there is a corresponding increase in intraoral pressure in the oral cavity. However, when the breath stream is released (voiced or voiceless), the air is forced through the constriction formed by the tongue and palate, creating a turbulent noise. (The constriction is similar to that formed during production of the palatal fricatives /ʃ/ and /ʒ/, that is, palatal, or postalveolar.)

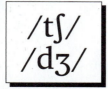

Description

/tʃ/   voiceless, palatal (postalveolar) affricate
/dʒ/   voiced, palatal (postalveolar) affricate

Sample Words

/tʃ/	/dʒ/
chick	jelly
righteous	adjoin
nature	injure
crutch	badger
chimney	Jake
hatchet	refrigerate
wretched	generous

Minimal Pairs

/tʃ/	/dʒ/	/tʃ/	/dʒ/
etch	edge	chin	gin
batch	badge	cherry	Jerri
match	Madge	cheap	jeep
rich	ridge	chalk	jock
"H"	age	choke	joke

Allographs

/tʃ/		/dʒ/	
Grapheme	*Example*	*Grapheme*	*Example*
ch	check	j	joke
tch	witch	g	gem
t	nature	gg	exaggerate
te	righteous	d	educate
ti	question	dg	lodge
		di	soldier

Discussion   Although English has only two phonemic affricates, different languages possess others, such as /ts/. This affricate combines the voiceless alveolar stop /t/ and the voiceless alveolar fricative /s/. The phonemes /t/ and /s/ do appear together in some English words and phrases such as "cats" /kæts/ and "let's go" /lɛtsgoʊ/. In these contexts, /ts/ is not a distinct phoneme. It is actually the result of the phoneme /t/ plus the morpheme /-s/. (In these contexts, /s/ is used as a plural morpheme in "cats" and as a contraction in "let's.") Be careful not to confuse the affricates /tʃ/ and /dʒ/ with the fricatives /ʃ/ and /ʒ/!

EXERCISE 5.4—THE AFFRICATE CONSONANTS

A. Indicate the words below that have /tʃ/ or /dʒ/ in their transcription. Write the correct phoneme next to the word.

✗ bon voyage	____ fantasia	✗ cabbage
✗ barrage	✗ touches	____ exertion
✗ arrange	✗ pasture	✗ sabotage
✗ charming	✗ nitrogen	✗ gender
✗ vulture	✗ riches	____ glacier
____ mushroom	____ charade	✗ eject
✗ gerbil	____ rigid	✗ unchained

B. For each item, create as many real words (or proper names) as possible by placing one of the following fricatives or affricates in the blank. Write your answers to the right of each item. More than one answer is possible for each item.

/f, v, θ, ð, s, z, ʃ, ʒ, h, tʃ, dʒ/

1. /__ɛr/   fair, there, share, hair, chair
2. /__æt/   fat, vat, that, sat, hat, chat
3. /__oʊ/   foe, though, few, show, Joe, hoe
4. /__ɑrm/   farm, harm, charm
5. /__ɪn/   fin, thin, then, shin, gen, chin, gin
6. /ri__/   rif, rich, ridge
7. /bæ__/   bath, bass, bash, batch, badge
8. /bi__/   beef, beach

C. For each item, select the word from the list that has the specified criterion in its transcription. More than one answer is possible for each item.

other   shrunk   none   jeans   hedge   churned   measure

1. Contains an initial voiced phoneme   _____
2. Contains a fricative   _____
3. Contains an affricate and a front vowel   _____
4. Contains an affricate and a nasal   _____
5. Contains a palatal obstruent   _____
6. Contains an obstruent and a central vowel   _____
7. Contains a stop, nasal, and affricate   _____
8. Contains all voiced sounds   _____

D. Circle the words that represent real English words.

1. /skrʌntʃ/	5. /muʒd/	9. /oʊðən/	13. /fæʃtɚ/
2. /pʊdʒɪ/	6. /kɪtʃən/	10. /dʒeɪd/	14. /gaʊtʃt/
3. /tʃɔrz/	7. /moʊtʃ/	11. /hʌdʒ/	15. /dʒʌmpɪ/
4. /hɑrʃɚ/	8. /ʃɑrm/	12. /tʃɝn/	16. /pɑrtʃt/

Continues

EXERCISE 5.4 (*cont.*)

E.   In the blanks, write each of the words using English orthography.

1. /tʃɝpt/ — chirped
2. /dʒʌŋk/ — junk
3. /tʃɪt tʃæt/ — chitchat
4. /wɪʃboʊn/ — wishbone
5. /ədʒɔɪnd/ — adjoined
6. /matʃoʊ/ — macho
7. /gəraʒ/ — garage
8. /pæstʃɚ/ — pasture
9. /ʃʊrlɪ/ — surely
10. /dʒɝzɪ/ — jersey
11. /pɝtʃəs/ — purchase
12. /tʃaklət/ — chocolate
13. /mətʃʊr/ — mature
14. /tʃʌmɪ/ — chummy
15. /ædʒəteɪt/ — adjatate
16. /dʒɛzəbɛl/ —

F.   For each item below, correct any vowel or consonant transcription errors by marking out the incorrect IPA symbol and placing the correct symbol above it. If no error is present, indicate by circling "no error."

1. major — /meɪʒɚ/ — no error   me·dʒɚ
2. March — /martʃ/ — (no error)
3. jumped — /dʒʌmpt/ — (no error)
4. Wichita — /wɪtʃita/ — (no error)
5. wedged — /wɛdʒt/ — no error   wɛdʒd
6. usher — /ʌʃɚ/ — (no error)   sardʒənt
7. sergeant — /sɝdʒənt/ — no error
8. massage — /məsaʒ/ — no error
9. gorge — /dʒɔrʒ/ — no error   gɔrdʒ
10. manger — /mændʒɚ/ — no error   ˈmendʒɚ

G.   Transcription Practice
Transcribe the following words using the IPA.

1. shocked — ʃakt
2. station — ˈsteʃən
3. butcher — bʊtʃɚ
4. knickers — ˈnɪkɚz
5. extra — ˈɛkstrə
6. tangent — tɛnʒɛnt
7. southern — ˈsʌðɚn
8. necktie — ˈnɛktaɪ
9. corsage — kɔrsadʒ
10. spirits — spɪrɪts
11. vivid — ˈvɪvɪd
12. shutter — ˈʃʌtɚ
13. excite — ɛksaɪt
14. axon — æksɑn
15. scoured — ˈskaʊərd
16. carved — karvd
17. outshine — aʊtˈʃaɪn
18. gender — ˈdʒɛndɚ
19. careless — kɛrlɛs
20. nurture — ˈnɝtʃɚ
21. cashmere — kæʒmɪr
22. chopping — tʃapɪn
23. cashbox — kæʃbaks
24. genders — ˈdʒɛndɚ
25. charming — ˈtʃarmɪn
26. sharpened — ʃarpend
27. cashier — kæʃɪr
28. garbage — ˈgarbɪdʒ
29. orchids — ɔrkɪdz
30. strengthen — ˈstrɛngθən
31. exists — ɛksɪts
32. ginger — ˈʒɪndʒɚ
33. thorny — θɔrnɪ
34. Egypt — idʒɪpt
35. chow mein — tʃaʊmeɪn
36. perverse — pɚˈvɝs
37. duchess — dʌtʃɛs
38. anxious — ˈɛnkʃəs
39. mischief — ˈmɪstʃɪf
40. capture — kæptʃɚ

Complete Assignment 5-4.

The Approximant Consonants: Glides and Liquids

Pronunciation Guide

Glides

/j/   as in "yet"   /jɛt/   /w/   as in "wet"   /wɛt/

Liquids

/r/   as in "rip"   /rɪp/   /l/   as in "lip"   /lɪp/

The **approximants**, the last group of consonants to be discussed, fall into a manner of production quite different from the others already discussed. In some respects, these four phonemes behave both like vowels, and in other respects like consonants. Even though these consonants are produced with an obstruction in the vocal tract, the articulators are merely approximated (not brought together) during their production; the constriction in the vocal tract is less than that associated with the English obstruent consonants.

Because the approximants do not usually form the nucleus of a syllable, they cannot be categorized as vowels. (The phoneme /l/ may become syllabic in some contexts, however.) In a manner similar to vowels, all of the approximants are voiced, so their sound source originates in the larynx. Also, all approximants are produced with a closed velopharyngeal port.

Phoneticians have given various names to this group of consonants. The approximants have been termed *semivowels, frictionless continuants,* and *oral resonants.* The approximants are generally subdivided into two groups: *glides* and *liquids.*

Glides, as their name suggests, involve a gliding motion of the articulators, in a manner similar to the production of a diphthong. For this reason, glides are often referred to as semivowels (although some individuals use this term to refer to *all* approximants). The duration of an approximant glide is shorter (faster) than the duration of a diphthongal glide. Glides are always prevocalic. The glides /j/ and /w/ are characterized by continued movement of the articulators throughout their production into the following vowel.

The term **liquid** is used to categorize the oral resonant consonants /r/ and /l/. Some phoneticians have categorized the liquids as semivowels and also as glides. The term *liquid* is in no way a reference to the way in which these phonemes are produced. *Liquid* is simply a general term that has been adopted by phoneticians to categorize these two phonemes.

Lowercase j

Description

/j/   voiced, palatal glide

Sample Words

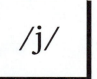

	/j/
your	feud
young	cured
yellow	mutate
Yale	onion
yes	fewer

Allographs

/j/

Grapheme	Example
y	yell
u	fuse
eu	feud
i	union

Discussion /j/ is produced by raising the tongue blade toward the palate (see Figure 5.7). The tongue and lips are in a position similar to that for production of the vowel /i/. The articulators then glide away from the articulation for /j/ to the lip and tongue position necessary for production of the following vowel. The continual motion of the articulators is what characterizes this consonant as a glide. Because the articulators change while gliding from /j/ to the following vowel, a corresponding change occurs in relation to the resonance of the vocal tract.

To demonstrate the similarity in articulation for the glide /j/ and the vowel /i/, say the word "yam" /jæm/. Prolong the initial /j/ phoneme as you say the word. You should hear the phoneme /j/ being produced as you glide from /i/ to /æ/ (/iiiiæm/).

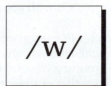

Lowercase w

Description

/w/	voiced, labiovelar glide

Sample Words

/w/

when	swill
weed	Kuwait
quick	away
twins	penguin
square	quartz

Allographs

/w/

Grapheme	Example
w	we
wh	why
qu	quit
u	language

Discussion The phoneme /w/ is characterized by its two simultaneous places of articulation, bilabial and velar. During the production of this phoneme, the lips become rounded, and at the same time, the back of the tongue approximates the soft palate. (Say a word beginning with /w/ and see for yourself.) In the production of this phoneme, the lips and tongue begin in the aforementioned position and continue their gliding movement into the following vowel. The beginning articulatory position for /w/ is quite similar to the position for the vowel /u/. Try saying the word "week" /wik/ by prolonging production of /w/. You should hear the glide /w/ being produced as you glide from /u/ to /i/ (/uuuuik/).

Some individuals differentiate between the voiced phoneme /w/ and the voiceless phoneme /ʍ/. The phoneme /ʍ/ is used by some speakers who pronounce the first two letters in words such as "when," "where," and "which" as "hw." For example, /ʍɛn/ would indicate a pronunciation of /hwɛn/ for "when." Most speakers of American English do not distinguish between the voiced and voiceless /w/ in their speech habits. In this text, only the voiced /w/ will be adopted.

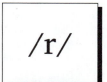

Lowercase r

Description

    /r/   voiced, palatal (postalveolar) liquid

Sample Words

/r/

red	car	rhesus	more
stress	fear	carrot	pure
brown	there	revolt	stork

Allographs

/r/

Grapheme	Example
r	rose
rr	barren
rh	rhododendron

Discussion   The official IPA symbol for this phoneme is actually /ɹ/ (known as "turned r"). As was mentioned earlier, /r/ is the symbol for a voiced alveolar trill, a sound found in Spanish and Finnish but not in English. As mentioned in Chapter 1, we will use the symbol /r/ to represent this particular phoneme. Because /r/ and /ɹ/ do not both exist in English, there will be no confusion as to its use. Also, /r/ is easier to write when doing transcription by hand. Of course, it is much easier to type /ɹ/ than it is to write it!

/r/ can be produced in one of two ways by English speakers even though they are both perceived the same. The production of **retroflex** /r/ involves raising the tip of the tongue and curling it back toward the rear of the alveolar ridge (or the anterior portion of the hard palate). That is why /r/ is referred to by some phoneticians as *postalveolar*. The front of the tongue lowers during production of retroflex /r/, causing the tongue body to become hollowed. The second method of producing /r/, the **bunched** articulation, involves lowering the tip of the tongue and raising (or bunching) the body of the tongue so that it closely approximates the hard palate. The voiced breath stream is forced through the constrictions formed by either method. Both the retroflex and bunched articulation of /r/ are often accompanied by lip rounding depending on the following vowel (Ball & Müller, 2005; Ladefoged & Johnson, 2011).

In Southern and Eastern American dialects, some speakers delete postvocalic /r/, as in "star" [stɑː] (note the lengthened vowel). Recall from Chapter 4 that in Southern and Eastern American dialects, some speakers *derhotacize* the central vowels /ɚ/ and /ɝ/, producing them without r-coloring as in "butter" /bʌɾə/ or "third" /θəd/, respectively. Similarly, Southern and Eastern speakers may vocalize postvocalic /r/ in the rhotic diphthongs /ɪr/, /ɛr/, /ʊr/, and /ɔr/ by substituting /ə/ for /r/. Some examples include "fair" /fɛə/ and "lure" /lʊə/. In these examples, the diphthong has become derhotacized (losing its r-coloring) due to the substitution of /ə/ for /r/.

Lowercase l

Description

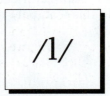

/l/	voiced, alveolar liquid

Sample Words

/l/

lawn	jello
split	mulch
bowl	hollow
black	pistol
bottle	allure

Allographs

/l/

Grapheme	Example
l	lend
ll	ball

Discussion   Because the airstream for /l/ flows over the sides of the tongue, /l/ is classified as a **lateral** consonant. The phoneme /l/ has two separate articulations depending on whether the phoneme is prevocalic or postvocalic. Each of these results in a different allophone of /l/. For prevocalic /l/ (as in "lip" or "slip"), the tongue tip is raised in order to approximate the alveolar ridge. In this position, the back of the tongue remains low in the oral cavity, and the airstream is diverted over both sides of the tongue. This is the production for the so-called *light* /l/. Other examples of *light* /l/ include "clue," "police," and both /l/s in "Lulu."

When /l/ occurs in the postvocalic position of words, the tongue tip is lowered, and the back of the tongue is raised to approximate the palate as the airstream passes over both sides of the tongue. This is the production for the *velarized*, or *dark*, /l/. This allophone of /l/ is found in the words "tall," "chorale," "until," and "welcome." In narrow transcription, dark /l/ is transcribed as [ɫ], as in "tall" [tɑɫ] and "chorale" [kɔræɫ], and *light* /l/ is transcribed as [l], as in "let" [lɛt]. For now, however, we will not distinguish between the two allophones, and we will transcribe them both using the same IPA symbol, namely, /l/. The use of diacritics in narrow transcription will be addressed in much greater detail in Chapter 8.

In many words, postvocalic /l/ becomes a syllabic consonant. Recall that a syllabic consonant serves as the nucleus of a syllable as in the words "rotten" /rɑʔn̩/ and "happen" /hæpm̩/. Unlike syllabic nasals, syllabic /l/ does *not* have to follow a homorganic consonant in order for it to be syllabic.

Examine the following examples of syllabic /l/. Listen to each of the words so that you are comfortable with its transcription.

legalize	/ligl̩ɑɪz/	bottled	/bɑɾl̩d/
hobble	/hɑbl̩/	hustle	/hʌsl̩/
cardinal	/kɑrdn̩l̩/	bundle	/bʌndl̩/

Note that all of the previous examples have a velarized (dark) l in their transcriptions even though it is not indicated (e.g., [hʌsɫ] and [bʌndɫ]).

In terms of dialectal variation, in African American English, word-final /l/ is sometimes replaced by /ʊ/ as in "nickel" /nɪkʊ/ or "bell" /bɛʊ/. Also, some Asian Indian speakers of English substitute /əl/ for syllabic /l/, as in "legal" /ligəl/.

EXERCISE 5.5—THE APPROXIMANT CONSONANTS

A. Indicate which of the following words has an approximant in its transcription. Write the correct phoneme, that is, /w, j, r, or l/, next to the word.

X awkward	X reasoned	___ suede	X jonquil
X bellow	X towered	X fewer	X screaming
X quick	___ Jupiter	X peril	X barley
___ today	X lazy	X swiped	X puny
___ torpedo	X repaid	X yawned	X fired

B. Indicate with an "X" which of the following words have /j/ in their transcription.

___ tune	___ hood	___ choosy
___ jealous	X piano	X compute
X putrid	___ maybe	X usual
___ loop	___ jar	X yours
X fuel	___ adjourn	___ daisy
___ keynote	X Cupid	___ boysenberry

C. Indicate with an "X" which of the following words have /w/ in their transcription.

___ awesome	X why	X warrior
X well	___ awry	X swept
X stalwart	___ wrath	X quirk
___ how	___ rowboat	___ borrowed
___ showed	X reward	___ wrist
X lower	X Howard	X wayward

Continues

EXERCISE 5.5 *(cont.)*

D. Indicate with an "X" the words that have /r/ in their transcription.

_____ lurk	__X__ surround	_____ purchase
__X__ barter	__X__ rewritten	_____ perfected
_____ burgundy	_____ tires	__X__ scorpion
__X__ unreal	__X__ fourth	_____ flirtatious
__X__ guarded	__X__ spirited	__X__ grandiose
__X__ grasp	_____ curvature	_____ divert

E. Circle the words that represent real English words.

1. (/dʒɛloʊ/)	6. /sɝklz̩/	11. /spjud/	16. /fjunts/
2. /blaɪð/	7. /fjɝt/	12. (/wɑlʃat/)	17. /jɛlɪ/
3. /riljə/	8. /kwɔrl̩d/	13. /swɪlz/	18. (/skjud/)
4. /ɚoʊlɚ/	9. /wʊln̩/	14. /riwɝd/	19. (/akwəd/)
5. (/dʒɑr/)	10. /pjaɪd/	15. /poʊləs/	20. /riɚən/

F. In the blanks, write each of the words using English orthography.

1. /jɛloʊ/	yellow	9. /lɪkwəd/	leakwud
2. /robʌst/	robust	10. /taɪld/	tiled
3. /warɪɚ/	warrior	11. /kəteɪld/	
4. /jɝnd/	yearned	12. /kwarl̩/	qvarrel
5. /biɾl̩z/	beetles	13. /lʌkl̩ɪ/	luckily
6. /graʊtʃt/	grouched	14. /læʔn̩/	Latin
7. /ripjut/	repute	15. /fjuʃə/	fushia
8. /gwavə/	guava	16. /kwɛstʃən/	question

G. For each item below, correct any vowel, diphthong, nasal, or stop consonant transcription errors by marking out the incorrect IPA symbol and placing the correct symbol above it. If no error is present, indicate by circling "no error."

1. bowling	/boʊwlɪŋ/	(no error)
2. wrongful	/wrɑŋfʊl/	no error
3. warbled	/warbl̩d/	no error
4. pewter	/piuɾɚ/	no error
5. quandary	/qwɑndrɪ/	no error
6. regional	/ridʒənl̩/	no error
7. lawyer	/l̩ɔjɚ/	no error
8. flurries	/fl̩ɝis/	no error
9. fuming	/fjumɪŋ/	no error
10. baloney	/bʌloʊnɪj/	no error
11. relish	/ɚɛlɪʃ/	no error
12. confusion	/kənfuʒən/	no error

Continues

EXERCISE 5.5 (*cont.*)

H. Transcription Practice
Transcribe the following two-syllable words, using the IPA.

1. quicksand   ˈkwɪksɛnd
2. slouched   ˈslaʊtʃd
3. jury   ʤɝi
4. acquaint   əˈkwent
5. shoulder   ˈʃoldɚ
6. slither   slɪðɚ
7. sergeant   sɑrʒɛnt
8. skewer   skjuɚ
9. cordial _____
10. useful _____
11. withdrew _____
12. worship _____
13. enshrined _____
14. fumed _____
15. luncheon _____
16. junior _____
17. unscathed _____
18. shrivel _____
19. Yankees _____
20. quarter _____

21. bugle _____
22. chisel _____
23. eunuch _____
24. Charles _____
25. belonging _____
26. rubric _____
27. unique _____
28. bequeathed _____
29. kayak _____
30. billiards _____
31. eyewash _____
32. lingual _____
33. quarreled _____
34. anguished _____
35. outward _____
36. rupture _____
37. shoe wax _____
38. quotient _____
39. strangler _____
40. allure _____

Complete Assignment 5-5.

Review Exercises

A. For the following words, determine whether a *tap* (ɾ), a *glottal stop* (ʔ), or *nasal plosion* (np) is found in its transcription. Fill in the blank with the appropriate answer. If none of these are apparent in the transcription, leave the answer blank.

____ 1. writin'
____ 2. rudder
____ 3. about
____ 4. nutty
____ 5. harden
____ 6. certain
____ 7. crater
____ 8. winter
____ 9. Martin
____ 10. sudden

B. Indicate with an "X" which of the following words or phrases have a syllabic consonant in their transcription.

_____	1. wheel	_____	6. pull
_____	2. written	_____	7. contagious
_____	3. regal	_____	8. that'll
_____	4. Seton Hall	_____	9. grab 'em by the neck
_____	5. candles	_____	10. hold 'er by the tail

C. For all of the consonant phonemes below, indicate their manner, place, and voicing.

	Manner	*Place*	*Voicing*
Example:			
/d/	stop	alveolar	voiced
/k/	_____	_____	_____
/r/	_____	_____	_____
/θ/	_____	_____	_____
/ŋ/	_____	_____	_____
/dʒ/	_____	_____	_____
/b/	_____	_____	_____
/ʃ/	_____	_____	_____
/j/	_____	_____	_____
/f/	_____	_____	_____
/n/	_____	_____	_____

D. Create at least two minimal pairs for the underlined phoneme so that they match the differing features given.

Differing Features

Example:

p̲it	mitt, wit	voice manner
1. s̲eed	_____	voice manner
2. cop̲e	_____	voice manner place
3. s̲ome	_____	place
4. z̲ip	_____	voice place
5. b̲ag	_____	place manner

E. Each of the following pairs of words differ by one phoneme. Determine how the phonemes differ in terms of manner, place, and/or voicing. Then list the differing features for each pair given.

Differing Features

Example:

none-ton   voice, manner

1. sin-sing
2. jaw-raw
3. sue-shoe
4. tin-tip
5. clue-crew
6. cop-mop
7. choke-joke
8. pet-met
9. done-gun
10. even-Eden
11. Yale-rail
12. late-lake
13. fame-shame
14. cat-cad
15. pass-pad

F. Identify the words that contain an affricate. If the word has an affricate, indicate the position in the word (prevocalic, postvocalic, or intervocalic), and whether the affricate is voiced or voiceless.

Word	Transcribed Affricate	Voicing	Position in Word
Example:			
charm	/tʃ/	voiceless	prevocalic
1. jester			
2. version			
3. itchy			
4. cash			
5. switched			
6. January			
7. regime			
8. mashing			
9. crush			
10. urgent			

G. Transcribe the underlined consonant allographs in the following words and indicate the appropriate voicing, place, and manner of articulation.

Word	Transcribed Phoneme	Voicing	Place	Manner
Example:				
c̲ab	/k/	voiceless	velar	stop
1. c̲elery				
2. bree̲c̲h				
3. p̲hase				
4. wr̲eck				
5. cal̲l̲				
6. me̲t̲hod				
7. y̲es				
8. cru̲d̲e				
9. c̲hasm				
10. ed̲g̲e				
11. w̲alk				
12. cohe̲s̲ion				

H. Transcription Practice

**CD #2
Track 1**

Transcribe the following words, using the IPA.

1. birthmarks _____
2. conjuring _____
3. beachcomber _____
4. otherwise _____
5. George Bush _____
6. Vatican _____
7. zinc oxide _____
8. handkerchief _____
9. expedite _____
10. foundation _____
11. admitted _____
12. thereafter _____
13. injunction _____
14. convergence _____
15. sabotage _____
16. physician _____
17. buttonhole _____
18. discouraged _____
19. evolved _____
20. indigent _____

21. cosmos _____
22. chimpanzees _____
23. discarded _____
24. prestigious _____
25. charming _____
26. Turkish bath _____
27. bothersome _____
28. jackknife _____
29. enzyme _____
30. tooth fairy _____
31. cherry pie _____
32. coauthor _____
33. hyacinth _____
34. enjoyment _____
35. pharmacist _____
36. unworthy _____
37. 100th _____
38. pasteurized _____
39. fidgety _____
40. Father's Day _____

I. Transcription Practice

Transcribe the following words (containing three syllables), using the IPA.

**CD #2
Track 2**

1. aorta _____
2. airliner _____
3. congealed _____
4. Caucasian _____
5. vocation _____
6. funeral _____
7. registered _____
8. yesterday _____
9. November _____
10. troublesome _____
11. upholstered _____
12. impudent _____
13. torrential _____
14. distribute _____
15. diaphragm _____
16. appetite _____
17. persevere _____
18. courageous _____
19. muscular _____
20. papyrus _____

21. sequential _____
22. portrayal _____
23. Thanksgiving _____
24. xylophone _____
25. artichoke _____
26. pigeonhole _____
27. Williamsburg _____
28. undergrowth _____
29. humorous _____
30. weariness _____
31. universe _____
32. ungathered _____
33. manuscript _____
34. obscurely _____
35. nucleus _____
36. quadrangle _____
37. harmonize _____
38. registrar _____
39. parboiled _____
40. structural _____

Complete Assignments 5-6 and 5-7.

Study Questions

1. What is a consonant? How do vowels and consonants differ?
2. Define the terms *sonorant* and *obstruent.*
3. Define the terms *manner, place,* and *voicing.*
4. Distinguish between *prevocalic, postvocalic,* and *intervocalic* consonants.
5. What is meant by the term *nasal plosion*?
6. What is a *syllabic* consonant? Which consonants can become syllabics in English? What are the rules that govern their usage?
7. When would you use a *tap* and a *glottal stop* in phonetic transcription?
8. Indicate the sound source for each of the following: vowels, stops, nasals, fricatives, affricates, and approximants.
9. Describe the actual ways in which the following consonant manners are produced: stops, fricatives, nasals, affricates, and approximants.

Online Resources

Hall, D. (n.d.). University of Toronto, interactive vocal tract. Retrieved from
  http://www.chass.utoronto.ca/~danhall/phonetics/sammy.html
  (interactive visual display of the vocal tract for all English phonemes)

University of Iowa Phonetics Flash Animation Project. (2001–2005). fənɛtɪks: the sounds of spoken English.
  Retrieved from *http://www.uiowa.edu/~acadtech/phonetics/#*
  (video and animation of English, German, and Spanish consonant production)

University of Victoria Department of Linguistics, Linguistics IPA Lab. (n.d.). *Public IPA chart.* Retrieved from
  http://web.uvic.ca/ling/resources/ipa/charts/IPAlab/IPAlab.htm
  (interactive IPA chart with pronunciations of all IPA consonant symbols)

Assignment 5-3   Name _____

Stop, nasal, and fricative consonant transcription.

Transcribe the following three- and four-syllable words.

CD #2
Track 5

1. succinctness	_____	26. seventeenth	_____
2. Alzheimer's	_____	27. thereabouts	_____
3. ambition	_____	28. homeopath	_____
4. commercial	_____	29. understanding	_____
5. unsanctioned	_____	30. uncertainty	_____
6. decomposed	_____	31. vaporizer	_____
7. visionary	_____	32. thermometer	_____
8. cathartic	_____	33. subconsciousness	_____
9. admonish	_____	34. sarcophagus	_____
10. systemic	_____	35. reservation	_____
11. ombudsman	_____	36. orthodontist	_____
12. redemption	_____	37. perversity	_____
13. Zambia	_____	38. subdivision	_____
14. schematic	_____	39. weatherbeaten	_____
15. horrific	_____	40. unconvincing	_____
16. aversion	_____	41. chauvinism	_____
17. vehemence	_____	42. innovative	_____
18. Venetian	_____	43. impersonate	_____
19. thoroughfare	_____	44. heterodyne	_____
20. orthodox	_____	45. catechism	_____
21. zucchini	_____	46. extortionist	_____
22. xenophobe	_____	47. disorganized	_____
23. fluorescent	_____	48. incandescence	_____
24. excavate	_____	49. criticism	_____
25. symphonic	_____	50. conversation	_____

Assignment 5-4

Name _____

Stop, nasal, fricative, and affricate consonant transcription.

Transcribe the following three- and four-syllable words.

CD #2
Track 6

1. repackaged _____
2. compassion _____
3. digestive _____
4. confiscate _____
5. injury _____
6. membranous _____
7. Egyptian _____
8. geosphere _____
9. foundation _____
10. intersperse _____
11. maturate _____
12. exertion _____
13. effervesce _____
14. matchmaker _____
15. chimpanzee _____
16. astonish _____
17. gestation _____
18. omniscient _____
19. amateur _____
20. chastisement _____
21. advantaged _____
22. pasteurized _____
23. x-axis _____
24. disparage _____
25. educate _____

26. affectionate _____
27. contortionist _____
28. menagerie _____
29. moisturizing _____
30. notorious _____
31. pessimistic _____
32. North Dakota _____
33. unimportant _____
34. terrifying _____
35. punctuation _____
36. potassium _____
37. jurisdiction _____
38. pedagogy _____
39. participant _____
40. overshadow _____
41. homogenized _____
42. indigestion _____
43. damaged goods _____
44. thundershower _____
45. graduation _____
46. juxtaposing _____
47. photogenic _____
48. designation _____
49. sandwiches _____
50. pathologies _____

Assignment 5-5   Name _____

Stop, nasal, fricative, affricate, glide, and liquid consonant transcription.

Transcribe the following three- and four-syllable words.

CD #2
Track 7

1. quietly _____
2. wondrous _____
3. Hercules _____
4. cultural _____
5. koala _____
6. rebellious _____
7. quantify _____
8. subsequent _____
9. withering _____
10. aquarium _____
11. inquiry _____
12. curious _____
13. worldly _____
14. strategy _____
15. pressurized _____
16. puberty _____
17. symbolic _____
18. refusal _____
19. wonderfully _____
20. journalism _____
21. disgruntled _____
22. visualize _____
23. Yosemite _____
24. malicious _____
25. illustrious _____
26. glorified _____
27. flamboyant _____
28. chromium _____
29. extrapolate _____
30. employee _____
31. legalized _____
32. delinquency _____
33. accumulate _____
34. chlorinated _____
35. Asiatic _____
36. ballerina _____
37. quagmire _____
38. inflammable _____
39. legislation _____
40. futuristic _____
41. burglarize _____
42. slovenly _____
43. nonchalant _____
44. liquidate _____
45. infuriate _____
46. bureaucracy _____
47. exquisitely _____
48. acquittal _____
49. bulimia _____
50. ridicule _____

Assignment 5-6

Name _____

Transcribe the following geographical locations in IPA.

1. Bowling Green, Kentucky _____
2. Wheeling, West Virginia _____
3. Albuquerque, New Mexico _____
4. Tallahassee, Florida _____
5. Chattanooga, Tennessee _____
6. Joplin, Missouri _____
7. Honolulu, Hawaii _____
8. Anaheim, California _____
9. Thunder Bay, Ontario _____
10. Rochester, Minnesota _____
11. Prague, Czechoslovakia _____
12. Helsinki, Finland _____
13. Raleigh, North Carolina _____
14. Tijuana, Mexico _____
15. Omaha, Nebraska _____
16. Denton, Texas _____
17. Geneva, Switzerland _____
18. Istanbul, Turkey _____
19. Johannesburg, South Africa _____
20. Hiroshima, Japan _____
21. Antwerp, Belgium _____
22. Montreal, Quebec _____
23. Boise, Idaho _____
24. Boston, Massachusetts _____
25. Stockholm, Sweden _____

Assignment 5-7

Name _____

Transcribe the following.

CD #2
Track 9

1. curious savage _____

2. transmission fluid _____

3. terrible twos _____

4. lightning 'n' thunder _____

5. persuasive argument _____

6. apparent dilemma _____

7. algebra equation _____

8. legal document _____

9. implausible idea _____

10. perplexed child _____

11. veritable fortune _____

12. grapefruit juice _____

13. watermelon rind _____

14. Wuthering Heights _____

15. torrential downpour _____

16. Scranton, PA _____

17. very tranquil _____

18. butterscotch pudding _____

19. patchwork quilts _____

20. oxygen cycle _____

21. anxious parent _____

22. earthquake rumble _____

23. pasteurized milk _____

24. privileged character _____

25. punitive damages _____

26. pharyngeal inflammation _____

Acoustic Characteristics of Vowels and Consonants

Learning Objectives

After reading this chapter you will be able to:

1. Identify and describe the acoustic characteristics of vowels and diphthongs.
2. Identify and describe the acoustic characteristics of stops, nasals, fricatives, affricates, glides, and liquids.
3. Describe the acoustic cues associated with manner, place, and voicing of consonants.
4. Identify the acoustic cues associated with vowels and consonants as seen on a spectrogram.

The purpose of this chapter is to introduce you to the acoustic characteristics associated with speech sound production. In Chapters 4 and 5, you learned about production of consonants and vowels and how to transcribe them using the IPA. The focus of those chapters was on speech *production* from an articulatory point of view. Little information was provided in relation to the acoustic information associated with each vowel and consonant. Each phoneme has a unique acoustic characteristic in terms of its perceived pitch, intensity, and duration. These acoustic differences help explain why one phoneme sounds completely different from any other phoneme. In other words, it is the acoustic specifications of individual speech sounds that alert a listener to the differences between individual consonants, between a consonant and a vowel, and between individual words and sentences.

Time, Frequency, and Intensity

In acoustics, three major physical parameters are used to describe the acoustic characteristic of any sound, including speech sounds. These three parameters are *time, frequency,* and *intensity*. The measurement of **time** in acoustics simply refers to the duration of any particular sound. Time is usually recorded in milliseconds (msec.) but also may be recorded in seconds (sec.; 1 sec. = 1000 msec.).

The **frequency** of a sound can be defined as the number of cycles a vibrating body completes in 1 second. Recall that in males, the vocal folds open and close approximately 125 times per second. Therefore, we can say that the fundamental frequency of the average male larynx is 125 cycles per second, or 125 Hertz (Hz), (named after Heinrich Hertz, a famous German physicist). Similarly, the tines of a 500-Hz tuning fork vibrate back and forth 500 times per second. *Hz*, as opposed to *cycles per second*, is more commonly used in speech and hearing science to represent the frequency characteristic of a sound. Acoustically, each phoneme of a language has unique frequency information associated with it, due not only to the movement of the vocal folds (fundamental frequency) but also to the resonances of the vocal tract linked to that phoneme. Frequency is perceived in terms of **pitch**. There is a direct relationship between frequency and pitch; as the frequency of a sound increases, so does its perceived pitch.

Intensity refers to the amplitude (magnitude) of energy associated with a particular sound. The greater the energy associated with a particular auditory event, the greater its intensity. As an example, clap your hands together. Now clap them more forcefully. In both cases you created a disturbance (movement) of air molecules on and surrounding your hands. The disturbance of air molecules was less when you lightly brought your hands together than when you clapped more forcefully. That is, the disturbance created a greater movement of air molecules when you clapped harder. The greater the movement of air molecules, the greater the energy expended, and the greater the intensity generated. Similarly, when a whisper escapes the lips, a disturbance of air molecules will result, creating a sound wave that will reach the listener's ear. The amplitude of the wave related to this disturbance in the air molecules would be appreciably less than the amplitude of a sound wave consistent with yelling. Typically, intensity is recorded in *decibels* (dB); however, other units of measurement also may be used (e.g., watts/meter^2). Note that the abbreviation "dB" is both singular *and* plural. If a sound measures 25 decibels, the correct notation is 25 dB, *not* 25 dBs. Intensity is perceived in terms of **loudness**. Similar to frequency and pitch, there is a direct relationship between intensity and loudness; as the intensity of a sound increases, so does its loudness.

In terms of the intensity of all English phonemes, the vowels and diphthongs are generally greater in intensity than the consonants. This is mainly because of the greater amplitude of acoustic energy associated with the resonance of the vocal tract during their production, when compared to consonants. This is due to the fact that the sound source is entirely from the vocal folds and the vocal tract is fairly open with no major constriction. The least intense vowel, /i/, is greater in intensity than /r/, the consonant with the greatest intensity. Next to vowels, sonorants have the greatest intensity, followed by the obstruents. The phoneme with the greatest acoustic energy, the vowel /ɔ/, is approximately 680 times more powerful than the voiceless fricative /θ/, the phoneme with the least acoustic energy (Fletcher, 1953). The difference in decibels between these two phonemes is approximately 28 dB. Keep in mind that these are average intensity values; the intensity of individual phonemes in connected speech varies considerably from utterance to utterance, from speaker to speaker, and from conversation to conversation. The intensity of connected speech also varies depending on whether a person is whispering (45 dB), speaking at a conversational level (65 dB), or talking loudly (85 dB) (Fletcher, 1953).

A **waveform** is a graphic representation of sound that displays time on the *abscissa* or *x*-axis, and intensity on the *ordinate* or *y*-axis. The waveform in Figure 6.1a displays a waveform of the word "attack" /ətæk/. The phonetic transcription has been provided to help you identify the individual phonemes.

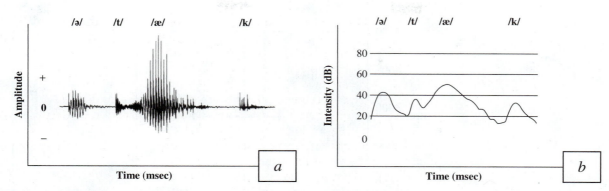

FIGURE 6.1 Speech waveform (*a*) and intensity contour (*b*) of the word "attack."

You already know that when sound occurs there is a disturbance in the air causing movement of air particles. The positive and negative fluctuations in the waveform given in Figure 6.1a simply reflect the back-and-forth movement of air particles during sound production.

Upon examination of the waveform, you should be able to see the differentiation of the four individual phonemes (corresponding to the phonetic symbols displayed directly above). You should have no trouble seeing that /æ/ has the greatest amplitude of all the phonemes in the word. This is because it is a stressed vowel, due to stress on the second syllable. Also notice that /ə/ has a greater amplitude than either of the two voiceless stops, even though it is in an unstressed syllable.

Figure 6.1b is a line drawing, called an *intensity contour,* that is derived from the waveform in Figure 6.1a. The contour shows the *average* intensity of the speech waveform at each moment in time from the beginning of the word until the end of the word. Notice that the *x*-axis still represents time; however, the *y*-axis is now labeled in decibels (dB). The average intensity of the four phonemes is 43 dB for /ə/, 37 dB for /t/, 51 dB for /æ/, and 34 dB for /k/. The intensity contour makes it easier to see that the vowels are more intense (in dB) than either of the consonants. When you compare all four phonemes, it becomes evident that there is a 17-dB variation in intensity among the 4 phonemes. This is a good example of how much the intensity of speech varies over time.

In regard to duration, vowels are generally longer than most consonants in any particular syllable. In Figure 6.1a, you can see that the two vowels are longer in duration than either /t/ or /k/. The actual length of any vowel or consonant phoneme is quite variable; phoneme length varies in relation to (1) whether the phoneme occurs in a stressed syllable, (2) the phonemic context (the other vowels and consonants that surround a particular phoneme in a word), and (3) the importance of the meaning of a word in an utterance that contains the phoneme. The speech waveform gives essential information related to the amplitude of speech over time. However, it is not possible to examine individual phonemes in terms of their frequency composition. *Spectrograms* are employed for just this purpose.

A **spectrogram** is a graphic representation of all three major physical parameters of sound: time, frequency, and intensity. Figure 6.2 shows individual spectrograms of the minimal pair "heed" /hid/ and "who'd" /hud/. Each of the spectrograms in Figure 6.2 is labeled phonetically at the top so

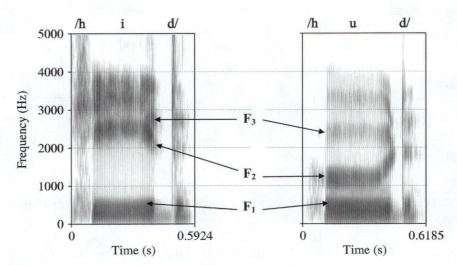

FIGURE 6.2   Spectrograms of the words /hid/ and /hud/.

that you can identify each phoneme with its corresponding acoustic representation. Similar to a waveform, time is indicated on the abscissa. The time it took the speaker to produce these two words is approximately 600 msec. (0.6 second). You can readily see that the vowel is longer in duration than the consonants in both spectrograms. On a spectrogram, frequency is indicated on the ordinate. You can see that the phonemes /h/ and /d/ have frequency tracings that cover a wide range of frequencies. This can be seen by examining the *vertical* marks that extend over a range of almost 5000 Hz from the bottom to the top of each spectrogram. Variations in intensity are indicated on a spectrogram as gradients in shading; sounds of greater intensity are darker than sounds of lesser intensity. Looking at Figure 6.2, you can see that the vowels /i/ and /u/ are greater in intensity (darker shading) than the consonants /h/ and /d/.

Spectrograms also provide evidence of voicing (i.e., vocal fold vibration during speech production). Look carefully at the vowels in the middle portion of each spectrogram. There are vertical striations that run from very low frequency to around 4000 Hz. These striations also can be seen in production of the consonant /d/. Each striation represents one abduction/adduction cycle of the vocal folds during production of voiced speech sounds. In the case of the /i/ vowel for this speaker, each striation occurs every 8 msec. (0.008 sec.). The time it takes a vibrating body to complete *one* cycle is called its **period**. Therefore, the period of vocal fold vibration in this case is 0.008 sec. The formula $f = 1/T$ is used to convert period to frequency (where T stands for time and f stands for frequency in Hz). Conversely, the formula $T = 1/f$ is used to convert frequency to period. For the speaker displayed in Figure 6.2, the fundamental frequency (basic rate of vibration) of the vocal folds is 125 Hz ($f = 1/0.008$).

In the next sections we will look more closely at how time, frequency, and intensity cues help characterize all of the English phonemes. We will first look at the acoustic characteristics of vowels and diphthongs and then turn our attention to consonants.

EXERCISE 6.1

1. Is the speaker in Figure 6.2 male or female? (Hint: You may need to refer back to Chapter 3.)

2. If the period of vocal fold vibration during production of /u/ is 0.004 second, what would be the fundamental frequency of the voice?

3. Your 4-year-old nephew has a fundamental frequency of 400 Hz. What would be the period of vibration of his vocal folds?

Vowels

It is easy to identify vowels on a spectrogram, due to not only their greater duration and intensity (when compared to consonants) but also to the dark *horizontal* bars indicated in each spectrogram (see Figure 6.2). These dark bars are known as **formants**. Formants are resonant frequencies of the vocal tract. Recall in our earlier discussion of the production of the front vowels in the words b*ead*, b*id*, b*ayed*, b*ed*, and b*ad* (Chapter 4), the tongue and lower jaw assume different positions for each vowel. Because the oral structures (including the shape of the pharynx) change during the production of each individual vowel, there is a corresponding change in the natural frequencies of vibration (resonances) of the vocal tract. Each vowel has a unique set of resonances or formant frequencies due to the specific positioning of the articulators necessary in production of each vowel. The formant pattern and accompanying resonance not only give each separate vowel a unique acoustic quality, they also provide acoustic cues to listeners so that each vowel can be recognized individually.

The resonances of the vocal tract associated with vowel production contain primarily low-frequency energy (although higher than the fundamental frequency of the voice). The frequency array, or energy pattern, associated with any sound is called its **spectrum**. Therefore, vowels are considered to have low-frequency spectra and are perceived as being low in spectral pitch. The sonorant consonants (nasals, glides, and liquids) also are characterized as having low-frequency spectra and, therefore, are perceived as low-pitched phonemes. The obstruents (especially the fricatives) have spectra higher in frequency than the vowels and sonorant consonants and are perceived as having higher spectral pitch. This is due to the high-frequency noise (turbulence) generally associated with obstruent production.

It should now be obvious when examining the two spectrograms in Figure 6.2 that the formant patterns associated with the two vowels are quite different because the shape of the vocal tract during their production is also different. The vowel /i/ is produced further forward in the oral cavity, whereas the vowel /u/ is produced further back in the oral cavity.

The first three formants in Figure 6.2 are numbered from F_1 to F_3, starting with the formant that is the lowest in frequency. Generally, the higher-frequency formants are less intense than the lower-frequency formants. Examine the shading of the three formants of the vowel /u/ in /hud/. You will see that the shading (intensity) of F_3 is considerably lighter when compared to the shading of F_1 and F_2. There does not appear to be a difference in intensity between the three marked formants for the vowel /i/ in /hid/. This is only because the formants were artificially darkened so that they would show up better in print.

Now, compare the second formant frequency of each vowel. Note how much higher in frequency the F_2 of /i/ is when compared to /u/. Careful inspection shows that the second formant of /i/ is greater than 2000 Hz, whereas the second formant of /u/ is closer to 1000 Hz. Generally, front vowels (such as /i/) have higher second formants than do the back vowels (such as /u/). Keep in mind that vowels do have more than three formants. See if you can identify F_4 for the vowels in both words in Figure 6.2. For the purpose of speech perception, listeners need to perceive only the lower formants, specifically F_1, F_2, and (sometimes) F_3 in order to be able to recognize and distinguish all of the vowels in English (that is, to be able to tell them apart).

Table 6.1 gives average values for the first two formants of 10 English vowels spoken by adult males. In Figure 6.3, the formant values from Table 6.1 are plotted with F_1 on the ordinate and F_2 on the abscissa. As you examine Figure 6.3, you will immediately see its resemblance to the traditional vowel quadrilateral displayed in Figure 6.4 (which is based on tongue height and advancement in production of vowels). The quadrilateral presented in Figure 6.3 is based on *acoustic* information (the F_1 and F_2 patterns of vowels), and is a much more accurate representation of the actual vowel space than the traditional quadrilateral displayed in Figure 6.4. In essence, then, the traditional vowel quadrilateral is only a schematic diagram of where the vowels *roughly* are located in the oral cavity during speech production.

TABLE 6.1 F_1 and F_2 Values (in Hz) for 10 Vowels, as Spoken by Adult Male Speakers.

	Vowels									
	/i/	/ɪ/	/ɛ/	/æ/	/ɑ/	/ɔ/	/ʊ/	/u/	/ʌ/	/ɝ/
F_1	270	390	530	660	730	570	440	300	640	490
F_2	2290	1990	1840	1720	1090	840	1020	870	1190	1350

Source: Data from Peterson & Barney, 1952.

Given the similarities of Figures 6.3 and 6.4, it appears there must be a relationship between tongue height, tongue advancement, and the formant values associated with each vowel. In fact, there are two rules that relate F_1 and F_2 to tongue height and tongue advancement, respectively:

1. F_1 is *inversely related to tongue height*. That is, the higher the tongue is elevated during vowel production, the lower the value of F_1. For example, the average F_1 of /i/ (a high vowel) is 270 Hz, whereas the average F_1 of /æ/ (a low vowel) is 660 Hz.
2. F_2 is *directly related to tongue advancement*. The more fronted the tongue placement during vowel production, the higher the value of F_2. For example, the average F_2 for the front vowel /i/ is 2290 Hz, whereas the average F_2 for the back vowel /u/ is 870 Hz.

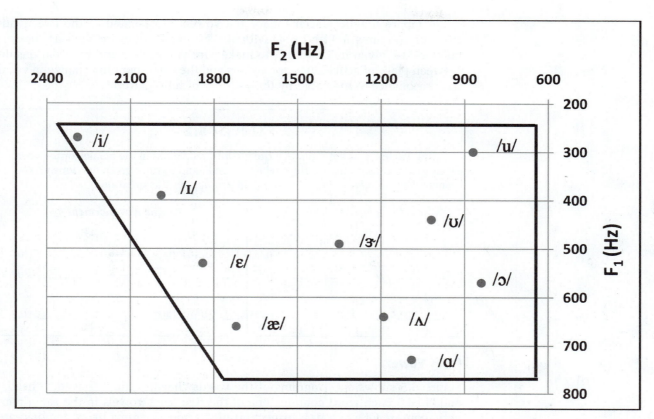

FIGURE 6.3 Plot of average male F$_1$ and F$_2$ values (in Hz) for 10 American English vowels.

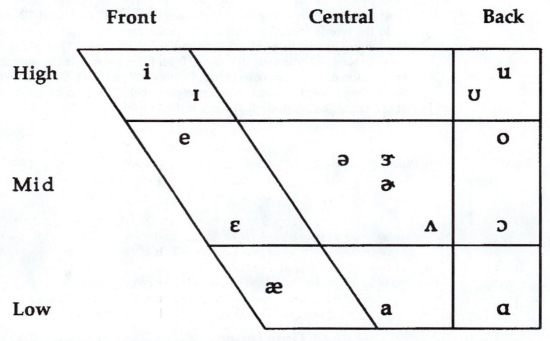

FIGURE 6.4 The traditional vowel quadrilateral showing tongue height and tongue advancement.

Compare tongue placement for the vowels represented in the two quadrilaterals (Figures 6.3 and 6.4) with the F_1 and F_2 rules, as well as the formant values given in Table 6.1, to make sure you understand the relationship between place of articulation for vowels and the corresponding change in vocal tract resonance as indicated by the varying formant patterns.

EXERCISE 6.2

Using Table 6.1 as your guide, write the formant values in the blanks for the vowels given. How do these values relate to the F_1 and F_2 rules given previously? You may want to refer to Figure 6.4 to help you answer this question.

Tongue Height				Tongue Advancement		
F_1		F_1		F_2		F_2
_____ /i/		_____ /u/		_____ /i/ →	_____ /u/
_____ /ɪ/		_____ /ʊ/		_____ /ɪ/ →	_____ /ʊ/
_____ /ɛ/		_____ /ɔ/		_____ /ɛ/ →	_____ /ɔ/
_____ /æ/		_____ /ɑ/		_____ /æ/ →	_____ /ɑ/

Front Vowels

Figure 6.5 shows spectrograms of the words "heed," "hid," "hayed," "head," and "had." Each word contains one of the five front vowels in the same phonetic context (i.e., /h_d/). Inspection of the spectrograms helps demonstrate the F_1 and F_2 formant rules discussed previously. Note the general *increase* in the frequency of the first formant for each of the vowels as the tongue lowers from production of /i/ in "heed" to /æ/ in "had." The change in F_1 is most evident when directly comparing the vowels in "heed" and "had." Now compare F_2 in the words "heed" and "had." Note the fact that F_2 *lowers* in frequency as the tongue lowers in production from "heed" to "had." This is due to the fact that the tongue systematically moves from front to back as the tongue lowers in production of the front vowels (see Figures 6.3 and 6.4). Obviously, then, each front vowel has a distinct resonance pattern linked to changes in vocal tract shape consistent with each vowel's articulation.

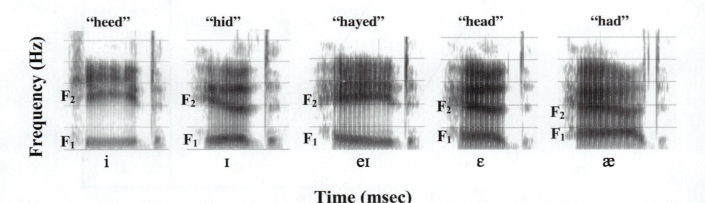

FIGURE 6.5   Spectrograms of the five front vowels in /h_d/ context.

Back Vowels

Figure 6.6 shows spectrograms of the five back vowels in /h_d/ context. Examine the acoustic characteristics of the five vowels, paying attention to changes in the formant patterns as the tongue lowers in production of the five back vowels. As predicted by the F_1 rule, as the tongue lowers in production from /u/ to /ɑ/, the frequency of F_1 rises. The second formant frequency is quite similar at the onset of each of the five vowels. This is because the back vowels are fairly consistent in terms of tongue advancement; they do not change as much in the front/back dimension as do the front vowels. Note, however, that the second formant rises throughout the production of each of the vowels. This is because each vowel begins with the tongue toward the back of the oral cavity (in the velar region) for production of the vowel. Then the tongue moves forward toward the alveolar ridge for production of /d/ at the end of each word. This dynamic change in the frequency of the formant from vowel to following consonant is known as a **formant transition**. The formant transition helps demonstrate how changes in tongue position alter the resonance of the vocal tract. Also, the formant transition is an acoustic cue that identifies the place of articulation of the postvocalic consonant (/d/ in this case). Formant transitions also occur between prevocalic consonants and vowels. More will be said about formant transitions in the section on stop consonants.

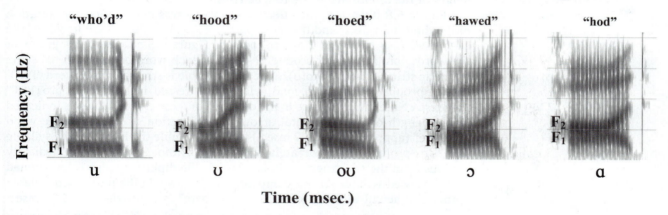

FIGURE 6.6 Spectrograms of the five back vowels in /h_d/context.

EXERCISE 6.3

Spectrograms a and b are of the words "dean" and "don." Which is which? How did you come to your conclusion?

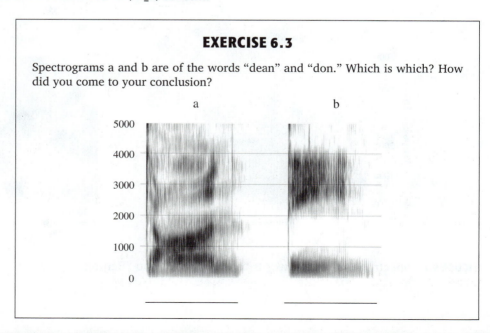

Diphthongs

/eɪ/ and /oʊ/

Recall that the diphthongs /eɪ/ and /oʊ/ were differentiated from the monoph-thongs /e/ and /o/ by their use in stressed syllables and at the end of words. Figure 6.7 demonstrates the effect of syllabic stress on the production of both the diphthong /eɪ/ and the vowel /e/ in the words "away" /əˈweɪ/ and "Bei-jing" /beˈʒɪŋ/, respectively. Note that both words have second-syllable stress. The vowel in the first syllable of "Beijing" would be transcribed with /e/ be-cause the syllable is unstressed. The second syllable in "away" contains the diphthong /eɪ/ because it is a stressed syllable. Note the difference in the dura-tion of these two vowels as indicated by the length of the horizontal arrows in Figure 6.7. The duration of /eɪ/ is 405 msec., whereas the duration of /e/ is only 226 msec. It is clear that stressed vowels are lengthened when compared to unstressed vowels. The diphthong in "away" is also lengthened due to the fact that it is in the final position of the word.

Figure 6.7 indicates that the F_2 of the onglide of /eɪ/ begins at approxi-mately 1000 Hz and rises to an offglide frequency greater than 2000 Hz. Also, consistent with the F_1 rule, note how the frequency of F_1 decreases over the length of the diphthong as the tongue rises from /e/ to /ɪ/.

Figure 6.8 illustrates the effect of syllabic stress not only on the duration of the diphthong /oʊ/ and the monophthong /o/, but also on the length of the entire syllables in which they are located. Figure 6.8 shows spectrograms of the words "probate" and "protest." Note that each word begins with the same phonetic string, that is, /pro(ʊ)/. The first syllable is stressed in the word "PRO-bate" /ˈproʊbet/ and the second syllable is stressed in the word "proTEST" /proˈtɛst/. Note the difference in the duration of these two syllables as indicated by the length of the horizontal arrows. The duration of /proʊ/ in the word "pr<u>o</u>bate" (approximately 292 msec.) is almost double the length of the syllable /pro/ in "pr<u>o</u>test" (approximately 156 msec.). Although it is not immediately obvious from the spectrograms in Figure 6.8, the diphthong also is lengthened in the stressed syllable /proʊ/ compared to the vowel in the unstressed syllable /pro/. The actual duration of /oʊ/ in "pr<u>o</u>bate" is approximately 129 msec.

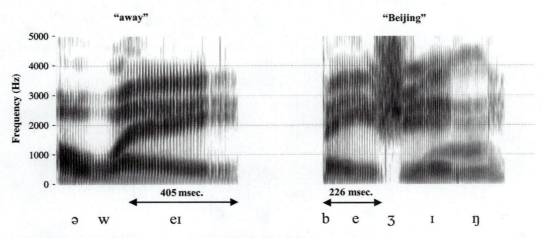

FIGURE 6.7   Spectrograms of the words "away" /əweɪ/ and "Beijing" /beʒɪŋ/.

"PRObate"

"proTEST"

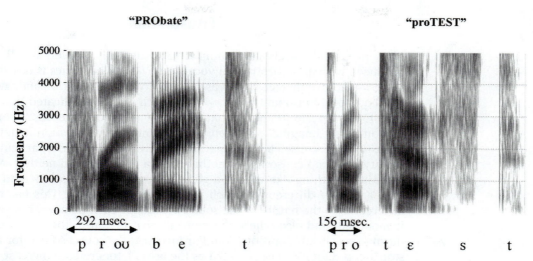

FIGURE 6.8 Spectrograms of the words "probate" /proʊbet/ and "protest" /protɛst/.

whereas the duration of /o/ in "pr<u>o</u>test" is approximately 76 msec. In either case, the vowel comprises almost 50 percent of the syllable.

/ɔɪ, aɪ, and aʊ/

The spectrogram of the words "boy" /bɔɪ/, "buy" /baɪ/, and "bough" /baʊ/ can be seen in Figure 6.9. Note that F_2 rises between the onglide and offglide of the diphthong in production of the words "boy" and "buy." This is predictable from the F_2 rule because the tongue moves forward in the oral cavity as the tongue glides from /ɔ/ to /ɪ/ in "boy" /bɔɪ/ and from /a/ to /ɪ/ in "buy" /baɪ/ (see Figure 6.9). The F_2 of the diphthong /aʊ/ in "bough" /baʊ/ behaves somewhat differently due to the fact that the offglide is a back vowel. As the tongue moves toward the back of the oral cavity as it changes position from /a/ to /ʊ/, there is a corresponding decrease in the frequency of F_2 as would be predicted by the F_2 rule.

For all three diphthongs, there is not much separation in frequency between F_1 and F_2 from the beginning of the word throughout the onglide. However, F_1 in /aɪ/ and /aʊ/ begins at a higher frequency than that seen in /ɔɪ/. The F_1 rule can explain this difference because /ɔ/, the onset of /ɔɪ/, is produced higher in the oral cavity than the onset /a/ in the diphthongs /aɪ/ and /aʊ/.

"boy"   "buy"   "bough"

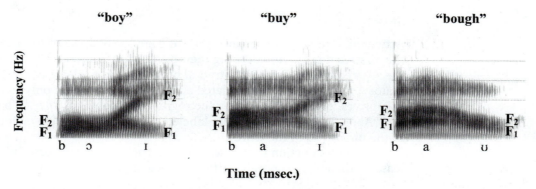

FIGURE 6.9 Spectrograms of "boy" /bɔɪ/, "buy" /baɪ/, and "bough" /baʊ/.

Consonants

Consonants and vowels are nothing alike acoustically. Vowels are all voiced and produced with an unobstructed vocal tract. Vowel acoustics is based primarily on resonances of the vocal tract as dictated by tongue position and jaw opening. As you know, consonant production is much more complicated than that, and therefore a description of consonant acoustics also becomes more complicated. As you might imagine, each consonant manner of production is quite distinct acoustically because each manner is quite distinct in terms of articulation. The quality of a stop consonant is nothing like a fricative, and neither of these has a quality anything like that of a glide since the time, intensity, and frequency cues are quite different for each manner of articulation. This has to do with differences in the nature of the sound source for each manner, how the airflow is modified, and also where the point of obstruction in the vocal tract occurs during speech sound production. For instance, the sound source for a voiceless stop is a brief noise burst created as the articulators release increased intraoral pressure from a point of constriction in the oral cavity formed at either the lips, alveolar ridge, or velum. Whereas the continuous noise associated with voiceless fricatives is generated when the airstream from the lungs is forced through a stricture at either the dental, labial, alveolar, palatal, or glottal places of articulation. The acoustic cues associated with these two very different noise sources are unique in terms of their acoustic specifications. Now add voicing to the equation and the inclusion of a second sound source completely changes the acoustic structure of both stops and fricatives. The nasal consonants also have unique acoustic specifications unlike any of the oral consonants due to the inclusion of the nasal cavity as part of the vocal tract during their production.

In the next section, the acoustic characteristics specific to each manner of production will be discussed. The obstruents will be discussed first, followed by the sonorants. Acoustic cues associated with voicing and place of articulation also will be discussed along with each manner of production.

Obstruent Consonants

The key acoustic feature of the obstruent consonants is the noise source associated with their production. Also, obstruents have voiced and voiceless cognates, unlike the sonorant consonants. As you inspect the acoustic features of the stops, fricatives, and affricates, pay particular attention to the differences in the time, intensity, and frequency cues that make their individual productions distinct from one another.

Stops

Articulation of stop consonants is quite complex because of the way in which the airstream is modified during their production. Stops involve obstruction of the airstream, an increase in intraoral pressure, and a release burst. These articulatory maneuvers have associated acoustic events specific only to production of plosives. Figure 6.10 shows spectrograms of the words "pay," "bay," "ape," and "Abe." The spectrograms are labeled phonetically to help you identify each of the phonemes in the words.

During production of *voiceless* stops, a frictional noise burst follows the release of the stop, especially in the prevocalic position. This frictional noise is

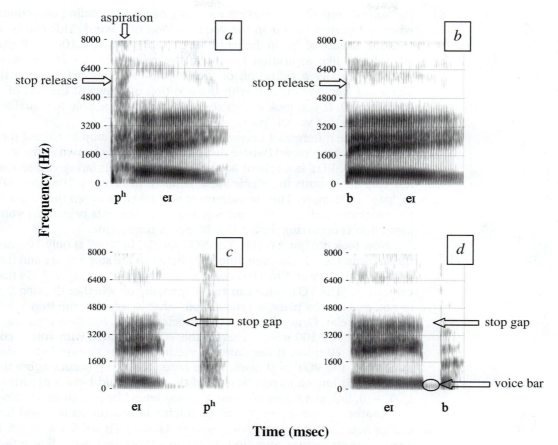

FIGURE 6.10 Spectrograms of the words (*a*) "pay," (*b*) "bay," (*c*) "ape," and (*d*) "Abe."

called **aspiration**. *Aspiration* is often defined as a burst of air associated with the production of voiceless stop consonants (Calvert, 1986; MacKay, 1987). This definition may be somewhat misleading, because all stop consonants have a noise burst associated with their production. Aspiration involves the production of a frictional noise (similar to the glottal phoneme /h/) following the release of a voiceless stop and preceding the following vowel. There is, in a sense, a second burst of noise associated with voiceless stops. Keep in mind that aspiration occurs only in the presence of the voiceless stop consonants /p/, /t/, and /k/. Although there is an audible release burst associated with voiced stops, aspiration (the second frictional noise) is absent. Narrow transcription would indicate aspiration of a voiceless stop as a "raised" [ʰ], as in "turn"[tʰɝn] and "pen" [pʰɛn].

In Figure 6.10a, "pay" [pʰeɪ], the stop /p/ begins with a hardly visible narrow spike of energy (stop release) followed by a long gray-shaded band that runs vertically up to 8000 Hz on the *y*-axis. This vertical band is a display of the aspiration that follows the release of the voiceless stop /p/ (indicated with a white arrow). Notice that in Figure 6.10b, "bay" /beɪ/, there is no such gap (aspiration) between the release of the stop and the following vowel. This is because aspiration does not occur during production of voiced stops. It appears as though the vowel begins almost immediately following the release of the voiced stop /b/. Aspiration also may occur (depending on pronunciation) when a voiceless stop is in the coda position of a word. This can be observed with the release of /p/ in the word "ape" [eɪpʰ] (Figure 6.10c). In Figure 6.10d, what looks like aspiration following the release of /b/ in the word "Abe" /eɪb/ is actually a reflection of the way the speaker pronounced the word. The word was pronounced with the addition of schwa at the end of the word (i.e., /eɪbə/). If you look at Figure 6.10d, you will be able to visualize the formants of the /ə/ vowel.

The time differential between the release of the stop burst and the onset of the voicing of the vowel (where the formants begin) is known as the **voice onset time (VOT)**. VOT is a salient acoustic cue in differentiating voiced from voiceless stop consonants in *syllable initial position*. In Figure 6.10a, the VOT for /p/ in "pay" is 86 msec. This measurement was taken between the stop release and the onset of voicing of the vowel (where the formants begin). As you can see, aspiration is occurring during this 86-msec. time frame.

Now look at Figure 6.10b. The VOT for /b/ in "bay" is only 10 msec. Again, this measurement is the time difference between the stop release and the onset of voicing of the vowel. Voiceless consonants always have longer VOTs than voiced consonants. The VOT value can vary depending on whether the stop is aspirated or not, and also by place of articulation—that is, whether the stop is bilabial, alveolar, or velar. Generally, the VOT associated with voiceless consonants ranges between 25 and 100 msec., whereas the VOT associated with voiced consonants is less than 20 msec. If the onset of voicing and the release burst occur at the same time, the VOT = 0 msec. If the onset of voicing occurs *before* the release burst, this is known as *prevoicing*, and the VOT would have a negative value. If VOT = 0, or has a negative value, the stop would be perceived as being voiced.

Another acoustic cue related to voicing of obstruents is vowel length preceding consonants in *word final position*. Look at Figure 6.10c and 6.10d once again. Pay particular attention to the length of /eɪ/ preceding either /p/ or /b/. What do you notice? It is clear that the vowel is longer in duration when it precedes /b/ (383 msec.) than when it precedes /p/ (222 msec.). Vowels will always be longer when they precede voiced stops than when they precede voiceless stops at the end of a word.

A **stop gap** is another defining characteristic of stop consonants that can be seen while viewing a spectrogram. Stop gaps precede the release of a stop, and can be seen in Figure 6.10c, "ape," and Figure 6.10d, "Abe." The stop gap is a silent interval that reflects the actual time (in milliseconds) when oral pressure is building up in the oral cavity prior to the stop release. Notice that the stop gap preceding /p/ is longer in duration (159 msec.) than the stop gap preceding /b/ (92 msec.). Because intraoral pressure is greater for voiceless than for voiced stops, it takes more time to build up the necessary intraoral pressure to achieve greater pressure. Voiceless stops are perceived as being louder than voiced stops because of the greater acoustic energy that is released with the burst.

During production of *voiced* stops, a low-frequency energy band occurs during the stop gap. This band of energy reflects vibration of the vocal folds during the period of the stop gap, and is called a **voice bar**. A voice bar can be seen in the circled area of Figure 6.10d, preceding the release of the /b/ in "Abe." Contrast this with the absence of the voice bar during production of the voiceless stop /p/ in Figure 6.10c.

To summarize, there are several acoustic cues that signal the presence or absence of voicing during stop consonant production. These include VOT, vowel length preceding a final stop, and the presence of voice bars. In addition, voiceless stops are perceived as being louder than voiced stops due to increased intraoral pressure and a louder release burst.

EXERCISE 6.4

Select the correct stop(s) for the description given.

Ex.	<u>/b/, /d/</u>	VOT = 0 msec.	/p/, /b/, /d/
1.	_____	perceived as being louder than the others	/t/, /d/, /g/
2.	_____	VOT = −5 msec.	/p/, /d/, /b/
3.	_____	VOT = +35 msec.	/p/, /b/, /t/
4.	_____	stop gap preceding the release	/p/, /k/, /d/
5.	_____	longer vowel preceding the stop in coda position	/t/, /p/, /g/

Acoustic information related to *place of articulation* of the stop consonants can also be seen when looking at a spectrogram. Place of articulation cues are located in the formant transitions associated with the vowel either preceding or following the consonant. Figure 6.11 shows spectrograms of the consonant–vowel (CV) syllables /bɑ/, /dɑ/, and /gɑ/. These syllables vary only by place of articulation of the consonant. These specialized spectrograms show mainly the vowel formants with most of the consonant information removed. You still can approximate where the stop burst is for each of the consonants. In these spectrograms, the formants have been highlighted with a series of dots that represent the average formant frequency value (in Hz) from the beginning to the end of each vowel. These dots make it easy to see the individual formants.

Notice that the F_1 for all three stops is quite similar, indicating the stop manner of articulation. However, when you compare F_2 and F_3 between the three syllables, differences will begin to emerge. First, look at the F_2 of /bɑ/. The formant transition begins at a frequency lower than 1000 Hz and rises slightly above 1000 Hz by the end of the vowel. In other words, the formant is making a transition from the consonant to the following vowel in /bɑ/.

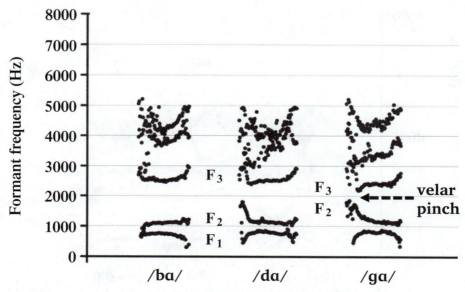

FIGURE 6.11   Formant transitions of the CV syllables /bɑ/, /dɑ/, and /gɑ/.

During production of /dɑ/, the F_2 transition begins close to 2000 Hz and then falls close to 1000 Hz for the remainder of the syllable. Now look at /gɑ/ (velar). The starting frequency of the formant transition associated with F_2 looks fairly similar to that of /dɑ/ (close to 2000 Hz). To see the difference between /dɑ/ and /gɑ/, you must look at the F_3 transition as well. Notice that in /gɑ/, the F_2 and F_3 transitions begin very close together in frequency at the beginning of the syllable (near 2000 Hz). This closeness of F_2 and F_3 is known as the **velar pinch**, and is associated only with velar stop consonant production. Note that there is over a 1000-Hz difference between the starting frequencies of the F_2 and F_3 transitions at the beginning of the syllable /dɑ/.

Figure 6.12 displays spectrograms of the vowel–consonant (VC) syllables "ebb" /ɛb/, "Ed" /ɛd/, and "egg" /ɛg/. When you examine the relationships of F_1, F_2, and F_3 among the three words, you should be able to see some patterns relating to place of articulation. In the word "ebb" (bilabial), the F_2 transition begins around 2000 Hz and falls throughout production of the word, so that it ends at its lowest frequency with articulation of /b/. Recall that in the CV syllable /bɑ/, F_2 also started at its lowest point with articulation of /b/, even though it was at the *beginning* of the word. In both cases, /b/ was associated with a low-frequency formant transition (less than 1000 Hz). In the word "Ed," F_2 drops only slightly from beginning to end and maintains a higher-frequency position (around 2000 Hz). Recall that in the CV syllable /dɑ/, F_2 *began* close to 2000 Hz as well. Finally, for "egg," the F_1 and F_2 transitions are similar to those seen for "Ed." But when F_3 is included, it is very easy to see the velar pinch at the *end* of the word, again indicating velar place of production. In both the CV /gɑ/ and the VC /ɛg/, the velar pinch was around 2000 Hz.

In summary, place of articulation cues for stops can be seen in the formant transitions either preceding or following a vowel in the same syllable. Formant transitions also serve as place of articulation cues for other consonant manners as well, including nasals and glides. F_2 and F_3 transition cues extend into frequencies greater than 1000 Hz (see Figures 6.11 and 6.12). It follows that place of articulation cues may be difficult for hearing-impaired individuals to hear, especially if their hearing loss extends to frequencies above 1000 Hz. This would result in perceptual confusions of minimal pairs such as "tone" and "cone" that differ only by place of articulation.

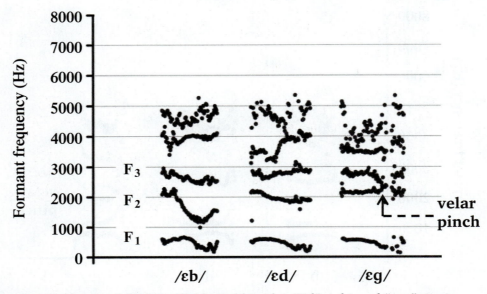

FIGURE 6.12 Formant transitions of the VC syllables "ebb" /ɛb/, "Ed" /ɛd/, and "egg" /ɛg/.

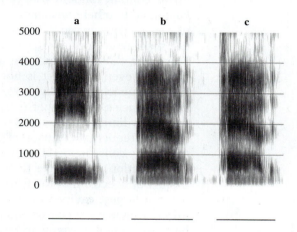

EXERCISE 6.5

The following spectrograms are of the words "pad," "bead," and "bad." Write the appropriate choice in the blank given below each spectrogram. What information did you use to make your decision?

Fricatives

Figure 6.13 shows waveforms and spectrograms of the words "shot" /ʃɔt/, "sought" /sɔt/, "fought" /fɔt/, and "thought" /θɔt/. You will immediately see that the fricatives look nothing like the spectrograms of stops. Note that fricatives appear as wide bands of energy (in terms of duration) that cover a wide range of frequencies. These wide bands of energy visually depict the turbulence created by forcing the breath stream through a narrow channel in the oral cavity. Unlike stops, the noise in fricatives is continuous. That is, it is possible to

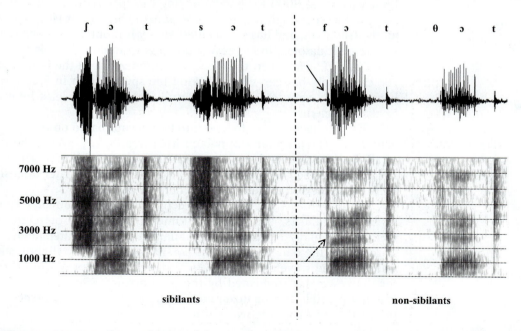

FIGURE 6.13   Spectrograms and waveforms of the words "shot" /ʃɔt/, "sought" /sɔt/, "fought" /fɔt/, and "thought" /θɔt/.

prolong the production of a fricative; it is not possible to prolong the production of a stop.

The forcing of the breath stream through the constriction generally results in production of phonemes that have high-frequency spectra. The turbulent sound associated with fricatives sounds something like *white noise* because fricatives contain random energy that spans a wide range of frequencies. When compared to other consonants, fricatives are among the highest-frequency phonemes. As you can see in Figure 6.13, the *primary* spectral energy for /ʃ/ (where the shading is the darkest) is between approximately 1700 and 5300 Hz. (It is evident that /ʃ/ does have additional resonance that extends up through 8000 Hz even though it is not as intense.) Now compare the primary resonant frequencies of /ʃ/ with /s/. The fricative /s/ has primary spectral energy at frequencies even higher than /ʃ/, that is, between 4600 and 9400 Hz. (The frequency limit was set at 8000 Hz when creating the spectrograms.)

The frequency spectrum of the individual fricatives is dictated by the location of the constriction in the vocal tract during their production (i.e., the place of production). The larger the cavity in front of the constriction, the lower the frequency spectrum of the fricative. Among all of the fricatives, the glottal /h/ has the largest cavity in front of the constriction, and consequently has the lowest-frequency spectrum. Conversely, /f/ and /v/, the labiodental fricatives, have the smallest cavity in front of the constriction and therefore have the highest-frequency spectra associated with them. Therefore, during production of fricatives, as the constriction in the oral cavity moves forward, the resonant frequencies of the frictional noise increase accordingly. It then follows that /s/ (alveolar place of production) would have higher-frequency resonance than /ʃ/ (palatal place of production).

In Figure 6.13, the frequency range for the labiodental fricative /f/ can be seen as a very light, thin band that occurs over a wide range of frequencies extending from close to 100 Hz up to almost 10,000 Hz (indicated with a dashed arrow). (The uppermost frequency range cannot be seen because the frequency limit was set at 8000 Hz when creating the spectrogram.) It is not surprising that /f/ has such high-frequency components because it is the most fronted of all the fricatives, and has the smallest cavity in front of the constriction formed by the articulators. Notice how much less in intensity /f/ is when compared to /s/ and /ʃ/. However, the frequency components of the interdental fricative /θ/ can barely be seen when viewing the spectrogram in Figure 6.13. This is because of its very low intensity. Recall that /θ/ is the least intense of all the English phonemes.

The fricatives can be divided into two groups based on their intensity characteristics. The alveolar and palatal fricatives /s, z, ʃ, ʒ/ are the most intense of all the fricatives and are known collectively as **sibilants**. The **non-sibilant** fricatives include /θ, ð, f, v, and h/. Because of their greater intensity, the sibilants are perceived as being louder than the non-sibilants.

The waveforms in Figure 6.13 confirm what you already know: the two sibilants /ʃ/ and /s/ show increased intensity when compared to the two non-sibilants /f/ and /θ/. Among the sibilants, /ʃ/ has greater intensity than /s/. In regard to the non-sibilants, it is possible to see a very slight peak in the amplitude of the waveform for /f/ in "fought," just prior to the onset of voicing for the vowel /ɔ/ (indicated by the solid arrow). Similar to the spectrogram, it is not possible to visualize much of the acoustic energy associated with the production of /θ/ in the waveform.

As mentioned, voiceless fricatives have greater airflow through the constriction during their production when compared to voiced fricatives. Therefore, voiceless fricatives (especially the sibilants) will appear darker on a spectrogram than voiced fricatives due to their greater intensity. Compare the two spectrograms of the words "leash" and "liege" in Figure 6.14. You can see by the darkness of the shading that /ʃ/ in "leash" is greater in intensity than /ʒ/ in "liege," especially in the higher frequencies.

It is not difficult to distinguish voiced from voiceless fricatives when viewing a spectrogram. This is because during production of voiced fricatives, it sometimes is possible to identify the vertical striations (consistent with vocal fold pulsing) throughout the period of noise. Observe the spectrogram of the fricatives /ʃ/ and /ʒ/ in Figure 6.14. You should be able to see evidence of vocal fold vibration during production of /ʒ/ in "liege," but not during the production of /ʃ/ in "leash" since /ʃ/ is voiceless. Recall that vowels preceding voiced consonants are longer than those preceding voiceless consonants. Figure 6.14 demonstrates this phenomenon with fricatives. When comparing "leash" and "liege," it is clear that /i/ is longer when it precedes /ʒ/ than when it precedes /ʃ/.

Individuals with hearing loss often have difficulty perceiving fricatives in words due to their high-frequency spectra. This is especially true if the hearing loss extends to the higher frequencies. Also, because the non-sibilant fricatives lack intensity (as seen in Figure 6.13), they may be especially difficult to hear. This would explain why hearing-impaired individuals have difficulty being able to tell the difference between minimal pairs such as "thin" /θɪn/ and "fin" /fɪn/, and "elf" /ɛlf/ and "else" /ɛls/.

Affricates

Figure 6.15 shows spectrograms of the two English affricates in the words "batch" /bætʃ/ and "badge" /bædʒ/. It should not be surprising that the acoustic cues for affricates include cues relating to both stop and fricative manners of production. First, note the expected presence of the stop gaps prior to the release of /t/ and /d/ in both words. Also, because the place of articulation is

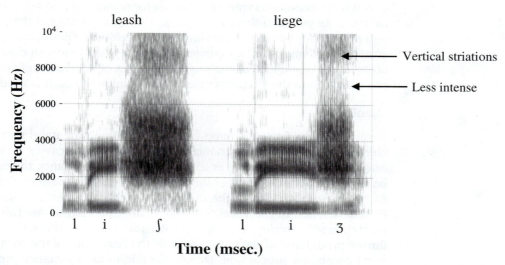

FIGURE 6.14 Spectrograms of the words "leash" /liʃ/ and "liege" /liʒ/.

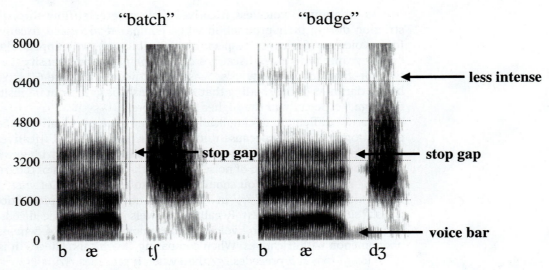

FIGURE 6.15   Spectrograms of the words "batch" /bætʃ/ and "badge" /bædʒ/.

the same for the two affricates, their frequency spectra are similar. A major difference in the two spectrograms is the greater intensity of the fricative component associated with the voiceless affricate when compared to the voiced affricate. This is due to greater airflow through the constriction in the oral cavity during production of /ʃ/. Also, as expected, the spectrogram of the voiced affricate in "badge" shows a voice bar prior to production of /dʒ/. As with stops and fricatives, the vowel is lengthened preceding the voiced affricate /dʒ/ in "badge," when compared to the voiceless affricate /tʃ/ in "batch."

Sonorant Consonants

The sonorant consonants are acoustically distinct from the obstruents in that they are produced with little or no constriction in the oral cavity and are produced with continuous voicing, allowing for resonance throughout the entire vocal tract. As you read through the acoustic characteristics of the sonorants, you will notice they are strikingly similar to the vowels. That is, they have formant structure and are generally greater in intensity and longer in duration than the obstruents. As you look at the acoustic features of the nasals, glides, and liquids, pay attention to the characteristics that are unique to each individual manner.

Nasals

Because airflow from the lungs is directed through the nasal port during nasal consonant production, resonance occurs in the nasal cavity as well as in the oral cavity and pharynx. In production of nasal consonants, the oral cavity can be considered a *sidebranch* of the vocal tract that now extends from the larynx to the nares. The size of the oral sidebranch decreases with the location of the constriction in the vocal tract from /m/ (bilabial) to /n/ (alveolar) to /ŋ/ (velar) (from anterior to posterior). Because the size of the oral cavity varies during production of the nasals, so does the resonance of the vocal tract during nasal consonant production. Due to the additional resonance provided by the nasal cavity, the nasal consonants have a sound quality quite different from the other phonemes in English.

Figure 6.16 shows spectrograms of the minimal pair "bay" /beɪ/ and "may" /meɪ/. The spectrograms allow you to contrast the differences in the production of a voiced bilabial *nasal* and a voiced bilabial *stop*. Examine the spectrogram of the word "may." Notice that the consonant /m/ looks somewhat like a vowel in that it has identifiable formants, unlike the spectrograms of stops. Also note the durational difference between production of a stop versus production of a nasal consonant. When viewing spectrograms of nasal consonants it is sometimes easy to see exactly where the nasal consonant begins or ends due to the abrupt shift in the resonance pattern of the vocal tract brought about by the constriction in the oral cavity and the lowering of the velum. In Figure 6.16, the black arrow indicates the separation of the nasal consonant and the following vowel.

When comparing /beɪ/ and /meɪ/, you may have noticed the slope of the formant transitions for the two words were almost identical. This is because /b/ and /m/ both are bilabial sounds. In this case, the F_2 transition rises from the consonant into the vowel which is consistent with bilabial consonant production in CV words (see the spectrogram of /bɑ/ in Figure 6.11). However, you may have noticed that the F_2 transitions for /beɪ/ and /meɪ/ begin and end at higher frequencies than the F_2 transition seen for the bilabial CV /bɑ/ shown in Figure 6.11. For both /beɪ/ and /meɪ/, F_2 increases in frequency from around 2000 to 2500 Hz, as the tongue rises from /e/ to /ɪ/. The formant transition for /bɑ/ begins and ends around 1000 Hz. Based on your knowledge of vowels and the F_2 rule, this should make sense to you. The diphthong in /beɪ/ and /meɪ/ contains two front vowels, explaining the high-frequency F_2 for those words. On the other hand, the vowel /ɑ/ in /bɑ/ is a low back vowel, with a low F_2.

When the velum lowers in production of a nasal consonant and the lips or tongue form an obstruction in the oral cavity, acoustic energy radiates outward through the nasal cavity. This acoustic radiation is known as **nasal murmur**. Nasal murmur is characterized by a series of formants. The first formant has the greatest energy and is comparable to the amplitude of vowel formants (Kent & Read, 2002). This first formant is called the **nasal formant**. The nasal formant easily can be seen on a spectrogram around 250 to 300 Hz for /m/, /n/, and /ŋ/. The nasal formant for /m/ in "may" is indicated in Figure 6.16 with a white arrow. Note that the nasal formant is lower in frequency than

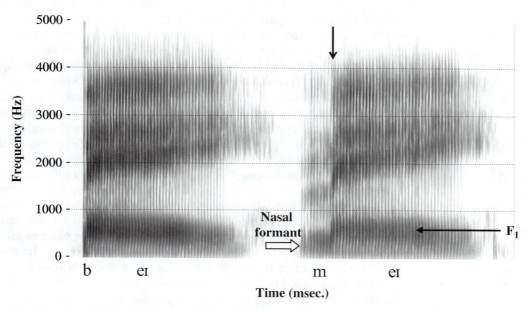

FIGURE 6.16 Spectrograms of "bay" /beɪ/ and "may" /meɪ/.

the F_1 of the vowel /eɪ/ in "may." Now, compare the formants of /m/ and /eɪ/. Notice that the higher-frequency formants of the nasal murmur have considerably less amplitude (lighter shading) than those associated with vowel production. This is because when the velum lowers in production of a nasal phoneme, the vocal tract resonances become less intense due to absorption of sound energy in the nasal cavity. The reduction in the amplitude of energy (intensity) of a vibrating system, brought about by sound absorption, is known as **damping**.

Damping explains only part of the reason why the higher formants associated with nasal murmur have less intensity. Recall that during production of a nasal consonant, the oral cavity is constricted or closed off (at either the lips for /m/, alveolar ridge for /n/, or velum for /ŋ/). No sound escapes through the oral cavity; instead all sound is diverted to the nares. As the velum lowers, *negative* resonances are created in the vocal tract. The negative resonances are referred to as *antiresonances* or **antiformants**. An antiformant arises from changes in the resonance patterns of the *oral cavity* when it becomes a side-branch of the vocal tract. Antiformants cause a general *decrease* in the intensity of the resonances of the vocal tract.

Now compare the diphthong /eɪ/ in the two words "bay" and "may" (Figure 6.16). It should be obvious that the formants of /eɪ/ in "may" appear markedly lighter than the formants of the same diphthong in the word "bay." The decrease in intensity of the formants indicates that the diphthong /eɪ/ has become *nasalized* due to creation of antiformants as the velum is lowered during its production. The word "may" would be transcribed as [meɪ̃] to indicate the diphthong has been nasalized due to the presence of the nasal consonant preceding it.

The velum lowers in production of the three nasal consonants about 100 msec. before the occlusion in the oral cavity begins, and remains lowered for an additional 100 msec. after the consonant has been produced. This leading and lagging of the lowered velum causes vowels occurring 100 msec. before and 100 msec. after the nasal consonant to become nasalized (Pickett, 1999). Therefore, antiformants of the vocal tract cause a decrease not only in the intensity of the formants of the nasal consonant itself but also in the formants of the vowel following it.

Figure 6.17 shows spectrograms of the minimal pair "nose" /noʊz/ and "doze" /doʊz/. Compare initial consonant production of the alveolar nasal /n/ and the alveolar stop /d/. The low-frequency nasal formant is easy to see at the beginning of the word "nose," as is the stop release at the beginning of "doze." You also can see the lighter shaded higher formants of the murmur (in the region of 1500 to 3000 Hz) associated with the /n/ in "nose." Other than at word onset, the major difference in the two spectrograms is the effects of nasalization on the diphthong /oʊ/ in "nose" [noʊ̃z]. Notice that the first four formants have less intensity than those seen for "doze." There is a significant decrease in intensity in the middle of the diphthong for F_3 and F_4. This is brought about by antiformants in the vocal tract during production of /n/. Also, note the almost complete absence of F_5 due to antiresonances. The two spectrograms are similar in terms of vowel formant transitions because the only difference in the two words is the difference in manner of the initial consonant (nasal vs. stop). The second formant transition for /n/ and /d/ both fall from approximately 2000 Hz to around 1200 Hz at the onglide of /o/ of the diphthong, signaling alveolar place of articulation. In addition to formant transition cues, the acoustic structure of the nasal murmur itself also plays a role in perception of *place of articulation* of all nasal consonants (Kent & Read, 2002). That is, the acoustic specification of the three nasals is distinct, alerting listeners to their differing place of articulation.

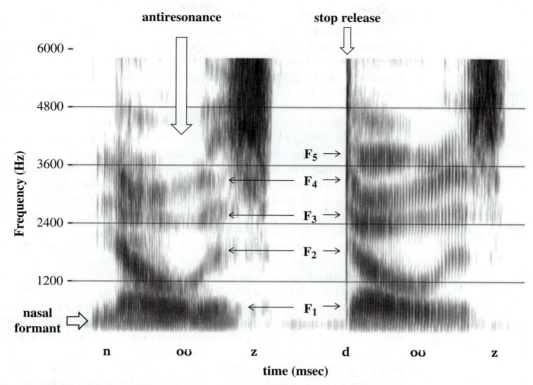

FIGURE 6.17   Spectrograms of the words "nose" /noʊz/ and "doze" /doʊz/.

EXERCISE 6.6

The spectrograms below are of the words "ban," "bat," and "bash." Write the appropriate choice in the blanks given below each spectrogram.

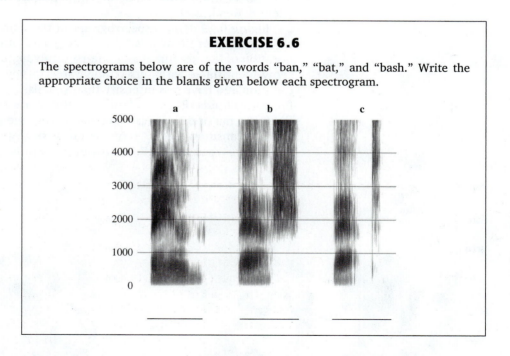

Approximants: Glides and Liquids

Figure 6.18 is a spectrogram of the glides /w/ and /j/ in the intervocalic position of the words "away" /əweɪ/ and "a yay" /əjeɪ/. Note the similarities in the two spectrograms. Because of their formant structure, the glides look very much like vowels or diphthongs. Nevertheless, glides generally are shorter in duration and less intense than vowels. The F_1 of both glides appear very similar on the spectrograms in terms of their low-frequency specifications. However, the frequency specification of F_2 for the two glides is quite different, reflecting the place of articulation associated with each. /w/ has a low F_2. This is not surprising since /w/ has a velar place of articulation similar to the vowel /u/. Recall that because /u/ is a back vowel it has a low F_2. On the other hand, the F_2 for /j/ is high because its place of articulation (palatal) is similar to the front vowel /i/, which has a high F_2. You will see a difference in the higher formants as seen on the spectrograms for these two phonemes. F_3 and F_4 are both visible on the spectrogram during production of /j/. Note that F_3 and F_4 are not visible during production of /w/ (the noticeable white gap above F_1 and F_2). This is because the upper formants have much less acoustic energy than F_1 and F_2.

Figure 6.18 shows a formant transition beginning around 500 Hz for the glide /w/ and rising to around 2000 Hz for production of /eɪ/. This rising transition pattern is consistent with production of other bilabial CV syllables (i.e., "bay" and "may" in Figure 6.16). On the other hand, the glide /j/ has a palatal place of articulation and shows an F_2 transition falling in frequency from approximately 2500 Hz to around 2000 Hz during production of /eɪ/. This falling formant transition is similar to the pattern observed in the CV syllable /dɑ/ in Figure 6.11. Even though /d/ is alveolar and /j/ is palatal, they both have a falling F_2 transition pattern from the consonant into the following vowel. Formant transitions for stop consonants are shorter in duration (they occur more quickly) than transitions for glides (Kent & Read, 2002).

Figure 6.19 depicts spectrograms of the liquids /l/ and /r/ in the intervocalic position of the words "allay" /əleɪ/ and "array" /əreɪ/, respectively. The duration of liquids and glides is fairly equivalent. Similar to glides, the liquids show identifiable formants (comparable to vowels), and they are shorter in duration and have less intensity than vowels. The frequency range of F_1 is low for both liquids. F_2 for /r/ and /l/ also share similar F_2 patterns. However, there is a major difference when comparing the F_3 transitions for /r/ and /l/. The F_3 transition for /l/ remains fairly steady at a high frequency (around 2500 Hz), whereas the F_3 transition for /r/ begins at a frequency less than

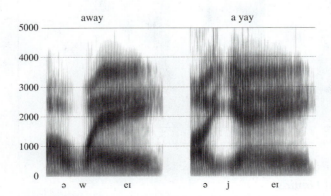

FIGURE 6.18 Spectrograms of the words "away" /əweɪ/ and "a yay" /əjeɪ/.

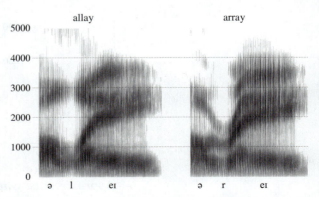

FIGURE 6.19 Spectrograms of the words "allay" /əleɪ/ and "array" /əreɪ/.

1500 Hz and rises to around 2500 Hz for production of the diphthong /eɪ/. This is due to the retroflexed articulation of /r/. The low-frequency F$_3$ associated with production of /r/ is a salient acoustic cue that distinguishes /r/ from /l/.

The lower-frequency F$_3$ transition is also evident when /r/ occurs in the *initial* position of words. Figure 6.20 shows spectrograms of the words "red" /rɛd/ and "led" /lɛd/. The F$_3$ transition associated with /l/ remains fairly stable around 2500 Hz, whereas the F$_3$ transition for /r/ begins at a frequency around 1600 Hz and rises to around 2800 Hz for production of /ɛ/.

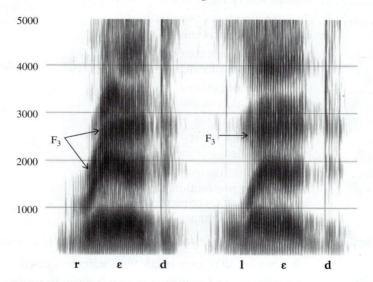

FIGURE 6.20 F$_3$ transitions in word initials /r/ and /l/.

Review Exercises

A. Fill in the blank with the appropriate answer.

1. A(n) _____ is a graphic representation of sound that displays intensity on the ordinate and time on the abscissa.

2. The difference in decibels between whispered speech and loud speech is approximately _____ dB.

3. A spectrogram shows frequency on the _____ -axis and time on the _____ -axis.

4. Aspiration occurs only in production of _____.

5. The frequency array or energy pattern associated with any sound is called its _____.

6. A(n) _____ is the silent interval that reflects the time during which intraoral pressure is increasing prior to its release.

7. A low-frequency energy band present during the period of a stop gap with production of /b/, /d/, or /g/ is called a(n) _____.

8. Of the fricatives, _____ has the lowest-*frequency* spectrum.

9. _____ is the phoneme with the least *intensity*.

B. Match each of the terms at the right with its correct description.

_____	1. negative resonances of the vocal tract	a. formant transition
_____	2. helps cue place of articulation	b. sibilants
_____	3. reduction in the amplitude of a vibrating system	c. aspiration
_____	4. resonances of the vocal tract	d. antiformants
_____	5. high-intensity fricatives	e. frequency
_____	6. time for a body to complete one cycle of vibration	f. damping
_____	7. time between release of a stop and onset of voicing	g. period
_____	8. the number of cycles a vibrating body completes in 1 second	h. VOT
_____	9. frictional noise burst following release of a stop	i. nasal murmur
_____	10. acoustic radiation from the nares during production of /m/, /n/, or /ŋ/, characterized by a series of formants	j. formants

C. Circle T or F to indicate whether you think the statement is true or false.

T   F   1. A negative VOT may occur with voiceless stops.

T   F   2. Another name for antiresonance is nasal murmur.

T   F   3. A low-frequency F_3 helps separate /r/ from /w/ perceptually.

T   F   4. On a spectrogram, intensity is located on the ordinate.

T   F   5. As the frequency of a tone increases, its period decreases.

T   F   6. As the tongue moves forward in the mouth during production of vowels, F_2 increases in frequency.

T   F   7. As the tongue lowers during vowel production, the frequency of F_1 increases.

T   F   8. Stop gaps do not occur during production of voiced stops.

T   F   9. Vowels are usually longer in duration when they precede voiced consonants.

T   F   10. The *velar pinch* can be seen on a spectrogram by examining F_1 and F_2.

T   F   11. /ʃ/ has a lower-frequency spectrum than /s/.

T   F   12. Formant transitions help cue place of articulation of sonorant consonants.

D. Compare each pair of vowels. Then indicate how F_1 and F_2 would vary as the tongue changes in production from the first vowel to the second vowel. Write either "rises" or "lowers" in the blanks.

Example:

/i/   /ɪ/ F_1 ___rises___

1. /u/   /ɑ/ F_1 _____

2. /ɛ/   /i/ F_1 _____

3. /o/   /e/ F_2 _____

4. /ɪ/   /ʊ/ F_2 _____

5. /æ/   /u/ F_1 _____ F_2 _____

E. Spectrogram Interpretation

   1a. The spectrogram below is of one of the CVC words listed at the right. Which
        word is it? How did you come to your conclusion?

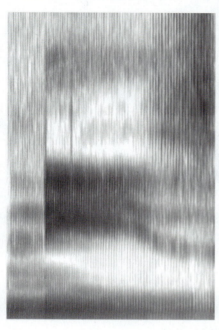

   a. cheese
   b. lease
   c. peace
   d. knees
   e. peas
   f. niece

   1b. The spectrogram below is of one of the CVC words listed at the right. Which
        word is it? How did you come to your conclusion?

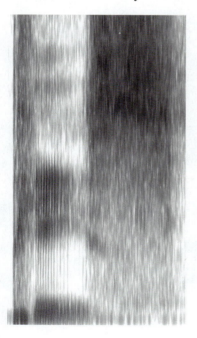

   a. cheese
   b. lease
   c. peace
   d. knees
   e. peas
   f. niece

2. Examine the two spectrograms of the words "rain" and "lane." Which is which? Which acoustic characteristics helped you make your decisions?

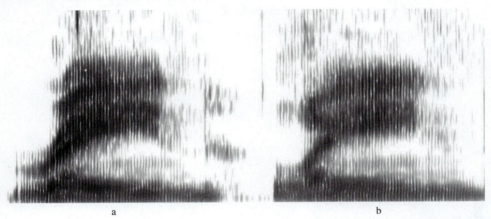

a   b

3. The following spectrogram is of the word "cod." Label each of the following directly on the spectrogram.

   a. a voice bar
   b. a formant transition
   c. F$_2$
   d. a stop gap
   e. aspiration

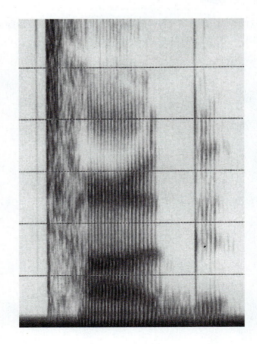

Study Questions

1. How do the F_1 and F_2 rules relate to tongue height and advancement during vowel production?
2. Which acoustic cues help differentiate voiced from voiceless stop consonants?
3. Contrast the terms *time, intensity,* and *frequency*. How are each indicated on a waveform and a spectrogram?
4. What are some ways in which vowels and consonants appear differently on a spectrogram?
5. What is a *formant*? What is its importance in speech acoustics?
6. How do *formant transitions* help cue differences in place of articulation when comparing bilabial, alveolar, and velar consonants?
7. Define the following terms in reference to production of plosives: *stop gap, aspiration, VOT,* and *voice bar*.
8. What are antiformants? What is the impact of antiformants on (a) nasal consonant production and (b) vowel nasalization?
9. What is the difference between a sibilant and a non-sibilant? Which consonants belong to each group?
10. What is the importance of F_3 in perception of liquids?

Online Resources

Boersma, P., & Weenink, D. (2014). Praat: Doing phonetics by computer. Retrieved from
   http://www.fon.hum.uva.nl/praat/
   (free downloadable speech analysis software for Windows, Macintosh, and other operating systems; record new speech samples or use existing speech sound files to create spectrograms and waveforms)

CHAPTER 7

Connected Speech

Learning Objectives

After reading this chapter you will be able to:

1. Explain the effects of assimilation as they relate to speech production and phonetic transcription.
2. Contrast the effects of *elision, epenthesis, metathesis,* and *vowel reduction* as they relate to connected speech.
3. Explain how the suprasegmental aspects of speech impact speech production and phonetic transcription.

The exercises in the previous chapters were designed so that you would learn to recognize all of the individual English speech sound segments and how to determine which IPA symbols best represent them. By now, you should feel fairly comfortable transcribing individual words using the correct IPA symbols in broad transcription. In Chapters 4 and 5, the words given in all of the examples and in all of the exercises were transcribed as isolated items, as if they were excised from a sentence. When a word is pronounced carefully as a single item, it is said to be spoken in its **citation form**. The identity of a word spoken in citation form may differ markedly from its identity in **connected speech**. Connected speech results from joining two or more words together in the creation of an utterance. In Chapter 5, some of the exercises involved transcription of items consisting of two words. However, these two-word utterances were transcribed as if each word was produced in citation form. The production of a particular utterance may vary drastically when comparing its citation form with its form in connected speech. In citation form, the word "him" would be transcribed as /hɪm/. The same word in connected speech might be transcribed as /əm/ as in the phrase "I caught him" /aɪkɔtəm/. Also, in connected speech, the production of any particular utterance will most likely vary from speaker to speaker due to differences in dialect and speaking style.

In clinical practice, speech-language pathologists transcribe isolated words when administering phonological tests to their clients to determine which speech sounds are in need of remediation. More often than not, clinicians need to transcribe entire utterances as spoken by their clients. For example, after obtaining a language sample from a child, a clinician will need to analyze the utterances not only in terms of the specific syntactic (grammatical) structures being used, but also in terms of the particular phonemes the child is using correctly or incorrectly. To perform a thorough phonological analysis of a client's speech patterns, the speech-language pathologist may need to transcribe entire utterances of connected speech.

Several major issues make transcribing connected or continuous speech much different from transcribing isolated words. In connected speech, the phonetic identity of words often changes. As already mentioned, the way a word sounds in citation form varies greatly from the way it might sound in a sentence. In connected speech, phonemes are eliminated and/or completely altered once words are strung together in an utterance. In addition, connected discourse is characterized by continuous changes in the stress, intonation, and timing of phonemes, words, and complete sentences. Listening to, and transcribing, words in continuous discourse requires a lot of concentration. It takes a good ear to be able to hear the subtle nuances associated with connected speech. This chapter will focus on two major issues associated with the transcription of connected speech: (1) assimilation and (2) the suprasegmental aspects of speech.

Assimilation

In citation form, each word is spoken in a fairly deliberate manner. That is, the phonemes are pronounced quite carefully, keeping the inherent length of each phoneme fairly intact. Once words are produced in conversation, the deliberateness of speech disappears. Phonemes are not produced in a strictly serial order as we speak; the onset of one phoneme will occur before the previous one has been completely articulated. This often results in an overlapping of the individual phonemes of English. For instance, the utterance "Where did you go?" might be produced as /wɛrdʒəgoʊ/. The question "What in the world are you going to do?" might be spoken as /wəʔn̩ðəwɜˑldəjəgʊnədu/. The syllable boundaries often become obscured in conversational, or casual, speech, even though listeners have little difficulty understanding what is being said. Also, notice that the quality of the vowels changes quite markedly in connected speech.

While we talk, it is necessary to overlap the production of the various phonemes to maintain the rapidity of connected speech. The overlapping of the articulators during speech production is termed **coarticulation**. Coarticulation is a time-efficient process; there is simply not enough time for the articulators to produce each phoneme in its intended isolated form. In addition, coarticulation makes connected speech easier for the speaker to produce. Speech would become quite laborious and slow, indeed, if each individual phoneme was produced in its full, isolated form in every syllable of every word.

An example of coarticulation can be found in the production of the word "soon." In this word, the lips are already rounded at the beginning of the word in anticipation of the rounded vowel /u/. That is, the normally unrounded phoneme /s/ becomes rounded due to the phonetic environment provided by the vowel. Say the word "soon," paying particular attention to the position of your lips for the phoneme /s/. This rounded version of /s/ (written as [sʷ] in narrow transcription) is an allophone of the /s/ phoneme. Another example of coarticulation can be seen by examining the articulation of the phoneme /n/ in the word "tenth." In "tenth," the tongue is placed against or between the teeth in production of /n/ instead of at the alveolar ridge. That is, /n/ will become *dentalized* in this particular phonetic environment. Dentalized /n/ is an allophone of /n/ indicated by the dental diacritic [̪], as in "tenth" [tɛn̪θ].

It should be apparent (from the previous examples) that a particular phoneme will be articulated differently if that phoneme is preceded or followed by a particular sequence of consonants and vowels. Also, the effects of rapid, continuous speech often will change the phonetic identity of phonemes. It is possible for a particular phonetic context to cause a phoneme to be replaced by a completely different phoneme. Sometimes it is even possible for the phonetic context to result in the complete deletion of a phoneme.

Examine the following utterance: /wʌz ʃi/ ("was she"). In conversation, this utterance is typically produced as /wʌʒ ʃi/. In this case, the /z/ phoneme is produced farther back in the mouth than normal due to the palatal fricative /ʃ/ found in the word "she." Notice that in this example, the change from /z/ to /ʒ/ (due to /ʃ/) occurs across the boundary between the two words. The process whereby phonemes take on the phonetic character of neighboring sounds is referred to as **assimilation**. Some phoneticians suggest that assimilation is brought about as a direct result of coarticulation during the production of connected speech (Calvert, 1986; Ohde & Sharf, 1992).

While some individuals support the notion that coarticulation and assimilation are two separate processes (MacKay, 1987), others use the terms synonymously (Cruttenden, 2008). When viewed as separate processes, coarticulation would be defined as a change in the phonetic identity of a sound that results only in an allophonic variation of a phoneme, whereas assimilation would refer specifically to articulatory changes that result in the production of a completely different phoneme.

In this text, coarticulation will be viewed as the articulatory process whereby individual phonemes overlap one another due to timing constraints and simplicity of production. Assimilation will be viewed as the realized changes in the identity of phonemes brought about by coarticulation. The term *assimilation* will be used here to refer to *both* allophonic changes and phonemic changes brought about by phonetic environment.

Regressive assimilation is one form of assimilation that occurs when the identity of a phoneme is modified due to a phoneme following it. This is also referred to as *right-to-left* or *anticipatory assimilation*. That is, the articulators anticipate the production of a phoneme occurring later in time. An example of regressive assimilation was given for the pronunciation of the phrase "was she" as /wʌʒ ʃi/. Recall that the /z/ in "was" /wʌz/ may be pronounced as /ʒ/ due to the influence of /ʃ/ in "she." This is illustrated in the following:

/wʌz ʃi/ → /wʌʒ ʃi/

Consider the utterance "Would you like to go?" How might you say this utterance? One acceptable pronunciation of this utterance might be /wʊdʒəlaɪkrəgoʊ/. Notice that "would you" is transcribed as /wʊdʒə/. The environment provided by the palatal glide /j/ of "you" alters the pronunciation of /d/ in the word "would," resulting in a right-to-left assimilation of /d/ to /dʒ/. In this case, the alveolar plosive /d/ becomes palatal, inducing articulation of the affricate /dʒ/. A similar example involves production of the word "question." This word can be pronounced one of two ways: /kwɛstʃən/ or /kwɛʃtʃən/. Notice that in the second example, the /s/ has been assimilated to /ʃ/ due to the palatal affricate /tʃ/ in the second syllable of the word. This is a clear demonstration of right-to-left assimilation.

Many of the assimilations brought about by phonetic environment are seen as a change in the *place of articulation* of a particular phoneme. Most of these assimilations are regressive; the phonemes become similar in place of articulation to later-occurring phonemes. The following examples demonstrate regressive assimilation resulting in a change in alveolar place of articulation (from Cruttenden, 2008).

that guy → /ðæk˺ gaɪ/   hat box → /hæp˺ bɑks/

bad boy → /bæb˺ bɔɪ/   road kill → [roʊɡ˺ kɪl]

tin cup → /tɪŋ kʌp/   win more → /wɪm mɔr/

cross check → /krɑʃ tʃɛk/   please share → /pliʒ ʃɛr/

I'll bet you → /aɪlbɛtʃə/   Miss Universe → /mɪʃunɪvɚs/

(Note: [˺] indicates an unreleased plosive.)

On the other hand, **progressive assimilation** occurs when a phoneme's identity changes as the result of a phoneme preceding it in time. This type of assimilation is also called *left-to-right* or *perseverative assimilation*. That is, the articulators persevere in their production of a particular phoneme and maintain a particular posture for a later phoneme. One example of progressive assimilation occurs when a nasal phoneme follows a plosive with the same place of articulation as in "happen" /hæpm̩/. In this case, the place of articulation of the plosive is preserved in production of the nasal in left-to-right assimilation (see Cruttenden, 2008) This is illustrated in the following:

/hæpən/ → /hæpm̩/

Another example of progressive, or left-to-right, assimilation can be seen when the plural morpheme "s" is pronounced as /z/ when it follows a voiced phoneme—for example, /dɑgz/ "dogs" or /ɑrmz/ "arms" (instead of /dɑgs/ or /ɑrms/). In these examples, the voiced phoneme has a left-to-right (progressive) effect on the following plural morpheme "s," causing it to be produced as /z/ instead of /s/. Similarly, production of the past-tense morpheme "ed" is produced as /t/ when preceded by a voiceless phoneme; for example, /wɑkt/ "walked" instead of /wɑkd/.

Elision

In English, it is common for phonemes to be entirely eliminated during production due to particular phonetic contexts. For instance, the word "exactly" may be spoken as /əgzækli/. Notice that the /t/ has been eliminated in this particular pronunciation. Omission of a phoneme during speech production is called **elision**. Another example of elision occurs in the word "camera." It is not uncommon for speakers to pronounce this word as /kæmrə/ as opposed to /kæmɚə/. Note that in /kæmrə/ an entire syllable has been deleted, or *elided*.

Elision often results as a historical process as a language develops over time. Elision also occurs as a result of coarticulation associated with connected speech. In addition, elision is found to occur across word boundaries due to certain phonetic environments. Examine the words and phrases (along with their transcriptions) in Table 7.1 to see the resultant elision brought about by effects of phonetic context.

TABLE 7.1 Examples of Elision.

Utterance	Transcription	Elided Phoneme
aptly	/æplɪ/	/t/
asthma	/æzmə/	/ð/
fifths	/fɪfs/	/θ/
glands	/glænz/	/d/
used to	/juztu/	/d/
cup of tea	/kʌpəti/	/v/
What's his name?	/wətsəzneɪm/	/h/
Give me that.	/gɪmɪðæt/	/v/

EXERCISE 7.1

Examine each of the following utterances and their transcriptions. Indicate in the blank the phoneme that has been elided.

1. lengths   /lɛŋks/   _____
2. friendship   /frɛnʃɪp/   _____
3. countess   /kaʊnəs/   _____
4. bands   /bænz/   _____
5. kept quiet   /kɛpkwaɪət/   _____
6. I caught her.   /aɪkɔɾɚ/   _____
7. word of mouth   /wɝɾəmaʊθ/   _____
8. Where did he go?   /wɛrdɪrigoʊ/   _____

Epenthesis

In connected speech, additional phonemes are sometimes inserted in words during their production. The addition of a phoneme to the production of a word is termed **epenthesis**. Epenthesis can be the result of factors related to (1) coarticulation, (2) variation in production, or (3) speech disorders.

In terms of coarticulation, the glides /j/ and /w/ may sometimes *seem* to appear between two adjacent vowels, either in the same word or in two different words. For example, it may *seem* that the glide /j/ is inserted after a front vowel (or diphthong) in words such as:

"Leo" /li(j)oʊ/   "Ohio" /ohaɪ(j)oʊ/   "we own" /wi(j)oʊn/

Similarly, it may seem that the glide /w/ is inserted after a back vowel, as in:

"cooing" /ku(w)ɪŋ/   "go in" /go(w)ɪn/   "to each" /tu(w)itʃ/

In these examples, the tongue is gliding in transition from one vowel nucleus to another. The addition of these "transitional" phonemes often result as "native speakers correctly pronounce their own language" (MacKay, 1987, p. 147). The glides /w/ and /j/ in these contexts are better thought of as *transitional phonemes*, as opposed to true phonemes. This can be demonstrated by comparing phrases that contrast a transitional /w/ with a phonemic /w/ as in "no axe" /no(w)æks/ versus "no wax" /no wæks/. Say these two phrases aloud, paying attention to your articulation as you say them. You clearly should be able to hear the difference between these two phrases when spoken aloud. Another example with transitional /j/ occurs in comparison of the phrases "my oak" /maɪ(j)oʊk/ versus "my yolk" /maɪ joʊk/ (see Cruttenden, 2008).

Epenthesis may occur in words in which a nasal consonant precedes a voiceless fricative as in:

"tense" /tɛn**t**s/   "lengths" /lɛŋ**k**θs/   "Amsterdam" /æ**m**pstɚdæm/

In production of these words, a homorganic voiceless stop (in bold) may be added during production, even though the stop does not actually occur in the word. These added phonemes are the result of physiological constraints on the articulators (due to coarticulation) when producing the phoneme sequence of nasal + fricative—that is, /ns/ (tense), /ŋθ/ (lengths), and /ms/ (Amsterdam).

Due to individual speaking style or dialectal variation, some speakers do not make a true distinction in production of words such as "chance"/"chants" or "tense"/"tents." For these individuals, both productions would be identical and therefore would be transcribed the same, that is, /tʃænts/ or /tɛnts/. However, many speakers *do,* in fact, make a clear distinction between the two pronunciations of these words: /tʃæns/ – /tʃænts/ or /tɛns/ – /tɛnts/. You will have to listen carefully during transcription to determine whether a speaker is actually inserting a stop following the nasal in these contexts.

Other examples of epenthesis occur in the idiosyncratic or dialectal production of certain words. For instance, the words "elm" and "film" are pronounced by some individuals (including my father) as /ɛləm/ and /fɪləm/. Also, some speakers in the southern United States insert the vowel /i/ before /u/ in words such as "Tuesday" /tiuzdeɪ/ or "due" /diu/. Also, some Asian Indian English speakers will insert a glide before a vowel, as in "okay" /wokeɪ/. The consonant clusters /sp/, /st/, or /sk/ do not occur in the initial position of words in many Asian Indian languages. Therefore, Asian Indian speakers of English may add /i/ or /ɪ/ to the initial portion of the cluster, creating two syllables as in "spot" /ɪspat/ or "school" /ɪskul/.

Finally, epenthesis is sometimes observed in individuals with speech sound disorders. For instance, some children will insert /ə/ in the middle of a consonant blend. Examples include "break" /bəreɪk/ and "glad" /gəlæd/. Schwa insertion is also prevalent in the speech of some deaf individuals.

EXERCISE 7.2

Examine each of the following words and their corresponding transcriptions. Indicate with an "X" the transcriptions that illustrate epenthesis.

1. noon   /nuən/   _____
2. pants   /pænts/   _____
3. choose   /tʃiuz/   _____
4. friends   /frɛnz/   _____
5. lamb   /læm/   _____
6. straw   /strɔr/   _____
7. rinse   /rɪns/   _____
8. milk   /mɛlk/   _____
9. clam   /kəlæm/   _____
10. Wednesday /wænzdeɪ/ _____

Metathesis

The transposition of sounds in a word is known as **metathesis**. Metathesis can occur as a result of a "slip of the tongue," personal speaking style, dialectal variation, or a speech disorder. Some examples include:

elephant	→ /ɛfələnt/	spaghetti	→ /pəsgɛɾi/
ask	→ /æks/	cinnamon	→ /sɪmənən/
realtor	→ /rilətɚ/	animal	→ /æmɪnl̩/

Vowel Reduction

Another issue commonly encountered when transcribing connected speech involves the phenomenon called **vowel reduction**. Often, the full form (full weight) of a vowel (such as /æ/) becomes more like the mid-central vowel /ə/ when spoken in connected speech. Compare the following transcriptions of the utterance "I can go."

/aɪ kæn goʊ/	*citation form with full vowel /æ/*
/aɪkəngoʊ/	*casual form with reduced vowel /ə/*

The first transcription would be indicative of very careful pronunciation, as if all three words were spoken in isolation. Contrast the citation form with the second transcription, the more casual form. Notice that the vowel /æ/ has been reduced to /ə/. In other words, the articulation of the vowel shifted from low front to mid-central. In this case, the tongue does not meet the true articulatory target for /æ/ in the low front portion of the mouth. Instead, the body of the tongue remains toward the center of the oral cavity. You have already experienced vowel reduction in certain isolated words such as "feasible." When transcribing this word, it would be possible to transcribe the second vowel with /ɪ/ as in /fizɪbl̩/ or with /ə/ as in /fizəbl̩/, depending on the pronunciation. In the second transcription, the /ɪ/ vowel reflects reduction to /ə/.

What causes vowel reduction? In connected speech, there is often not time for the articulators to achieve their target positions because speech occurs so rapidly. Therefore, the articulators adopt new positions that are still acceptable to the ear. These vowel reductions are not considered to be "bad," "lazy," or "sloppy" articulations. They are simply considered to be the product of connected speech. Following is a list of words demonstrating the process of vowel reduction. Each word is transcribed twice, first using a particular vowel in its full form, and second using the reduced vowel form. Notice that the two pronunciations for each word are acceptable depending on the way a person might say the words.

Examples of Vowel Reduction

	Full Vowel	*Reduced Vowel*
tomorrow	/tumɑroʊ/	/təmɑroʊ/
decide	/disaɪd/	/dəsaɪd/
tribunal	/traɪbjunl̩/	/trəbjunl̩/
obscene	/ɑbsin/	/əbsin/
excel	/ɛksɛl/	/əksɛl/
domestic	/domɛstɪk/	/dəmɛstɪk/

The following six word pairs are composed of words sharing the same morpheme. Note the difference in pronunciation between the vowels (in bold) in each pair. The first word in each pair has a vowel with full weight, that is, not reduced. The second word of each pair has the reduced form of the vowel. In each pair, the change in vowel form from full to reduced is due to a change in primary word stress *away from the syllable* in question.

transform	/trænsˈfɔrm/	concept	/ˈkɑnsɛpt/
transformation	/trænsfɚˈmeɪʃən/	conception	/kənˈsɛpʃən/
excrete	/ɛksˈkrit/	impose	/ɪmˈpoʊz/
excretory	/ˈɛkskrətɔrɪ/	imposition	/ɪmpəˈzɪʃən/
sequence	/ˈsikwəns/	condemn	/kənˈdɛm/
sequential	/səˈkwɛnʃəl/	condemnation	/kɑndəmˈneɪʃən/

Each of the following word pairs demonstrates more than one vowel undergoing a change in vowel quality. Examine each pair in order to see the changes from the full to the reduced vowel form, or vice versa.

demon	/ˈdimən/	geometry	/dʒiˈɑmətri/
demonic	/dəˈmɑnək/	geometric	/dʒiəˈmɛtrɪk/
metabolism	/məˈtæbəlɪzm̩/	parameter	/pɚˈæmɚɚ/
metabolic	/mɛtəˈbɑlɪk/	parametric	/pɛrəˈmɛtrɪk/

EXERCISE 7.3

Transcribe each of the following word pairs, paying attention to the changes in vowel quality (for the bold letters) inherent in their pronunciations.

Example:

valid	/vælɪd/
validity	/vəlɪdɪɾɪ/

1. m**i**racle _____

   m**i**raculous _____

2. **a**ccuse _____

   accusation _____

3. auth**o**rize _____

   auth**o**rity _____

4. dem**o**lish _____

   dem**o**lition _____

5. mech**a**nical _____

   mech**a**nistic _____

In connected speech, several English monosyllabic words undergo a change in pronunciation when compared to the way they might be spoken in isolation. The change in pronunciation of these words is brought about by vowel reduction associated with changes in word stress. An example can be demonstrated with the pronunciation of the word "as," as in the phrase *as soon as possible* (/əz sun əz pɑsəbl̩/). The reason for this change in the pronunciation of "as" (from /æz/ to /əz/) is due to the fact that, in isolation, the word "as" could be spoken as a stressed monosyllable. In connected, casual speech, it would rarely be stressed. The change in the pronunciation of "as" demonstrates a shift from what is called the *strong form* of the word (/æz/) to the *weak form* of the word (/əz/) (Cruttenden, 2008). The strong form would indicate the word has been stressed. In conversational speech, these words rarely receive stress. For example, the word "the" is rarely pronounced with full stress on the vowel, as in /ðʌ/. More commonly, the pronunciation would be unstressed: /ðə/. Some other examples of weak forms of words include /n̩/ for "and" as in /ðɪs n̩ ðæt/ /jə/ for "you" as in /jə θɪŋk/, /fɚ/ for "for" as in /fɚ mi/, and /ɪ/ for "his" as in /wʌts ɪz nem/.

CD #2
Track 10

EXERCISE 7.4

Transcribe each phrase twice: first in citation form and then in casual form.

Example:

bigger than me	/bɪgɚ ðæn mi/	/bɪgɚ ðən mi/
1. your mother	_____	_____
2. right and left	_____	_____
3. food for thought	_____	_____

Continues

EXERCISE 7.4 (*cont.*)

4. What will they do?   _____   _____
5. Thank him.   _____   _____
6. as big as   _____   _____
7. of mice and men   _____   _____
8. What is her name?   _____   _____

The following examples help demonstrate more clearly pronunciation changes inherent in continuous speech. Compare the first transcription, the citation form of each utterance, with the second transcription, the more casual pronunciation. Keep in mind that the examples given are only *one* possible way of saying each utterance in connected speech. Pay particular attention to the inherent vowel reduction, as well as the assimilation, associated with the more casual form. Note the use of the double-bar symbol in the following transcriptions. It is used to represent punctuation marks in transcription of connected speech. Specifically, the double bar /‖/ replaces semicolons, periods, and question marks.

Did you eat yet? I could eat a horse.

[dɪd ju it jɛt ‖ aɪ kʊd it eɪ hɔrs ‖]

[dʒitjɛt ‖ aɪkədirəhɔrs ‖]

What in the world are you going to do?

[wʌt ɪn ðə wɜld ɑr ju goʊɪŋ tu du ‖]

[wə?n̩ðəwɜldəjəgʊnədu ‖]

What has your brother done with my cat and dog?

[wʌt hæz jɔr brʌðɚ dʌn wɪθ maɪ kæt ænd dɑg ‖]

[wətʃɚbrəðɚdʌnwɪθmaɪkæ?n̩dɔg ‖]

When does the train arrive with her luggage?

[wɛn dʌz ðʌ treɪn əraɪv wɪθ hɝ lʌgədʒ ‖]

[wɛnzðətrenəraɪvwɪðɚlʌgədʒ ‖]

CD #2
Track 11

EXERCISE 7.5

Transcribe the following utterances, first in citation form and then in casual form.

1. I bet you I can help them get out of that mess.

    _____

    _____

2. I caught you cheating on that test. I am going to tell the teacher.

    _____

    _____

3. What is his reason for not being able to come to the party?

    _____

    _____

Continues

EXERCISE 7.5 (*cont.*)

4. What's the matter with Thelma? Let me see if I can cheer her up.

   _____

   _____

5. What did you do to your car? I should be able to get it going.

   _____

   _____

Complete Assignment 7-1.

Suprasegmental Aspects of Speech

In contrast with isolated words, connected speech is characterized by continual modifications or alterations in stress, in the timing of words, and in intonation. It is these alterations that give connected speech its natural characteristic rhythm. Stress, timing, and intonation variations do not affect solely the individual speech sound segments of words. These modifications span entire syllables, words, phrases, and sentences. For this reason, stress, timing, and intonation are generally referred to as the **suprasegmental** aspects of speech production. The prefix *supra-* means *above, beyond,* or *to transcend.* Therefore, the suprasegmental features of speech go beyond or transcend the boundaries of the individual speech sound segment or phoneme, affecting an entire utterance.

Stress Revisited

The preceding discussion should not imply that isolated words are immune from the effects of the suprasegmental features of speech. In Chapter 2, the importance of identifying word stress for purposes of phonetic transcription was discussed. As you recall, a stressed syllable in a word is generally spoken with more articulatory force, resulting in a syllable that is louder, longer in duration, and higher in pitch than an unstressed syllable. Word stress is a suprasegmental feature of speech because entire syllables are stressed, not just individual phonemes. Your transcription practice in the previous chapters has helped you clearly understand the importance of being able to identify the syllables with primary stress in any word. During transcription, you know when to accurately use /ə/ versus /ʌ/ and /ɚ/ versus /ɝ/. Without this knowledge, it would not be possible to transcribe English accurately using the IPA.

In Chapter 2, we were concerned only with identifying primary stress in words. It is time to turn our attention to the other degrees of word stress. Multisyllabic words have syllables with more than one degree or level of stress. For instance, the word "pretense" has two levels of stress: primary and secondary. This word would be transcribed as /ˈpriˌtɛns/. Note that the IPA symbol for indicating secondary stress is a small mark below and to the left of the syllable receiving secondary stress. The following two-syllable words each have two levels of stress.

ˌmainˈtain	ˌtranˈscend	ˈvalˌue
ˌinˈclude	ˌalˈthough	ˈproˌnoun
ˌtranˈscribe	ˈeˌgo	ˈcouˌpon
ˌsarˈdine	ˈmoˌped	ˈpayˌroll

CD #2
Track 12

EXERCISE 7.6

The following words have two levels of stress, primary and secondary. Mark each syllable's stress pattern accordingly, using the appropriate IPA symbols for stress.

1. intense
2. falsehood
3. Lucite
4. rosette

5. teabag
6. frostbite
7. obese
8. entree

9. erode
10. handshake
11. react
12. household

Not all multisyllabic words have syllables with both primary and secondary stress. Some multisyllabic words have only one (primary) stressed syllable. When the nucleus of the other syllable (or syllables) contains either /ə/, /ɚ/, /m̩/, /n̩/, or /l̩/ (or sometimes /ɪ/ and /ʊ/ when produced in a reduced form), the syllable is said to be unstressed. We already know that /ə/ and /ɚ/ are never found in a syllable receiving primary stress. According to Carrell and Tiffany (1960), the schwa vowel is considered an indefinite vowel because it is more of a "murmur" than a full vowel. Its indefinite status makes it a non-prominent nucleus, so much so that it receives no stress at all. The following bisyllabic words have only one stressed syllable (marked appropriately). The other syllable is unstressed.

ˈriddle	ˈperson	surˈround
ˈbutton	ˈzebra	preˈtend
ˈmelon	ˈhappy	conˈtain
ˈmanage	seˈdate	reˈmind

Note that when /ɪ/ is the nucleus of a final open syllable (as in "happy") or the nucleus of the syllable /ɪŋ/, it is unstressed (and lax) as well.

CD #2
Track 13

EXERCISE 7.7

The following bisyllabic words have only one syllable that receives stress; the other syllable is unstressed. Mark the stressed syllable using the correct IPA symbol for primary stress.

1. leopard
2. sweater
3. rhythm
4. contend

5. murky
6. anoint
7. magnet
8. belief

9. scary
10. naked
11. extreme
12. parade

The following three-syllable words have only one stressed syllable:

conˈtagious	baˈloney	aˈlerted
ferˈocious	ˈcalendar	ˈconstable
aˈversion	ˈterrible	ˈshivering
conˈcession	beˈhavior	ˈinterval

The following four-syllable words also have only one stressed syllable:

ˈliteracy	ˈpassionately	volˈuminous
ˈdefinitely	ˈknowledgeable	chroˈnology
ˈspeculative	chryˈsanthemum	couˈrageously
ˈpersonable	toˈgetherness	exˈperience

CD #2
Track 14

EXERCISE 7.8

The following three- and four-syllable words have only one stressed syllable. Mark each one correctly using the IPA symbol for primary stress.

1. measuring
2. statistics
3. laryngeal
4. warranted
5. courageous
6. Germany
7. unbearable
8. Canadian
9. sorority
10. fraternity
11. Albuquerque
12. dysphonia

Now contrast the following three- and four-syllable words that each have syllables with primary and secondary stress (in addition to unstressed syllables).

ˌplanˈtation	ˌreimˈburse	ˌmorˈphemic
ˈinterˌnet	ˌtranˈsistor	ˈtantaˌmount
ˌtranˈscription	ˌMonˈtana	ˈpeneˌtrate
ˈsaxoˌphone	ˈtermiˌnate	ˈzodiˌac
ˈmandaˌtory	ˌparaˈplegia	disˈcrimiˌnate
ˈrepliˌcate	ˌeduˈcation	ˈgeneraˌlize

CD #2
Track 15

EXERCISE 7.9

The following three- and four-syllable words have two levels of stress (in addition to some unstressed syllables). Mark primary and secondary stress using the appropriate IPA symbols.

1. myopic
2. cyberspace
3. architect
4. idea
5. citation
6. circumstance
7. bacteria
8. effervescent
9. alimony
10. communicate
11. elevator
12. Indiana

Complete Assignment 7-2.

Sentence Stress

In addition to word stress, each sentence a speaker produces also has inherent **sentence stress**. Examine the following: "Donna drove to school." Say this sentence aloud in a natural manner, the way you might say it while conversing with a friend. In this manner, you may have noticed that the last word in the sentence tends to stand out or have more emphasis. Say the sentence again, and see if you notice the emphasis on the last word, "Donna drove to 'school." Many sentences and phrases are spoken with the primary emphasis or stress on the last word. Look at the following phrases and sentences. Listen for the emphasis on the final word in each phrase or sentence. Notice the words that receive primary stress, especially in the last two examples.

> I like his 'style.
> Keith and Dick went 'home.
> If I get 'caught, I will get in 'trouble.
> In order to get good 'grades, you will have to study 'harder.

Phrases and sentences do not always end with a stressed word. Certain words in a sentence will usually receive emphasis or stress depending on (1) the level of importance of that word in the sentence and (2) the speaker's intent of the message being conveyed. Words that contain salient information in a sentence are called **content words**. Content words are generally nouns, verbs, adjectives, and adverbs. The less important words in a sentence, including pronouns, articles, prepositions, and conjunctions, are called **function words**. Content words tend to (but do not always) receive sentence stress; function words usually do not receive stress. In the sentence "Donna drove to school," the content words are "Donna," "drove," and "school." Although "school" tends to receive stress when this sentence is produced in a neutral manner, it would be possible to stress the other content words, depending on the speaker's intent. When the final word of the sentence, "school," is stressed, the speaker denotes the location to which Donna drove—she drove to school, not the library. Compare these variations of the sentence:

> Donna 'drove to school.   'Donna drove to school.

What is the speaker's intent in each of these sentences? In the first sentence, the speaker stressed the word "drove" to indicate Donna's mode of transportation—Donna drove to school; she did not walk. In the second sentence, the speaker stressed the word "Donna" to indicate that Donna, not her husband Roger, drove to school. Notice that in each case, stress was placed on a content word.

The use of sentence stress to indicate a speaker's particular intent is termed *contrastive stress*. Examine the stress shifts in the following statements. In each case, the speaker uses stress contrastively to indicate the particular intent desired.

Sentence:	Intent:
Katie purchased a new red sedan.	*Kennedi* didn't buy the car.
Katie *purchased* a new red sedan.	Katie didn't *sell* the car.
Katie purchased a *new* red sedan.	Katie didn't buy a *used* car.
Katie purchased a new *red* sedan.	Katie didn't buy the *green* car.
Katie purchased a new red *sedan*.	Katie didn't buy the *SUV*.

EXERCISE 7.10

<u>Underline</u> the word in each of the following sentences that would receive primary sentence stress, based upon the given intent.

Example:

	Intent:	I didn't buy pants.
	Sentence:	I bought a <u>shirt</u> last week.

1. Intent: We did not go to a play last night.

    Sentence: Aunt Carol and I went to a matinee.

2. Intent: David doesn't live on West Brooklyn.

    Sentence: My neighbor David lives at 4555 East Brooklyn Avenue.

3. Intent: Sam doesn't care for taffy.

    Sentence: Flo ate the taffy from the circus.

4. Intent: Billy and Jennifer talked to their grandmother.

    Sentence: Billy and Jennifer did not get a chance to talk to their uncle.

5. Intent: They liked Mrs. Harlan's husband.

    Sentence: The third graders really liked Mr. Harlan.

**CD #2
Track 16**

EXERCISE 7.11

Listen to each of the following sentences. <u>Underline</u> the word that is given primary sentence stress. Then write the intent of the utterance on the blank line.

Example:

    Mary had a little <u>lamb</u>.

    <u>She didn't have a goat.</u>

1. The girl's name was Chris.

    _____

2. Jared only forgot to get the toothpaste at the store.

    _____

3. Why did they walk to the playground?

    _____

4. Why did they walk to the playground?

    _____

5. Mark got a new blue bike for his birthday.

    _____

6. Mark got a new blue bike for his birthday.

    _____

7. Mark got a new blue bike for his birthday.

    _____

Sentence stress also plays an important role in distinguishing the *type* of information being presented by a speaker. When conversing with someone, the conversation usually volleys back and forth between the two participants. Two types of information are provided during a conversation, **given information** and **new information**. When people converse, each person typically will provide new information to the conversation, adding to the given (old) information previously discussed. For instance, a friend might ask, "What did you have for lunch?" Your reply might be, "I had a hamburger and french fries for lunch." *Hamburger* and *french fries* would be considered new information, since this is your addition to the conversation. Because these words provide new information to the listener, these words would typically be stressed. The phrases "I had a . . ." and "for lunch" would be given information since the information refers back to the prior question; these phrases would not receive stress. Suppose your friend responds, "Oh, I only had a cheeseburger." In this case *cheeseburger* would be the new information in the dialog; it would correspondingly receive stress.

Examine the following conversation between Janet and Robin. They are discussing Janet's most recent purchase. As you read the dialogue, it is easy to see that each participant's response advances the conversation. New information is in italic.

Janet: You got a new *purse.*

Robin: Yeah, I got it at the *mall.*

Janet: *Which* mall?

Robin: The one *downtown.*

Janet: Which *store*?

Robin: Oh. I got it at *Green's.*

Janet: Was it *expensive*?

Robin: It was on *sale.*

Janet: Was it more than *fifty dollars*?

Robin: It was only *twenty*!

As the conversation ensues, each participant stresses or emphasizes the new information she wishes to convey. Of course, neither participant is consciously stressing these words; it happens as a result of knowing how sentence stress is utilized in conversation. The use of sentence stress (as well as other suprasegmental features) is behavior that is the direct consequence of learning language and being familiar with the way language operates in conversation.

CD #2
Track 17

EXERCISE 7.12

The following dialogue is between a waitress and a customer in a restaurant. Circle the words in the dialogue that are stressed in order to convey new information.

Waitress: Would you like something to drink?

Customer: Lemonade, please. I would also like to order.

Waitress: Would you like an appetizer?

Customer: No, thank you.

Continues

EXERCISE 7.12 (*cont.*)

Waitress: Would you like to hear about our specials?
Customer: Please.
Waitress: We have grilled salmon and fettuccine alfredo.
Customer: I'll have the fettuccine.
Waitress: Would you like our house dressing on your salad? It's Italian.
Customer: I would like to have blue cheese, please.
Waitress: I'll also bring out some fresh rolls.
Customer: Thank you.
Waitress: You're welcome.

When marking sentence stress in transcription, you will first need to identify the one word that receives primary sentence stress. Then you will need to identify the other content words in the utterance. The word receiving primary sentence stress will be marked with the traditional IPA symbol (ˈ) preceding the syllable that normally receives word stress. The stressed syllables of the other content words will be marked using the IPA symbol for secondary stress (ˌ). For example, the sentence "I want iced coffee" would be marked for sentence stress in the following manner (depending on the speaker's intent):

ˌI want ˈiced ˌcoffee. (I want cold coffee.)
ˌI want ˌiced ˈcoffee. (I do not want tea.)

Now contrast the following sentence pairs:

The **boys** jumped into the pool.   **Olivia** will be married in September.
The ˈboys ˌjumped into the ˌpool.   ˈOlivia will be ˌmarried in Sepˌtember.

The boys **jumped** into the pool.   Olivia will be **married** in September.
The ˌboys ˈjumped into the ˌpool.   ˌOlivia will be ˈmarried in Sepˌtember.

The boys jumped into the **pool**.   Olivia will be married in **September**.
The ˌboys ˌjumped into the ˈpool.   ˌOlivia will be ˌmarried in Sepˈtember.

Foreign speakers who are learning English as a second language may have trouble with English stress patterns, both in words and in sentences. Word stress is not predictable in English as it is in some other languages. Therefore, it is difficult for new users of English to learn to use stress patterns correctly. Improper use of word and sentence stress may add to the "accent" of an individual learning English as a second language.

Individuals who have a severe or profound hearing loss may experience difficulties producing stress patterns correctly because their auditory channel is diminished. One common characteristic of "deaf speech" is incorrect placement of stress on function words, because the rules of stress placement are not fully understood. A speaker who stresses function words has speech patterns that appear unintelligible to normal hearing listeners because normal listeners are not accustomed to hearing this type of spoken stress pattern.

CD #2
Track 18

EXERCISE 7.13

Mark sentence stress for each of the following items using the appropriate IPA notation. Each sentence will be spoken by two different speakers. Pay attention to differences in stress between the two speakers. You will need the audio CD for this exercise.

Example:

    a. The ˌcow ˌjumped over the ˈmoon.

    b. The ˌcow ˈjumped over the ˌmoon.

1. a. Steve's roommate is from Minneapolis.
   b. Steve's roommate is from Minneapolis.

2. a. Tim went skydiving on Saturday.
   b. Tim went skydiving on Saturday.

3. a. The answer on the exam was "false."
   b. The answer on the exam was "false."

4. a. Mary's birthday is next Tuesday.
   b. Mary's birthday is next Tuesday.

5. a. I'd like a steak for dinner.
   b. I'd like a steak for dinner.

6. a. I went to New York City to see some plays.
   b. I went to New York City to see some plays.

7. a. My professor shaved his mustache.
   b. My professor shaved his mustache.

8. a. I need potatoes from the store.
   b. I need potatoes from the store.

Intonation

It is often difficult to talk about sentence stress without addressing the topic of intonation, another suprasegmental feature of speech. Because stress involves changes in voice pitch, speakers continually modify the fundamental frequency of their voice while speaking in order to stress particular words in an utterance. The modification of voice pitch is known as **intonation**. A speaker's intonation pattern cues a listener as to the type of utterance being spoken, that is, a statement of fact, a question, an exclamation, and so forth. When someone asks a question requiring a yes/no answer, voice pitch generally rises at the end of the utterance. Intonation is also responsible, at least in part, for indicating a speaker's particular mood.

Consider the short sentence "I did." This statement can be spoken in several ways, depending upon the speaker's intent and the corresponding intonation pattern. For instance, "I did" could be spoken as a casual, matter-of-fact reply to the question "Did you read the paper today?" The statement could be spoken with emphasis on the word "did" in response to the never-ending parental question "Have you cleaned your room yet?" In response to "Who ate the pie?" a speaker would probably emphasize the word "I." With each change in speaker intent, there would be a corresponding change in the intonation applied to the utterance. Note that in each version of the utterance, there is not only a change in sentence stress, but also a corresponding increase in the fundamental frequency of the voice, which would be perceived as a higher pitch.

An **intonational phrase** is made up of all changes in fundamental frequency spanning the length of a meaningful utterance. An intonational phrase may consist of an entire sentence, a phrase, or simply one word. Long sentences will usually have more than one intonational phrase. Intonational phrases in longer sentences are signaled by a slight pause in the utterance (indicated in writing with a comma, hyphen, or semicolon). Following are several utterances comprised of one, two, and three intonational phrases.

One intonational phrase:	*Two intonational phrases:*
Yes!	You took my umbrella, didn't you?
I want to go home.	I got a blue scarf, not a red one.

Three intonational phrases:

The boys, who ate the candy, got sick.
Lauren, who is my best friend, took me to the ball game.

There are two intonational phrases in the accusation "*You* took my umbrella, *didn't* you?" The words in italic type would most likely have the highest voice pitch. Say the sentence out loud, paying particular attention to the changes in the pitch of the voice. You will notice that the highest voice pitch occurs on the words "you" and "didn't." Similarly, in the sentence "The boys, who ate the candy, got sick," there are three distinct intonational phrases (separated by commas). You should notice that the highest voice pitch occurs on the words "boys," "candy," and "sick."

The syllable that receives the greatest pitch change in any particular intonational phrase is called the **tonic syllable** (Ladefoged & Johnson, 2011) or **nuclear syllable** (Fudge, 1984). Likewise, the emphasis given to this syllable is referred to as the **tonic accent** or the **nuclear accent**. Each intonational phrase is characterized by only one tonic accent. In the question "Are you done?" the tonic accent would fall on the final word "done." The tonic accent would be located on the second syllable of the word "confused" in the statement "He was confused," because word stress is normally found on the second syllable of that word.

The tonic accent most often is located at the end of an intonational phrase (Ladefoged & Johnson, 2011). However, when a speaker uses contrastive stress to draw attention to a particular word in an utterance, the tonic accent would be located on the stressed syllable. Compare the two pronunciations of the following sentence.

It won't rain *today*.

It *won't* rain today.

In the first example, the tonic accent would be located on the last syllable of the utterance ("It won't rain toˈday"). In the second example, the tonic accent would be located on the second word ("It ˈwon't rain today").

Intonational phrases are characterized by the *direction* of their pitch change; they are generally classified as falling or rising. If the receptionist at your doctor's office asks you, "Do you have an appointment?" you would hear a rise in intonation at the end of the question. If the receptionist states "The doctor will see you in a few minutes" you would probably not hear a rising intonation pattern. The voice pitch would most likely fall at the end of the utterance.

Falling intonational phrases accompany complete statements and commands and are indicative of the finality of an utterance (Jones, 1963). In the sentence "The boys went home" (spoken as an unemotional statement), the voice pitch falls throughout the utterance. There is a general fall, or declination, in the pitch of the voice over the length of most neutrally spoken statements. Some other examples of falling intonational phrases would be evident in utterances such as the following:

I guess.   That should do it.   It's time to go.   I like riding roller coasters.

Falling intonational phrases also are typical in utterances comprised of Wh-questions. Wh-questions are those that begin an utterance with the words "where," "what," "why," "when," "which," and "how." Examples include:

Why did you go?	What's your favorite color?
Where is your friend?	When did you arrive?

Rising intonational phrases (typical of questions and incomplete thoughts) usually indicate some uncertainty on the speaker's part (Jones, 1963; Pike, 1945). As previously indicated, yes/no questions have a rising intonation pattern. Examples include:

Are you coming?	Is it time yet?
He did?	Can you?

Rising intonational phrases also occur with *tag questions*.

His name is Bill, isn't it?	They're watching reruns again, aren't they?
I am gonna just hang out, okay?	He likes Lady Gaga, doesn't he?

Rising intonational phrases also are common when reciting a list of items. For example:

My favorite colors are red, blue, and green.

Say the previous sentence aloud. Listen to the rise in the pitch of your voice, following the words "red" and "blue." Each rise in pitch alerts the listener that more information is forthcoming in the utterance. The voice pitch then falls toward the end of the sentence.

The examples given represent only a few of the more common intonation patterns seen in American English. In addition, the various examples given are only suggestions of the way the utterances could be spoken. It would be possible to pronounce any of the examples in a variety of ways. For instance, the sentence "I can't." could be spoken as a statement (falling intonation) or as a yes/no question (rising intonation)—that is, "I can't?"—depending on the speaker's intent.

CD #2
Track 19

EXERCISE 7.14

Indicate whether the intonational phrases in the following utterances are generally rising or falling. Circle the appropriate response.

1. When will you leave?   Rising   Falling
2. Is your brother home?   Rising   Falling
3. I need to go the library.   Rising   Falling
4. What's your favorite season?   Rising   Falling
5. Did you get paid yet?   Rising   Falling
6. The dog ran away.   Rising   Falling
7. Sophie is my oldest friend.   Rising   Falling
8. How did you know about that?   Rising   Falling
9. Honest?!?   Rising   Falling
10. I'm sure!!!   Rising   Falling

Tempo

Tempo is the term used to describe the durational aspect of connected speech. Because timing, or duration of articulatory events, affects entire utterances, tempo also is considered to be a suprasegmental feature of speech. Obviously, the overall rate of speech plays a role in determining the tempo of speech. For adults, the average speech rate is on the order of approximately 5 to 5.5 syllables per second (Calvert, 1986). Tempo also is determined by the duration of individual phonemes and the duration of pauses located between syllables, words, phrases, and sentences.

Duration of Individual Phonemes

Each of the phonemes in English, when spoken in isolation, has an inherent duration. As a rule, diphthongs have a greater duration than vowels, and vowels have a greater duration than the consonants. Among the consonants, the glides and liquids have the greatest duration; the stop consonants have the shortest duration. The duration of any individual phoneme will change once placed in connected speech. For instance, you already know that the stressed syllable of a word is longer in duration than an unstressed syllable due to the increased duration of its individual phonemes. Refer back to Figure 6.8 in Chapter 6. This figure shows spectrograms of the words ['probate] and [pro'tɛst]. Recall that the diphthong in the first (stressed) syllable of "probate" is longer in duration (129 msec.) than the vowel in the first (unstressed) syllable of "protest" (76 msec.). It follows that the first syllable in "probate" would be longer in duration than the first syllable in the word "protest."

The inherent length of individual phonemes also varies depending upon phonetic context. Recall from Chapter 6 that vowels preceding voiceless consonants are shorter in duration than vowels preceding voiced consonants. For example, the vowel /æ/ in "batch" is shorter than /æ/ in the word "badge" (refer to the spectrograms in Figure 6.15).

Vowels in open syllables also are longer than vowels in closed syllables. Compare the length of the vowel /i/ in the words "beet" and "bee" by saying them aloud. It should be evident that /i/ in the open syllable "bee" is longer in duration. Figure 7.1 shows spectrograms of the words "beet" and "bee." The duration of /i/ in "beet" is 245 msec., approximately one-half the duration of /i/ in "bee" (457 msec.). Clearly, the vowel in the open syllable is longer. The IPA uses a colon to indicate that a phoneme has been lengthened. Therefore, the words "batch" and "badge" could be transcribed as [bætʃ] and [bæːdʒ], respectively. Similarly, the words "beet" and "bee" could be transcribed as [bit] and [biː].

In connected speech, the final phoneme of one word and the initial phoneme of the following word may often be the same, as in "Yes, Susie." Say this phrase aloud. You will notice that there is really no break in the production of the two /s/ phonemes. Instead, you most likely hear a prolonged /s/ phoneme. This phrase would be transcribed [jɛsːuzɪ] using the lengthening diacritic to indicate the elongated /s/ phoneme. Note that the syllable boundary disappears due to the prolonged /s/. Some other examples of this phenomenon include:

but, Terry	[bʌtːɛrɪ]	with them	[wɪðːɛm]
men know	[mɛnːoʊ]	call Linda	[kɑlːɪndə]

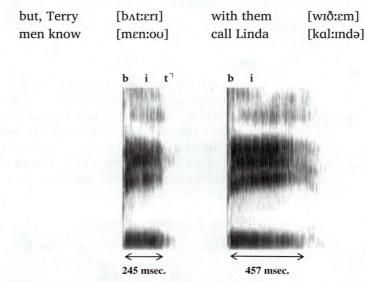

FIGURE 7.1   Comparison of vowel length in open and closed syllables.

EXERCISE 7.15

Select the one word from each pair that would have the longer vowel. Transcribe that word using the [ː] diacritic.

Example:

   key   keep   [kiː]

1. peace	peas	_____	4. spa	spot	_____
2. leave	leaf	_____	5. lack	lag	_____
3. rude	root	_____	6. toot	too	_____

CD #2
Track 20

EXERCISE 7.16

Transcribe the following utterances, using the [ː] diacritic where appropriate.

Example:

kite tail	[kaɪtːeɪl]

1. rice soup _____
2. cotton netting _____
3. big guns _____
4. tail light _____
5. calm morning _____
6. bar room _____
7. leaf fire _____
8. push Sherri _____

Pauses and Juncture in Connected Speech

Pauses occur in connected speech for a number of reasons. First, a pause may simply indicate that the speaker is taking a breath. Second, pauses may indicate hesitations on the part of a speaker as in the following, "His name was . . . um . . . um . . . oh, I remember . . . Joe." Third, pauses are used in conversation to indicate the presence of a new thought or to emphasize a particular point. Examine the utterance "I want to go to the movies, but I don't have any money." The comma, which separates the two clauses, marks a pause in the utterance when it is said aloud. The speaker pauses because two ideas are being presented. The speaker needs to emphasize the importance of each idea, especially the latter. Similarly, there would be a pause at each of the commas in the utterance "I need to buy shampoo, tissue, bath soap, and deodorant," signaling the identity of each of the items. Recall that each comma also indicates the beginning of a separate phrase, with an accompanying change in intonation.

Juncture is the term used to indicate the way in which syllables and words are linked together in connected speech. **External juncture** is the term given to a pause that connects two intonational phrases. (That is, the connecting pause is external to the phrase.) The IPA symbols [|] and [‖] are used to mark external juncture in connected speech. These symbols replace the commas, semicolons, and periods that mark the juncture on the printed page. The single-bar IPA symbol [|] is used to indicate the presence of a short pause (represented in print as a comma). As you recall, longer pauses, represented in print by a period, question mark, or semicolon, would be represented with a double bar [‖]. The sentence "Yes, I would like to go, but I can't" would be transcribed as [jɛs | aɪ wʊd laɪk tə goʊ | bət aɪ kænt ‖].

When transcribing connected speech, it sometimes becomes necessary to indicate the presence of a pause between words in the same intonational phrase because the transition between syllables may become blurred. Consider the utterances "I scream" and "ice cream." They share an identical phoneme string (i.e., /aɪskrim/). To indicate the pause between "I" and "scream" in the first utterance, the [+] diacritic is used: [aɪ + skrim]. The syllables [aɪ + skrim] are said to have **open internal juncture** because there is a pause between the syllables. The transcription of the second utterance, "ice cream" [aɪskrim], has no pause between the two syllables. Therefore, [aɪskrim] has **close internal**

juncture. No special symbols are needed to indicate close internal juncture because there is no pause between the syllables. Another example of open and close internal juncture occurs with the utterances, *night rate* → [naɪt + reɪt] (open) and *nitrate* → [naɪtreɪt] (close).

Now examine the following three phrase pairs:

Ex. A:	"it's tongue"	[ɪts + tʌŋ]	"it stung"	[ɪt + stʌŋ]
Ex. B:	"why cheat"	[waɪ + tʃit]	"white sheet"	[waɪt + ʃit]
Ex. C:	"grade A"	[greɪd + eɪ]	"gray day"	[greɪ + deɪ]

Each example illustrates two phrases with a shift in *open internal juncture*. Note that a plus sign diacritic is warranted in all cases to indicate the pause between syllables. In each example, the syllable boundary (where the pause is taken) is determined by the intent of the utterance.

CD #2
Track 21

EXERCISE 7.17

Use the single-bar [|] and double-bar diacritics [‖] to indicate external juncture in the following utterances. All punctuation marks have been omitted.

Example:

[When I'm sleepy | I go to bed ‖]

1. I want hot dogs ice cream and cotton candy
2. They left didn't they
3. The family who lived next door moved away
4. What is her problem
5. My uncle the dentist is 34 years old

Complete Assignment 7-3.

Review Exercises

A. For each of the following pronunciations, indicate the phonemic change that occurred as a result of assimilation. Also indicate the change in place in articulation.

Example:	Pronunciation	Phoneme change	Change from alveolar to:
bad boy	[bæb:ɔɪ]	b/d	bilabial
1. can make	[kæm:eɪk]	_____	_____
2. How's your mother?	/haʊʒɚ mʌðɚ/	_____	_____
3. gin game	/dʒɪŋ geɪm/	_____	_____
4. lead pipe	[lɛbˀ paɪp]	_____	_____
5. has shaken	/hæʒ ʃeɪkn̩/	_____	_____
6. red gown	[rɛgˀ gaʊn]	_____	_____

B. Transcribe each of the following items after eliding the indicated phoneme.

Example:	**Elided phoneme**	**Transcription**
aptly	/t/	/æplɪ/

1. bends   /d/   _____
2. winter   /t/   _____
3. land mine   /d/   _____
4. can of worms   /f/   _____
5. counter   /t/   _____
6. twelfths   /θ/   _____
7. What's her problem?   /h/   _____
8. wept loudly   /t/   _____

C. Transcribe each of the following utterances, first in citation form and then in casual form.

CD #3
Track 1

1. I want to go home.

   _____

   _____

2. Let me see your book.

   _____

   _____

3. Could you move a little to the right?

   _____

   _____

4. Did John ever get paid?

   _____

   _____

5. Why did she leave so early?

   _____

   _____

6. It is raining cats and dogs.

   _____

   _____

7. When are you going to leave?

   _____

   _____

8. You have got to be kidding!

   _____

   _____

9. Who is going to rake the leaves tonight?

_____

_____

10. I want to wax my truck tomorrow morning.

_____

_____

D. Rewrite each of the following in English orthography (citation form).

1. [dʒɛvɚgoɾəðəsɝkəs ‖]

_____

2. [wɛndədʃilivdʒɔrdʒə ‖]

_____

3. [maɪsɪsɾɚgɑɾənubɔɪfrɛnd ‖]

_____

4. [gɪmɪədeɪɚtutədəsaɪd ‖]

_____

5. [aɪmgʊnəhæftəseɪmofɚnaʊ ‖]

_____

6. [aɪθɪŋkɪtsgʊnəreɪnɪðɚtədeɪɚtəmɑroʊ ‖]

_____

7. [wʊdʒɚɛvɚθɪŋkəduənðætfɚmi ‖]

_____

8. [dujəθɪŋkðətsuzn̩tʊkənəfɚvəm ‖]

_____

9. [əmʃɚðətðɛrgʊnətɛljəwətʃənidtəduət ‖]

_____

10. [traɪəzimaɪt|hidʒɚstkʊdəntduwətʃiwɑnəd ‖]

_____

E. Indicate primary and secondary stress, where appropriate, for each of the following three- and four-syllable words. Keep in mind that some syllables in the words are unstressed. Use a dictionary to help identify any syllable boundaries of which you are unsure.

**CD #3
Track 2**

1. courageous
2. terrified
3. majestic
4. asthmatic
5. Plexiglas
6. plurality
7. mandatory
8. clandestine
9. flamboyant
10. creation

11. computation
12. cranberry
13. bulletin
14. surrendered
15. semantics
16. colonial
17. mercenary
18. independent
19. October
20. ballerina

F. 1. Transcribe each of the following word pairs. Be sure to indicate primary and secondary stress.

2. Compare your vowel transcriptions in each pair (for the vowels represented by the bold letters). If vowel reduction results when going from the first to the second word, place an "X" in the "reduced" column. If your transcription indicates a change from a reduced vowel to the full form of the vowel, place an "X" in the "full" column.

		Reduced	Full
Example:			
valid	validity		
/ˈvælɪd/	/vəˈlɪdɪɾɪ/	X	
1. or**i**gin	or**i**ginate		
2. micr**o**scope	micr**o**scopy		
3. arist**o**crat	arist**o**cracy		
4. strat**e**gy	strat**e**gic		
5. man**i**ac	man**i**acal		
6. homog**e**nous	homog**e**neous		
7. par**a**lyze	par**a**lysis		
8. fel**o**ny	fel**o**nious		

9. perspire	perspiration	
10. repeat	repetitious	

G. Indicate with an "X" whether the following utterances have an overall rising or falling intonation contour.

	Rising	Falling
1. I got a sweater for my birthday.	_____	_____
2. Are you happy?	_____	_____
3. The girls had spaghetti for supper.	_____	_____
4. Are you positive?	_____	_____
5. When you're finished, go to bed.	_____	_____
6. Were you late for work today?	_____	_____
7. Let me get back to you.	_____	_____
8. Did you buy a new CD?	_____	_____
9. What do you mean?	_____	_____
10. Is that your idea of a joke?	_____	_____

CD #3 Track 3

H. Use the diacritical markings [|] or [‖] to indicate external juncture for each of the following utterances. All punctuation marks have been omitted.

1. If I want your help you'll be the first to know
2. Maybe I will maybe I won't
3. They bought a new house didn't they
4. The girls who went swimming all got a cold
5. I can't really make up my mind
6. I scream you scream we all scream for ice cream
7. When are you leaving on vacation
8. Are your cousins coming for a visit or not
9. Do you have ants in your pants
10. I quit my job but only when I was sure I could get another

CD #3 Track 4

I. Transcribe each of the following utterances in casual form, indicating a lengthened phoneme [ː] when necessary. Also use the diacritical markings [|] or [‖] to indicate external juncture when necessary.

Example:

Did you have a good day?

[dɪdʒəhævəgʊdːdeɪ ‖]

CD #3 Track 5

1. I caught my cat Tom by the tail.

2. Which shampoo did you buy at the store?

3. Would you put the white tablecloth on the table, please?

_____

4. Mom might take me shopping, if I get good grades.

_____

5. Have you finished taping the TV special yet?

_____

6. With them, it's hard to tell what they are thinking.

_____

7. Please give me your phone number before you leave.

_____

8. Clem made a home run at the big game last Tuesday.

_____

9. Teddy and Farrell love to play outside with the water sprinkler.

_____

10. I won't take any more of the junk Ken hands out.

_____

J. Each of the following sentences will be spoken by two different speakers. Transcribe each of the utterances in casual form. Be sure to use single-bar or double-bar diacritics to indicate external juncture.

CD #3
Track 6

1. Why can't you ever act your age?

_____

_____

2. Why, oh why did I ever leave Iowa?

_____

_____

3. When did they say their flight was?

_____

_____

4. I will probably go home tomorrow, or the day after.

_____

_____

5. Where did she ever get an idea like that?

_____

_____

6. You have got to be pulling my leg.

_____

_____

7. My friends S.B. and Dale are going to pick me up at 3:00.

_____

_____

8. Why did you repaint the barn already?

_____

_____

9. They are going to tell you what you need.

_____

_____

10. Did she take two of them? Nah, she took four.

_____

_____

K. Mark sentence stress for each of the following sentences using the appropriate IPA notation. Each sentence will be spoken twice, with varying sentence stress. Pay attention to the differences in stress between the two pronunciations. You will need the audio CDs for this exercise.

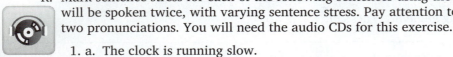

**CD #3
Track 7**

1. a. The clock is running slow.
   b. The clock is running slow.
2. a. Allison got married in New York.
   b. Allison got married in New York.
3. a. Christina bought a new backpack.
   b. Christina bought a new backpack.
4. a. Dr. Mills is my favorite professor.
   b. Dr. Mills is my favorite professor.
5. a. The report is due in five weeks.
   b. The report is due in five weeks.
6. a. Ryan and Mindy went to Hawaii for their honeymoon.
   b. Ryan and Mindy went to Hawaii for their honeymoon.
7. a. Patti's favorite jeans are ripped in the knees.
   b. Patti's favorite jeans are ripped in the knees.
8. a. Did you ride the new roller coaster?
   b. Did you ride the new roller coaster?
9. a. Sid got new skis for his vacation in Utah.
   b. Sid got new skis for his vacation in Utah.
10. a. I want to see that movie tonight at 8.
    b. I want to see that movie tonight at 8.

Study Questions

1. What is coarticulation, and what is assimilation? What is the difference between these two processes?
2. What is the difference between regressive and progressive assimilation? What are other terms that could be used to represent the same processes?
3. Define the following processes associated with connected speech:
   a. elision   b. epenthesis   c. metathesis

4. Describe the process of vowel reduction.

5. What is the cause of the change in the casual pronunciation of the following words?

   was shared → /wʌʒ ʃɛrd/   tan car → /tæŋ kɑr/

   bat girl → /bæk gɝl/   would you → /wʊd ʒu/

6. What is the difference between a syllable that receives secondary stress and a syllable that is unstressed? What is the difference in the way these levels of stress are marked?

7. How is sentence stress marked?

8. What is the difference between given and new information?

9. What is a content word? What is a function word?

10. Define the terms *intonation* and *intonational phrase.*

11. When would you observe (1) a rising intonational phrase and (2) a falling intonational phrase?

12. How does phonetic environment affect vowel duration?

13. What is the difference between internal and external juncture?

14. What is the difference between open and close internal juncture?

15. What role do pauses play in connected speech?

Online Resources

Beare, K. (2014). *Intonation and stress: Key to understanding and being understood.* Retrieved from
   http://esl.about.com/od/speakingadvanced/a/timestress.htm
   (basic introduction to stress and intonation in English)

Power, T. (n.d.). *Teaching English intonation and stress patterns.* Retrieved from
   http://www.tedpower.co.uk/esl0108.html
   (resource guide for teachers of English as a second language)

Assignment 7-1   Name _____

CD #3
Track 8

Transcribe each of the following utterances, first in citation form and then in casual form. Only the casual form will be presented on the CD.

1. I bet you that you are going to win the race.

   _____

   _____

2. We really have to study tonight for the phonetics test.

   _____

   _____

3. Tell Sherry that she will have to go to the store to get some bacon and eggs.

   _____

   _____

4. My friend Caroline is having a party on the third of next month.

   _____

   _____

5. Bob can always finish his homework when he gets home.

   _____

   _____

6. Let me think about your answer for a minute.

   _____

   _____

7. We have just got to clean the house tomorrow.

   _____

   _____

8. Don't forget to pick up our cleaning on the way to work.

   _____

   _____

9. I am going to miss you when you move to the country.

   _____

   _____

10. Please share those ideas with the rest of the group.

   _____

   _____

Assignment 7-2

Name _____

Indicate primary and secondary stress (where appropriate) for the following words:

CD #3
Track 9

1. stethoscope
2. zoology
3. synchronized
4. latitude
5. execute
6. conversion
7. voyager
8. triangle
9. nomadic
10. infinite
11. fluoridate
12. December
13. detonate
14. vulcanize
15. bronchitis

16. automate
17. symmetrical
18. stupendous
19. flirtatious
20. distribute
21. chlorinate
22. magazine
23. openness
24. kitchenette
25. gullible
26. flamingo
27. evasive
28. caravan
29. modernize
30. comprehend

Assignment 7-3

Name _____

Each of the following items will be spoken by two different speakers. Transcribe the following utterances in casual form. Be sure to use single-bar and/or double-bar diacritics to indicate external juncture. Also use the lengthening diacritic [:] when appropriate.

CD #3
Track 10

1. You can lead a horse to water, but you can't make him drink.
   _____
   _____

2. I am not sure we have those shoes in your size; they only come in sizes seven, eight and one-half, or nine.
   _____
   _____

3. That man said he would drive around back to pick up his packages.
   _____
   _____

4. My professor remembered to bring in the model of the larynx; it was really helpful.
   _____
   _____

5. When you are finished typing the paper, remember to come over so we can celebrate.
   _____
   _____

6. Miss Smith thinks that her cousin Neil will be coming over for a visit today.
   _____
   _____

7. My niece Sarah's favorite colors have always been magenta, turquoise, and chartreuse.
   _____
   _____

8. Don't tell her I told you, but Jeannene said she has always been neutral when it comes to that topic.
   _____
   _____

9. If you stay a little while longer, I'll give you a piece of that terrific carrot cake.
   _____
   _____

10. Now, remember, the game begins sharply at 4:30. Don't forget to bring your bat and glove.
    _____
    _____

Assignment 7-4   Name _____

Rewrite each of the following questions in English orthography. Then write your answer to each one, both in IPA and in English orthography.

1. [ðə nʌmbɚ əv deɪz wɪtʃ əkɝ ɪn ə lip jɪr ɪz .....‖]

   _____

   _____

2. [ðə sɪɾi ɪn wɪtʃ ðə stætʃu əv lɪbɚɾi ɪz loʊkeɾəd ɪz noʊn əz .....‖]

   _____

   _____

3. [karɾialədʒɪsts | dəmətalədʒɪsts | ænəsθizialədʒɪsts | n̩ːɚalədʒɪsts | ɚ al taɪps əv .....‖]

   _____

   _____

4. [ɪn ə tɛn dɪdʒɪt foʊn nʌmbɚ | ðə fɝst θri nʌmbɚz ar rəfɝ d tu æz ðə .....‖]

   _____

   _____

5. [əsum ju səksɛfʊli fɪnɪʃ jɚ frɛʃmən jɪr əv kalədʒ | ju wɪl rətɝ n jɚ sɛkənd jɪr æz ə .....‖]

   _____

   _____

6. [ðə nem əv ðə halɪdeɪ wɛn tʃɪldrən go trɪkɚtriɾɪŋ ɪz noʊn əz .....‖]

   _____

   _____

7. əv ældʒəbrə | hɪstɚi | dʒiɔgrəfi | ænd saɪkɔlədʒi | ðə sʌbdʒɛkt wɪtʃ ɪnvalvz ðə stʌdi əv mæθəmæriks ɪz .....‖]

   _____

   _____

8. [ðə sɛkənd mʌnθ əv ɛni kæləndɚ jɪr ɪz .....‖]

   _____

   _____

9. [wɛn ju æd ðə nʌmbɚz twɛni θri plʌs əlɛvən təgɛðɚ | ðə rəzalt ikwəlz .....‖]

   _____

   _____

10. [ə træfɪk saɪn wɪtʃ ɪz ʃeɪpt laɪk ən aktəgan ɪz kamənli rəfɝd tu æz ə .....‖]

    _____

    _____

11. [ðə siẓn əv ðə jɪr | wɛn ðə livz tʃeɪndʒ ðɛr kʌlɚz ɪz kald iðɚ fal ɔr .....‖]

    _____

    _____

12. [ðə skwɛrːut əv eɪɾi wʌn ikwəlz .....‖]

    _____

    _____

Assignment 7-4 (cont.)

13. [ɪf jə mɪks ðə kʌləz blu n̩ jɛloʊ təgɛðɚ | ju ʃʊd gɛt .....‖]

_____

_____

14. [eɪprəl ʃaʊəz most ɔfn̩ brɪŋ meɪ .....‖]

_____

_____

15. [ðə pɑrt əv ðə tʌŋ | dʒʌst bəhaɪnd ðə tɪp | ɪz kɑld ðə .....‖]

_____

_____

Clinical Phonetics: Transcription of Speech Sound Disorders

Learning Objectives

After reading this chapter you will be able to:

1. Describe and transcribe substitution, syllable structure, and assimilation phonological processes.
2. Perform narrow (allophonic) transcription of disordered speech utilizing appropriate diacritics and non-English IPA symbols.
3. List and discuss factors you need to consider to ensure accuracy in the practice of phonetic transcription.

The purpose of this chapter is to introduce you to the application of phonetics in a clinical setting. The focus of the book thus far has been to acquaint you with the process of transcribing typically developing speech patterns (at least what is considered to be typical in Standard American English). As future clinicians, you will be faced with the task of evaluating a client's speech behavior to determine whether that client is in need of intervention. Therefore, you should have an understanding of the process of typical speech-language development. In addition, you will need to know how to evaluate your client to determine whether there is a problem with speech-language production. Ultimately, if the client is in need of intervention, you will need to know how to generate a plan for treatment. These topics will be briefly introduced in this chapter. A thorough discussion of these topics is beyond the scope of this text, however. This material will be covered in other courses in your curriculum that focus on phonological development and disorders.

The terms **articulation disorder** and **phonological disorder** both have been used by hearing and speech professionals over the years to characterize a client who experiences difficulty with speech sound production. The term *articulation disorder* usually refers to a person who has a problem producing only a few phonemes, or whose speech errors are tied to the motoric aspects of speech production. *Phonological disorder,* on the other hand, generally refers to an individual who has difficulty with the sound system of a language and utilizing the rules that govern the combination and order of phonemes in words (Elbert & Gierut, 1986). More recently, professionals have adopted the use of the term **speech sound disorder** to include *all* disorders involving speech sound production. In this text, the term *speech sound disorder* will be used in this manner.

Speech-language pathologists typically administer a battery of tests to assess speech production ability. Articulation tests attempt to systematically identify the correct or incorrect usage of phonemes in a child's repertoire by having the child name objects, or pictures of objects, with which they are familiar. Consonants and consonant clusters (and sometimes vowels) are evaluated in various positions of words to determine whether the individual phonemes of English can be produced correctly in differing phonetic contexts in an age-appropriate manner. Spontaneous, connected speech samples are elicited by engaging the client in conversation about hobbies, favorite activities, or a favorite TV show or movie. With very young children, spontaneous speech samples may be obtained while children describe pictures in a book or while they play with toys. The spontaneous, connected speech samples are transcribed and analyzed for age-appropriate behavior. Once testing is completed, it is possible to analyze a client's speech productions in utterances of varying lengths (i.e., syllables, words, phrases, and sentences). The results of testing will ultimately help determine the therapeutic approach selected.

Articulation tests are usually scored on a phoneme-by-phoneme basis to determine whether the client displays any speech errors, or **misarticulations**. The errors are then categorized as errors of *substitution, omission, distortion,* and/or *addition*. An example of a **substitution** would be producing the word "hello" as /hɛwoʊ/, substituting /w/ for /l/; this would be written as a w/l substitution. An example of an **omission** would be producing the word "big" as /bɪ/, leaving off the final /g/. A **distortion** would involve the production of an allophone of the intended phoneme. If a client produced the word "sit" with a *dentalized* /s/, that is [s̪ɪt] (which sounds somewhat like /θɪt/), it would be considered a distortion. An **addition** error involves the insertion of an extra phoneme in a word, as in /dɑgə/ for "dog." Analyzing speech sound errors on a phoneme-by-phoneme basis may be appropriate when a child displays only a few phonemic errors. Should a child have several speech sound errors, other methods of analysis may prove to be more favorable. One such method would involve analyzing speech sound errors in terms of the *phonological processes* the child is exhibiting.

Phonological Processes

Over the past 80 years, many large-scale studies attempted to delineate the order of phoneme acquisition in typically developing children (Poole, 1934; Prather, Hedrick, & Kern, 1975; Sander, 1972; Smit, Hand, Freilinger, Bernthal, & Bird, 1990; Templin, 1957; Wellman, Case, Mengert, & Bradbury, 1931). These developmental studies all examined a large number of young children in order to answer a basic question: "What is the age at which children typically develop and master individual English speech sounds?"

When comparing the findings from these different developmental studies, it becomes apparent that the ages cited for typical development of individual phonemes vary. For instance, according to Sander (1972), /r/ is mastered by the age of 6;0 (meaning 6 years; 0 months). However, the research of Smit et al. (1990) indicates that /r/ is not accurately produced until the age of 8;0. The disparity in findings between developmental studies is common and may be due to several factors including (1) differences in the socioeconomic status of the children being examined, (2) differences in the number of subjects being studied, and (3) the way in which a speech sample is obtained by the experimenter. For example, children's speech productions may be obtained spontaneously (in response to questions asked by the experimenter or by naming pictures or objects) or by imitating words spoken by the examiner.

Also, these older developmental studies are problematic in that if a child produced a sound correctly by naming a picture or object, it does not guarantee that the child can produce the same sound correctly in spontaneous speech. Also, determining a child's phonetic inventory to define the age at which individual speech sounds are developed is not the same thing as determining the status of the child's developing phonological rule system (Bauman-Waengler, 2012).

In analyzing typical phonological development in children, it may be more advantageous to look at the underlying patterns or processes children use in the production of speech sounds. Stampe (1969) proposed a theory of **natural phonology** that supports the idea that young children are born with innate processes necessary for the production of speech. Because young children are not capable of producing adult speech patterns, they often simplify the adult form. These simplifications are termed **phonological processes**. As children mature, they learn to suppress these processes. When this happens, children then are able to produce the more appropriate adult form of the articulation. If only segmental development is considered, a child who is not capable of producing a certain phoneme may be viewed as not having that sound in her phonetic inventory. When viewed in terms of phonological processes, the child may be using a phonological process that results in the deletion or modification of that sound. Adults may have difficulty understanding the speech patterns of a young child with whom they are not familiar. This is often due not to missing sounds in the child's phonetic repertoire, but is most likely due to the fact that adults are not accustomed to the simplifications, or processes, being produced by the child (Hodson & Paden, 1991).

Many phonological processes are found to occur in the speech patterns of typically developing children. These processes can be divided into three general categories: **syllable structure processes**, **substitution processes**, and **assimilatory processes** (Ingram, 1976). Some of the more common processes associated with these subdivisions are presented in the following sections and are summarized in Table 8.1. Developmental data (the age when specific processes are suppressed) are from Grunwell (1987). Make sure to pay particular attention to the examples given *in terms of their phonetic transcription.*

Syllable Structure Processes

These processes, as a group, affect the production of syllables so that they are simplified, usually into a consonant–vowel (CV) pattern (Ingram, 1976). CV patterns are among the first syllable types to be used in the speech patterns of developing infants.

Weak Syllable Deletion
Weak syllable deletion, or simply *syllable deletion,* is a phonological process that involves the omission of an unstressed (weak) syllable either preceding or following a stressed syllable. This process may persist until a child is nearly 4;0. It is also common in some adult productions (Hodson & Paden, 1991). Examples include:

telephone → /tɛfon/   probably → /prɑblɪ/ or /prɑlɪ/
tomato → /meɪro/   above → /bʌv/

TABLE 8.1   Examples of Some Common Phonological Processes of Children.

Syllable Structure Processes	Example Word	Production
Weak syllable deletion	surprise	/praɪz/
Final consonant deletion	look	/lʊ/
Reduplication	baby	/bibi/
Cluster reduction	clean	/kin/
Substitution Processes		
Stopping	sand	/tænd/
Fronting	kite	/taɪt/
Deaffrication	jump	/ʒʌmp/
Gliding	lake	/weɪk/
Vocalization	help	/hɛʊp/
Assimilatory Processes		
Labial assimilation	put	/pʊp/
Alveolar assimilation	mine	/naɪn/
Velar assimilation	garden	/gɑrgən/
Prevocalic voicing	cop	/gɑp/
Devoicing	ride	/raɪt/

EXERCISE 8.1

Indicate with an "X" examples of weak syllable deletion.

Examples:

	Intended Word	Transcription
_____	ˈplease	/piz/
X	elephant	/ɛfənt/

		Intended Word	Transcription
_____	1.	ˈscissors 2	/sɪ/
X	2.	ˈbaby 2	/beɪ/
X	3.	baˈnana 3	/nænə/
_____	4.	ˈmama 2	/mə/
X	5.	toˈday 2	/deɪ/
_____	6.	ˈmilk 1	/mɪk/
X	7.	ˈmitten 2	/mɪt/
_____	8.	ˈlady	/di/

Final Consonant Deletion

Final consonant deletion effectively reduces a syllable to a CV pattern, that is, to an open syllable. Typically developing children begin to use most consonants in the coda position of words by the time they reach the age of 3;0. This process is generally suppressed completely by age 3;6. Examples include:

bake → /beɪ/ mouse → /maʊ/ cat → /kæ/

EXERCISE 8.2

Which of the following words could be affected by final consonant deletion? Indicate those words with an "X" and then transcribe the word in IPA, applying the process of final consonant deletion.

Examples:

shoe _____ _____

foot X /fʊ/

away 1. _____ _____

cup 2. X /cʌ/

through 3. _____ _____

bread 4. X /brɛ/

say 5. _____ _____

phone 6. X /fo/

black 7. X /blæ/

stop 8. X /sta/

Reduplication

Reduplication involves the repetition of a syllable of a word. Total reduplication involves a repetition of an entire syllable, as in "mommy" → /mɑmɑ/. Partial reduplication involves repetition of just a consonant or vowel, as in "bottle" → /bɑdɑ/ (Lowe, 1996). Reduplication is common in the early speech development of some children. It is generally suppressed before 2;6. Other examples include:

daddy → /dædæ/ or /dɑdɑ/ doggy → /dɑgɑ/
movie → /mumu/ baby → /bibi/

EXERCISE 8.3

For the words given, indicate with an "X" the transcriptions that indicate the process of reduplication.

_____ 1. wagon /wægə/ __X__ 4. pencil /pɛpɛ/

__X__ 2. children /dɪdɪ/ __X__ 5. water /wɑwɑ/

_____ 3. jacket /dækɪ/ _____ 6. yellow /jɛdo/

Cluster Reduction

Cluster reduction results in the deletion of a consonant from a consonant cluster (adjacent consonants in the same syllable). If the cluster contains three consonants, one or two of the consonants may be deleted, as in "spray" → /preɪ/ or /reɪ/. Cluster reduction in typically developing children may persist until 4;0 or 5;0 (Smit, 1993). Other examples include:

snow → /noʊ/   play → /peɪ/   stripe → /traɪp/, /taɪp/, or /raɪp/

EXERCISE 8.4

For the words given, indicate with an "X" the transcriptions that indicate the process of cluster reduction.

X	1. blue	/bu/		X	5. stop	/tɑp/
___	2. spot	/spɑ/		___	6. crayon	/keɪɑn/
___	3. path	/pæt/		X	7. milk	/mɪk/
X	4. spring	/rɪŋ/		___	8. wish	/wɪs/

Substitution Processes

Substitution processes involve the replacement of one class of phonemes for another. For instance, the phonological process known as **stopping** involves the substitution of a stop for a fricative or affricate. Similarly, the process known as **fronting** involves the substitution of an alveolar phoneme for a velar or palatal articulation.

Stopping

As just mentioned, stopping involves the substitution of a stop for a fricative or an affricate. This is a commonly occurring process because stops are acquired before most fricatives in typically developing speech. The substitution is usually for a stop produced with the same, or similar, place of articulation:

Fricative/Affricate		Substituted Stop	Fricative		Substituted Stop
/s, ʃ, tʃ, θ/	→	/t/	/f/	→	/p/
/z, ʒ, dʒ, ð/	→	/d/	/v/	→	/b/

Sometimes children produce a stop for a fricative or affricate along with a change in voicing, for example, /sɪp/ → /dɪp/. The change in voicing is a phonological process called *prevocalic voicing* and will be discussed in more detail in the following text. Stopping of fricatives and affricates may continue for some phonemes until 4;0 or 5;0. Examples include:

sake → /teɪk/   (voiceless alveolar fricative → voiceless alveolar stop)
zoo → /du/   (voiced alveolar fricative → voiced alveolar stop)
fat → /pæt/   (voiceless labiodental fricative → voiceless bilabial stop)
ship → /tɪp/   (voiceless palatal fricative → voiceless alveolar stop)

The last example ("ship") demonstrates not only stopping, but also a more forward place of production of the affected consonant phoneme. That is, place of production shifted from palatal to alveolar. This process is called *fronting* and is discussed in the next section.

EXERCISE 8.5

Place an "X" in front of the following transcriptions that represent an example of stopping.

_____	1. shoe	→	/zu/ ʃ→z		_____	5. comb	→	/goʊm/ k→g
X	2. thank	→	/tæŋk/ θ→t		X	6. summer	→	/tʌmɚ/ s→t
_____	3. raisin	→	/weɪzn̩/ r→w		_____	7. yellow	→	/wɛloʊ/ j→w
X	4. march	→	/mɑrt/ tʃ→t		X	8. shop	→	/tɑp/ ʃ→t

Fronting

It is common for young children to substitute velar and palatal consonants with an alveolar place of articulation. This substitution process is commonly referred to as *fronting*. The alveolar substitutions typical of fronting are given below:

Velar		*Alveolar*	*Palatal*		*Alveolar*
/k/	→	/t/	/ʃ/	→	/s/
/g/	→	/d/	/tʃ/	→	/ts/
/ŋ/	→	/n/	/ʒ/	→	/z/
			/dʒ/	→	/dz/

Fronting usually disappears in typically developing children's speech by the age of 2;6 to 3;0. Examples include:

cat → /tæt/   (voiceless velar stop → voiceless alveolar stop)

wash → /wɑs/   (voiceless palatal fricative → voiceless alveolar fricative)

juice → /dzus/   (voiced palatal affricate → voiced alveolar affricate)

mash → /mæt/   (voiceless palatal fricative → voiceless alveolar stop)

The affricate /dz/ (in /dzus/) is not a phoneme of English, but may occur in disordered speech patterns. Also note that the pronunciation of /mæt/ for "mash" displays both fronting and stopping of the final phoneme:

mash /mæʃ/ → /mæs/ (fronting, i.e., palatal /ʃ/ → alveolar /s/)

and

/mæs/ → /mæt/ (stopping, i.e., fricative /s/ → stop /t/)

EXERCISE 8.6

Place an "X" in front of the following transcriptions that are indicative of fronting.

_____	1. candy	→	/gændɪ/ k-g		X	5. brush	→	/brʌs/ ʃ→s
X	2. rake	→	/reɪt/ k-t		_____	6. paper	→	/teɪpɚ/
X	3. bring	→	/brɪn/ ŋ→n		X	7. goose	→	/dus/
_____	4. clown	→	/kraʊn/ r-l		_____	8. sing	→	/tɪŋ/

Deaffrication

Deaffrication occurs when a child substitutes a fricative for an affricate. Examples include:

> chip → /ʃɪp/   (voiceless, palatal affricate → voiceless, palatal fricative)
>
> juice → /ʒus/   (voiced, palatal affricate → voiced, palatal fricative)
>
> ledge → /lɛz/   (voiced, palatal affricate → voiced, alveolar fricative)

The last example, ledge → /lɛz/, demonstrates two substitution processes: (1) deaffrication and (2) fronting. In addition to the substitution of the fricative for an affricate, that is, /dʒ/ → /ʒ/ (deaffrication), the palatal /ʒ/ is produced as the alveolar /z/ (fronting).

Suppose a child produced the word "June" as /dun/. How many substitution processes are occurring in this production? If you answered "three," you are correct. A change from /dʒ → d/ involves deaffrication, fronting, and stopping. Study this example to make sure you understand the three processes that are occurring:

> June   /dʒun/ →   /ʒun/ (deaffrication)
>
>   /ʒun/ →   /zun/ (fronting)
>
>   /zun/ →   /dun/ (stopping)

EXERCISE 8.7

Place an "X" in front of the following transcriptions that are indicative of deaffrication.

_____ 1. shake → /seɪk/   _____ 5. gem → /tʃɛm/

_____ 2. choose → /tsuz/   _____ 6. witch → /wɪʃ/

_____ 3. Jack → /ʒæk/   _____ 7. chalk → /sɔk/

_____ 4. mesh → /mɛs/   _____ 8. chase → /ʃeɪs/

Gliding

Gliding is a substitution process that involves the substitution of the glides /w/ or /j/ for the liquids /l/ and /r/. Gliding is common in children displaying typical developmental patterns as well as in those with phonological disorders. This process is overused in some cartoons to depict characters with disordered speech, for example, /wæbɪt/ for "rabbit." This phonological process is seen in children as young as 2;0, and may persist until a child is 5;0 or older. Examples include:

> red → /wɛd/   blue → /bwu/
>
> like → /jaɪk/   grow → /gwoʊ/

EXERCISE 8.8

Place an "X" in front of the following transcriptions that are indicative of gliding.

_____ 1. soap → /woʊp/   _____ 5. rice → /laɪs/

_____ 2. leaf → /wif/   _____ 6. yes → /wɛs/

_____ 3. ring → /jɪŋ/   _____ 7. grow → /gwoʊ/

_____ 4. lazy → /jeɪzɪ/   _____ 8. free → /fli/

Vocalization

Vocalization involves the substitution of a vowel for postvocalic /r/ or /l/, including syllabic /l/. The vowels commonly substituted include /ʊ/, /ɔ/, and /o/ (or /oʊ/). Vocalization also refers to *derhotacization* of the central rhotic vowels /ɚ/ and /ɜ/ (as discussed in Chapter 4) as well as derhotacization of postvocalic /r/ when it loses its r-coloring due to a vowel substitution. (Recall from Chapter 5 that some speakers from the South and East derhotacize post-vocalic /r/—"here" /hɪə/ and "square" /skwɛə/.) Vocalization of postvocalic /r/ and the rhotic vowels will be discussed in more detail in relation to dialects in Chapter 9. Some examples of vocalization include:

			Substitution
tiger	→	/tigʊ/	ʊ/ɚ *
turn	→	/tɔn/	ɔ/ɜ *
third	→	/θʊd/	ʊ/ɜ *
bear	→	/bɛʊ/	ʊ/r *
help	→	/hɛʊp/	ʊ/l
fell	→	/fɛo/	o/l
little	→	/wɪɾo/ or /wɪɾol/	o/l̩ *or* ol/l̩

*Examples of derhotacization.

Note that the last example (little → /wɪɾo/) demonstrates both vocalization of the final /l/ *and* gliding of the initial /l/.

Some children may still produce the final /l/ following the vowel as in /wɪɾol/. You will have to listen carefully to determine if the /l/ was maintained in the child's articulation. This is a production especially prone to transcription error (see Louko & Edwards, 2001).

EXERCISE 8.9

Place an "X" in front of the transcriptions that are indicative of *vocalization*.

X 1. middle → /mɪdo/		X 5. belt → /bɛʊt/
X 2. answer → /ænsʊ/		___ 6. telephone → /tɛfon/
X 3. work → /wɔk/		X 7. curtain → /kʊʔn̩/
___ 4. could → /kɔd/		___ 8. bark → /bɑk/

Assimilatory Processes

Assimilatory processes involve an alteration in phoneme production due to phonetic environment (see Chapter 7 for a review of assimilation). Assimilatory processes involve labial, velar, nasal, and/or voicing assimilation. The assimilation in any of these instances may be either progressive or regressive. These processes are not present in all typically developing children. When they occur, they usually disappear before the age of 3. The assimilation processes associated with consonant production are also referred to as *consonant harmony*.

Labial Assimilation

Labial assimilation occurs when a non-labial phoneme is produced with a labial place of articulation. This is due to the presence of a labial phoneme elsewhere in the word. For example:

book → /bʊp/   (progressive assimilation)

(In this case, the non-labial /k/ is produced with a labial articulation due to the presence of the /b/ phoneme at the beginning of the word.)

mad   → /mæb/   (progressive assimilation)

cap   → /pæp/   (regressive assimilation)

swing → /ɸwɪŋ/   (regressive assimilation)

/ɸ/ is a voiceless bilabial fricative, a phoneme found on the IPA chart, but not common to English. It is found in African languages such as Hausa and Ewe. To produce /ɸ/, place your lips together and blow out so air escapes (but don't whistle). Pretend you are softly blowing out a candle. (Don't push air from the glottis, otherwise you will produce /h/.) Another way to produce /ɸ/ is to say the word "whew." When producing the word "swing" as /ɸwɪŋ/, the alveolar fricative /s/ undergoes labial assimilation due to the presence of /w/.

EXERCISE 8.10

Place an "X" in front of the words that correctly indicate the process of labial assimilation.

_____ 1. pie   → /baɪ/   _____ 5. boat   → /boʊp/

_____ 2. tap   → /pæp/   _____ 6. train → /preɪn/

_____ 3. lip   → /lɪb/   _____ 7. cause → /pɔz/

_____ 4. numb   → /mʌm/   _____ 8. big   → /bɪb/

Alveolar Assimilation

Alveolar assimilation occurs when a non-alveolar phoneme is produced with an alveolar place of articulation due to the presence of an alveolar phoneme elsewhere in the word. Examples include:

time → /taɪn/   (progressive assimilation)

shut → /sʌt/   (regressive assimilation)

bat → /dæt/   (regressive assimilation)

EXERCISE 8.11

Place an "X" in front of the words that correctly indicate the process of alveolar assimilation.

_____ 1. pat   → /tæt/   _____ 5. knife → /naɪs/

_____ 2. short → /sɔrt/   _____ 6. that   → /zæt/

_____ 3. Tom   → /mɔm/   _____ 7. phone → /soʊn/

_____ 4. tune   → /dun/   _____ 8. vat   → /væp/

It is not always easy to determine whether a child's speech productions are a result of assimilation or of a substitution process. For instance, a child who produces the word "cat" as /tæt/ might be demonstrating alveolar assimilation or may be fronting the /k/ phoneme. To determine whether a child is using assimilatory processes, it is necessary to evaluate several productions from the child's speech sample. In this manner, a particular phonological pattern may emerge. Examine two different children's productions of the following six words. What phonological pattern do you see?

Child #1		**Child #2**	
kite	/taɪt/	kite	/taɪt/
dog	/dɑd/	dog	/dɑd/
should	/sʊd/	should	/sʊd/
push	/pʊs/	push	/pʊʃ/
go	/doʊ/	go	/goʊ/
bike	/baɪt/	bike	/baɪk/

Child #1's productions of "kite," "dog," and "should" could be suggestive of either alveolar assimilation or fronting. However, productions of the words "push," "go," and "bike" reflect only fronting because no alveolar phonemes exist in these words. Therefore, this child appears to be demonstrating the process of fronting. Contrast this pattern with child #2, who mispronounces only the first three words, words with alveolar phonemes. Child #2 appears to be demonstrating alveolar assimilation.

Velar Assimilation

Velar assimilation occurs when a non-velar phoneme is produced with a velar place of articulation due to the presence of a velar phoneme elsewhere in the word. Examples include:

cup	→ /kʌk/	(progressive assimilation)
gone	→ /gɔŋ/	(progressive assimilation)
take	→ /keɪk/	(regressive assimilation)

EXERCISE 8.12

Place an "X" in front of the words that correctly indicate the process of velar assimilation.

_____ 1. turkey → /kɝkɪ/	_____ 5. bang → /gæŋ/
_____ 2. kill → /gɪl/	_____ 6. shook → /ʃʊg/
_____ 3. grass → /kræs/	_____ 7. cap → /kæk/
_____ 4. fake → /keɪk/	_____ 8. brag → /græg/

Voicing Assimilation

There are two types of voicing assimilation. The first type, **prevocalic voicing**, involves voicing of a normally unvoiced consonant. This occurs when the consonant precedes the nucleus of a syllable. That is, the unvoiced consonant assimilates to the (voiced) nucleus. Examples include:

pig → /bɪg/ (regressive assimilation)
cup → /gʌp/ (regressive assimilation)

Another type of voicing assimilation involves the **devoicing** of syllable-final voiced phonemes that either precede a pause or silence between words, or occur at the end of an utterance. That is, the final phoneme "assimilates to the silence" following the word (Ingram, 1976, p. 35). Examples include:

bad → /bæt/ (regressive assimilation)
hose → /hos/ (regressive assimilation)

EXERCISE 8.13

Indicate whether the transcriptions of the following words involve prevocalic voicing (P) or devoicing (D). Write P or D in the blanks. If neither process is demonstrated, leave the item blank.

_____ 1. pear → /bɛr/   _____ 5. gone → /kɔn/
_____ 2. led → /lɛt/   _____ 6. flag → /flæk/
_____ 3. fair → /vɛr/   _____ 7. shoe → /ʒu/
_____ 4. card → /kɑrt/   _____ 8. chair → /ʃɛr/

Complete Assignment 8-1.

Not all of the processes outlined previously necessarily occur in the speech patterns of all typically developing children. The processes that are most common in typical children's speech patterns include weak syllable deletion, final consonant deletion, gliding, and cluster reduction (Stoel-Gammon & Dunn, 1985). Also, suppression of a particular process does not happen all at once. Suppression may initially occur for only certain phonemes in a class. For instance, children who demonstrate stopping may suppress the process for /f/ and /s/ before they suppress it for the fricatives /v, z, ʃ, ð, and θ/ and also for the affricates /tʃ/ and /dʒ/ (Grunwell, 1987).

Suppose you just evaluated a 7-year-old child using a picture-naming task, and you transcribed the following responses for seven of the words presented:

Picture	Child's Production	Picture	Child's Production
stove	/toʊb/	zipper	/dɪpʊ/
bird	/bʊd/	blue	/bu/
bath	/bæt/	drum	/dʌm/
sun	/tʌn/		

A phoneme-by-phoneme analysis would reveal several errors, including the following:

omission /s/ (stove)
/l/ (blue)
/r/ (drum)

substitution	d/z	(zipper)	ʊ/ɚ	(zipper)
	t/θ	(bath)	ʊ/ɝ	(bird)
	t/s	(sun)	b/v	(stove)
distortions	none			
additions	none			

Because there are several speech sound errors present, a clearer picture of this child's phonological system may emerge if the speech productions are scrutinized in terms of phonological processes the child is demonstrating:

Picture	Child's Production	Phonemic Substitution	Phonemic Process(es)
stove	/toʊb/	st → t; v → b	cluster reduction; stopping
bird	/bʊd/	ɝ → ʊ	vocalization
bath	/bæt/	θ → t	stopping
sun	/tʌn/	s → t	stopping
zipper	/dɪpʊ/	z → d; ɚ → ʊ	stopping; vocalization
blue	/bu/	bl → b	cluster reduction
drum	/dʌm/	dr → d	cluster reduction

Upon analysis of the child's responses, it now becomes evident that the child still has not suppressed the processes of *vocalization, stopping,* and *cluster reduction.* These process are suppressed in typical children by age 5. Therefore, therapeutic remediation most likely would be indicated for this 7-year-old child.

Children with Phonological Disorders

Children with speech sound disorders often display some of the same types of phonological processes as typically developing children. However, the processes would be suppressed *later* than typically observed, as in the previous example. The phonological processes used most consistently by children with speech sound disorders include cluster reduction, stopping, and liquid simplification (a combination of gliding and vocalization) (Stoel-Gammon & Dunn, 1985). These specific processes are among those consistently seen in typically developing children as well.

Children with disordered phonology also display several processes not usually found in the speech of typically developing children. These processes are called **idiosyncratic processes.** Several idiosyncratic processes include (from Stoel-Gammon & Dunn, 1985):

1. *Glottal replacement*—the substitution of a glottal stop for another consonant.

   pick → /pɪʔ/   butter → /bʌʔʊ/ (with vocalization)   lip → /ʔɪp/

   When the initial sound of a word is replaced with a glottal stop, it may sound as if the intial sound is simply deleted. You will need to listen carefully to make sure.

2. *Initial consonant deletion*—the omission of a single consonant at the beginning of a word.

   cut → /ʌt/   game → /eɪm/

In the case of initial consonant deletion, you will need to determine whether the initial consonant truly is being deleted or is being replaced with a glottal stop.

3. *Backing*—the substitution of a velar stop consonant for consonants usually produced more anterior in the oral cavity. Backing usually involves alveolars and palatals; however, labial sounds may be affected.

time → /kaɪm/   zoom → /gum/   push → /pʊk/

4. *Stops replacing a glide*—the substitution of a stop for a glide.

yes → /dɛs/   wait → /beɪt/

5. *Fricatives replacing a stop*—the substitution of a fricative for a stop (frication).

sit → /sɪs/   doll → /zɔl/

EXERCISE 8.14

For each of the given transcriptions, fill in the blank with the name of the appropriate idiosyncratic process just described. There may be more than one answer for each item.

Example:

cat   → /kæʔ/   _____ glottal replacement _____

1. chairs → /ɛrz/   _____
2. letter → /lɛsɚ/   _____
3. witch → /dɪtʃ/   _____
4. tape → /keɪp/   _____
5. bunny → /ʌʔɪ/   _____
6. bad → /gæʔ/   _____

Another method of phonological assessment, quite different from phonological process analysis, is known as **nonlinear phonology**. Nonlinear phonology involves performing an inventory of a child's speech sound system on *multiple levels* (hence the name *nonlinear*), including production of individual speech sounds, syllables, stress patterns, and words. In nonlinear phonology, the child's speech sample can come from both administration of phonological tests (naming pictures) and/or from elicitation of spontaneous speech (e.g., telling a story). The clinician then takes the recorded sample and transcribes each word the child produces. Some of the information the clinician can gather from a nonlinear analysis includes:

1. A complete inventory of the individual consonants and vowels the child produces.
2. An inventory of syllable shapes used by the child; in other words, whether a child produces open and/or closed syllables and consonant clusters at the beginning and/or end of syllables.

3. The combination of consonants (C) and vowels (V) the child uses to produce various syllable types: CV, VC, CVC, CCVC, CVCC, and so on.
4. The word shapes the child produces—the number and types of syllables in a word. (That is, can a child produce only one-syllable words, or can he also produce two-, three-, and four-syllable words?)
5. The stress patterns the child produces in bisyllabic and multisyllabic words with varying stress patterns, such as lion, giraffe, elephant, orangutan.

This type of analysis is important because the child's sound system is evaluated not just in terms of the phonemes that are produced correctly or incorrectly relative to the adult model, but it is also analyzed independently, as a functional system in its own right in terms of phoneme production in words varying in phonetic composition, stress, and number of syllables. In other words, phonemes are identified without consideration of what is phonemic or contrastive in the target language (adult system), but rather which consonants and vowels are used contrastively in particular contexts in the child's system.

How does nonlinear phonology help in remediation of a child with a phonological disorder? A simple example may help answer this question. Suppose a child produces the word "cat" as /kae/. At first glance, it appears that she may have problems producing the final /t/ phoneme (final consonant deletion). However, does she really have problems with final /t/, or does she generally have problems producing a coda in all CVC words? Because nonlinear phonology looks at phoneme production at several levels, the answer may become more evident by analyzing the child's speech sample and looking for patterns of production across a number of words. If it is determined that the child cannot produce final consonants in words, it could be considered a *constraint* on a particular level or tier of her phonological system, whereas the absence of /t/ in "cat" but the presence of other consonants in coda position would be a constraint on a different tier. In order for the child's phonology to improve, therapy would need to consider what constraints exist and how remediation aimed at different tiers would improve her ability to produce the adult pattern.

Complete Assignments 8-2 and 8-3.

Transcription of Speech Sound Disorders: Diacritics

So far in this text we have been using *broad transcription* as a method of transcribing phonemes in words and sentences; we have paid little attention to allophonic variation in phoneme production. In this chapter, we will turn our attention to the use of *narrow transcription* in order to more accurately describe the utterances of individuals who exhibit speech sound disorders. In the last chapter, you were introduced to some diacritics used in the transcription of some suprasegmental aspects of speech, including those for timing of phonemes, i.e., [:], and for juncture, i.e., [|] and [‖]. This chapter will introduce diacritics used in the transcription of *segmental* aspects of speech, that is, for transcribing vowels and consonants. It is important that you become familiar with allophonic transcription of individual phonemes. Often, when transcribing individuals with speech sound disorders, the use of broad transcription will not suffice because broad transcription does not allow for transcription of allophonic variation in phoneme production. If a child pronounces the word "red" as /wɛd/ (gliding), broad transcription would be adequate in capturing the production on paper. Now consider the speech patterns of a child who has difficulty with velopharyngeal closure and has a concomitant problem with nasal emission (air escaping through the nasal cavity). Broad transcription of the child's production of the word "smile," /smaɪl/, would not indicate the occurrence of nasal emission. Narrow transcription of this word, [s̃maɪl], reveals that nasal emission occurred during production of /s/. (The symbol [͂] represents an allophone of [s], [s] with nasal emission.)

In the following section, several diacritics will be introduced as they relate to allophonic variants of speech sounds associated with (1) stop consonant production, (2) nasality, (3) voicing, and (4) changes in place of articulation. Only some of the more commonly used diacritics will be discussed on the following pages. The diacritic markings adopted in this text are from the 2005 revision of the IPA. Refer to Figure 2.1 for the complete list of the IPA diacritics.

Some of the diacritics can be used in transcribing typical pronunciation patterns. As you know, all voiceless stop consonants are aspirated when they occur in the initial position of a syllable. Narrow transcription of the word "teen" [tʰin] shows a raised "h" indicating that it has been produced with aspiration. In transcribing individuals with speech sound disorders, it might not be necessary to show the occurrence of aspiration in contexts where aspiration is expected to occur, as in the word "teen." Instead, you would need to indicate aspiration in transcription of phonetic contexts where it is not expected to occur. Also, you would need to indicate missing aspiration when it is expected to occur.

Stop Consonant Production

In Chapter 6 you learned that stop consonants are composed of an articulatory closure, an increase in intraoral pressure, and a release burst at one of three points of articulation: bilabial, alveolar, or velar. The manner in which stop consonants are produced (released, unreleased, aspirated, unaspirated) varies as a function of phonetic environment, dialect, and whether a person has a speech sound disorder.

Unreleased Stops [p˺]

An **unreleased** stop consonant is one that has no audible release burst associated with it. Unreleased stops occur quite often in English at the ends of words as in "leak," "put," "map," "hog," and "red." Contrast the production of the word "stop" first by releasing the final /p/ and then by not releasing it. The transcription of the unreleased production would be [stɑp˺]. Likewise, contrast the two productions of the word "bid," that is, [bɪd˺] and [bɪd]. When two voiceless stop consonants occur one after the other in the same syllable, the first one is not released, as in the words "stacked" [stæk˺t] and "reaped" [rip˺t].

Aspiration of Stops [pʰ]

Recall from Chapter 6 that *aspiration* is a frictional noise burst associated with the release of *voiceless* plosives. Aspiration occurs only in stops in the initial position of stressed syllables. Examples of aspiration occur in the words "pass" [pʰæs], "torn" [tʰɔrn], "kiss" [kʰɪs], "atone" [ətʰoʊn], and "repay" [rəpʰeɪ]. Released voiceless stops at the ends of words may be aspirated as well, as in "leap" [lipʰ], "snake" [sneɪkʰ], and "right" [raɪtʰ]. Aspiration does *not* normally occur when a voiceless stop follows the fricative /s/, as in "spoon," "scat," or "stood."

If an aspirated stop does occur in this phonetic environment due to a speech sound disorder, it should be marked appropriately, as in "spoon" [spʰun].

Unaspirated Stops [p⁼]   *reduced aspiration p⁼*
The symbol [⁼] is placed above and to the right of unaspirated voiceless stops. Unaspirated stops are most common when they occur immediately following the fricative /s/ as in the words "spin" [sp⁼ɪn] or "escape" [əsk⁼eɪp˺]. Although stops may be unaspirated, they may still be released. Both of the unaspirated stops in "spin" and "escape" are released.

Young children and children with phonological disorders may not aspirate initial stop consonants at the beginning of words as expected. When an aspirated stop is produced without aspiration, it may sound to a listener as a voiced stop. For instance, "pan" [p⁼æn] might sound like "ban" /bæn/. Therefore, it is important to listen carefully to make sure your transcription is adequate. This is a misperception quite prone to transcription error (Louko & Edwards, 2001). Additionally, unaspirated stops are typically seen in the initial position of voiceless stops in some Asian languages such as Vietnamese and Filipino. This will be discussed further in Chapter 9.

EXERCISE 8.15

Place an "X" next to each of the following words that normally contain an unaspirated phoneme.

1. _____ slack
2. _____ praised
3. _____ scorn
4. _____ despite
5. _____ excuse
6. _____ surprise
7. _____ stripe
8. _____ smooth

EXERCISE 8.16

Place an "X" next to the words that are *possible* transcriptions for the words given, using the diacritics for unreleased, unaspirated, and aspirated productions. If a transcription is given that is not typical in a particular phonetic context, correct it.

Examples:

| X | licked | [lɪk˺tʰ] | |
| --- | cap | [kæp˺] | [kʰæp˺] |

1. _____ skunk   [sk⁼ʌŋkʰ]   _____
2. _____ snacked   [snæk˺tʰ]   _____
3. _____ target   [tɑrgət˺]   _____
4. _____ brave   [bʰreɪv]   _____
5. _____ toga   [tʰoʊgʰə]   _____
6. _____ guarded   [gɑrdəd˺]   _____
7. _____ person   [pɝsʰən]   _____
8. _____ carefully [kʰɛrfʊlɪ]   _____

Nasality

Several diacritics are used in narrow transcription to indicate changes in nasality associated with speech production. These include nasalization, nasal emission, and denasality.

Nasalization [æ̃]

Recall from Chapter 6 that vowels may become nasalized in the presence of nasal consonants. For example, in the word "mean," the vowel /i/ is surrounded by two nasal phonemes. The velum lowers during the production of the initial consonant /m/ and remains lowered throughout the word (for articulatory efficiency) because the final phoneme /n/ also is a nasal. The result is a nasalized vowel, as in [mĩn]. The following words also have nasalized vowels due to the nasal environment provided by /m/, /n/, or /ŋ/: "hang" [hæ̃ŋ], "in" [ĩn], "mom" [mɑ̃m], and both vowels in "roomy" [rũmĩ] and "any" [ẽnĩ]. The effects of nasalization can also be seen across word boundaries as in "I can eat" [aɪ kæn ĩt]. Note that nasalization can be regressive, progressive, or a combination of both (as in the word "mom"). Some children with cochlear implants will show vowel nasalization preceding a nasal consonant, as predicted, but delete the consonant, as in "comb" [kʰo͡ʊ] (Teoh & Chin, 2009).

In the transcription of disordered speech, this diacritic is also used to indicate the presence of excessive nasality associated with the production of non-nasal phonemes. This condition is known as hypernasal resonance or **hypernasality**. Hypernasality may be due to improper velopharyngeal closure. The presence of hypernasality may be evident throughout an entire production of a word or an utterance.

Some individuals with severe or profound hearing loss may display hypernasality in their speech. In fact, deaf speech is often described as sounding "nasal." The problem in this case is not a physical one, because there is no structural deviation in the speech organs associated with velopharyngeal closure. Improper use of nasality is more likely due to faulty learning associated with the hearing loss. The auditory cues associated with nasality are difficult for deaf individuals to hear (Erber, 1983). Without having an appropriate auditory model of how oral versus nasal consonants should sound, it is difficult for some deaf individuals to produce nasality correctly.

EXERCISE 8.17

Place an "X" next to the words where you might expect nasalization based upon the given phonetic context.

1. _____ mean [mĩn]
2. _____ boon [bũn]
3. _____ buddy [bʌdĩ]
4. _____ strung [strʌ̃ŋ]
5. _____ slam [s̃læm]
6. _____ thong [θɑ̃ŋ]

Nasal Emission [˜]

Nasal emission is the audible escape of air through the nares due to improper velopharyngeal closure. Airflow may escape through the velopharyngeal port itself or may escape through a cleft in the palate or velum. Individuals with cleft palate may exhibit nasal emission especially during the production of stops and fricatives (which require greater intraoral pressure) even if the cleft has been repaired. This is usually due to speaking habits learned prior to the surgery (Trost-Cardemone, 2009). The diacritic [˜] is used when nasal emission accompanies a phoneme that is *not* normally nasalized. Examples include "snail" [sněɪl], "nice" [naɪš], "zoo" [žu], and "pie" [p̃aɪ]. Keep in mind that nasal emission is not the same as nasalization. Nasalization of speech results when the velum is lowered in production of oral sounds, resulting in nasal resonance. Nasal emission is a process in which air escapes through the nares.

Denasality [˜]

Another condition related to nasality is **denasality**, also known as **hyponasality**. Denasality results when the nasal phonemes /m, n, and ŋ/ are produced *without* nasalization. Denasality is most often associated with the speech patterns of a person with a cold or upper respiratory tract infection. The utterance "My name is Matt" would sound like "By dabe is Batt" when spoken denasalized. Using the diacritic [˜] to indicate denasality, this utterance would be transcribed as [m̃aɪ ñeɪm̃ɪz m̃æt]. Children who do not have a cold but consistently sound like they do should probably be evaluated by a physician to determine whether a structural abnormality exists that may interfere with the production of nasal phonemes.

Voicing

These diacritics indicate a change in the manner of vocal fold vibration during the production of consonants and vowels. These changes include voicing and devoicing.

Voicing [t̬]

This diacritic is used when a voiceless phoneme is produced with partial voicing. A good example of voicing occurs when using the tap [ɾ] in the transcription of words such as "better" [bɛɾɚ] and "kitty" [kɪɾɪ]. In these words, the voiceless /t/ becomes partially voiced due to the voiced environment provided by the surrounding phonemes. However, the assimilation does not result in production of the voiced phoneme /d/. Some people use the diacritic for voicing instead of a tap when transcribing words such as "better" [bɛt̬ɚ] or "kitty" [kɪt̬ɪ]. Another example of partial voicing may occur in some pronunciations of the words "pester" [pɛs̬tɚ], "mister" [mɪs̬tɚ], and "Leslie" [lɛs̬lɪ].

EXERCISE 8.18

Transcribe the following words, using the diacritic for voicing instead of a tap (when necessary).

1. kettle   _____   4. attempt   _____

2. written _____   5. baton   _____

3. water   _____   6. battled   _____

Devoicing [ɹ̥] / [ʒ̥]

In certain phonetic environments, phonemes that are normally voiced become less voiced. This phenomenon is known as *devoicing*. Phonemes that become devoiced still have some voicing associated with them; they are not completely voiceless. The concept of devoicing is not really new to you. Recall that a word such as "ladder" is transcribed with the tap /ɾ/, indicating devoicing of the /d/ phoneme. You may recall that this assimilation results when /t/ or /d/ is intervocalic.

Devoicing also occurs when one of the approximants /w, l, r, or j/ follows a voiceless consonant. Examples include "fray" [fɹ̥eɪ], "pew" [pj̊u], "slip" [sl̥ɪp], and "queen" [kw̥in]. Devoicing also may occur across word boundaries as in "thank you" [θæŋkj̊u]. (Note that the devoicing diacritic is placed *above* descending IPA symbols such as /j̊/ and /ʒ̊/.)

Words ending with a voiced fricative or affricate may become devoiced if silence follows the word, that is, if they are at the end of an utterance (Cruttenden, 2008). Examples include [bæd̥ʒ̊], [wʌz̥], and [lʌy̥]. In connected speech, when a word that ends with a voiced fricative is followed by a word that begins with a voiceless consonant, the fricative also may become devoiced (Cruttenden, 2008). For instance, the phrase "has seen" may be pronounced as [həz̥sin]. Other examples include "of course" [əyk̥ɔrs], "she's sorry" [ʃiz̥sɑɹɪ], and "I've passed" [aɪy̥pæst].

If a client is devoicing phonemes in contexts that are not expected, make sure to indicate that in your transcription using the [̥] diacritic. For example, in cleft palate speech, voiceless plosives and fricatives may be produced as *voiceless* nasals (Grunwell & Harding, 1996) such as "sun" [ŋ̊õn] or "pan" [m̥æ̃n].

EXERCISE 8.19

Using the diacritic for devoicing [̥], transcribe the following utterances.

1. pewter   _____   5. he does   _____
2. clearly   _____   6. Ridge Street _____
3. he's stubborn _____   7. I lose   _____
4. bathe Pam   _____   8. they've played _____

Place of Articulation

Several IPA diacritics are used to indicate allophonic variants related to changes in place of articulation of consonants and vowels. Some of these changes occur as a result of assimilation processes. Others occur as a result of dialect or phonological disorder.

Advanced/Retracted [k̟] / [t̠]

These two symbols are used to indicate a variation in tongue position associated with phoneme production. For example, when a consonant is produced with the tongue more forward in the oral cavity than normal (advanced), the symbol [̟] is used. Narrow transcription of the word "key" would be [k̟i] because the /k/ (normally produced with the body of the tongue in the velar region) is produced closer to the palate due to the environment provided by the front vowel /i/ (regressive assimilation).

When a consonant is produced with the tongue farther back than normal (retracted), the symbol [_] is used. When the alveolar stops /t/ or /d/ precede /r/, their place of articulation becomes postalveolar (closer to the palate) because /r/ is a palatal phoneme. Some examples include "true" [t̠ru] and "dry" [d̠raɪ] (regressive assimilation). Because of the backed articulation of these consonants, the words "true" and "dry" may appear to sound like /tʃru/ and /dʒraɪ/, respectively.

These two symbols may also be used to indicate a variation in tongue advancement associated with vowel production. The change in articulation may be due to dialectal variation or a speech sound disorder. The change would involve the front/back dimension. For example, a retracted production of /æ/ would be transcribed as [æ̠], indicating that the vowel is farther back than would be expected, but not so far back as to result in the production of the vowel /ɑ/. Similarly, an advanced production of /ɑ/, that is [ɑ̟], would be farther forward than normal, but not enough to result in production of /æ/.

EXERCISE 8.20

Place an "X" by the words that have a correct transcription using the diacritics [̟] and [_].

_____ 1. could [k̟ʊd]   _____ 3. drop [d̠rɑp]   _____ 5. keep [k̟ip]

_____ 2. kiss [k̠ɪs]   _____ 4. clam [k̠læm]   _____ 6. comb [koʊm̟]

Raised, Lowered [̝ , ̞]

These diacritics can be placed beneath a vowel when there is a change in the height dimension associated with that vowel. The change in tongue height may be the result of a particular dialectal pronunciation of a vowel or as a result of a speech disorder. The symbol [̝] indicates that a vowel is produced with the body of the tongue raised more than expected for that particular vowel. For instance, if an adult attempts to produce the vowel /ɛ/, but raises the tongue higher than expected (but not so high as to produce /ɪ/), the transcription would be [ɛ̝]. Likewise, production of /ʊ/ with a lowered tongue position would be transcribed as [ʊ̞], as long as the production does not result in articulation of the vowel /o/.

EXERCISE 8.21

Examine each of the following vowels and their transcriptions. Then indicate which vowel would result if the articulation was raised, lowered, advanced, or retracted (depending on the diacritic used).

Examples:

vowel produced:		resultant vowel is closer to:
[i̞]		/ɪ/
[ɑ̟]		/æ/

1. [ɛ̝] _____   5. [ʊ̞] _____

2. [æ̠] _____   6. [ɛ̞] _____

3. [o̝] _____   7. [ɪ̝] _____

4. [o̟] _____   8. [ʊ̟] _____

Labialized [ʷ]

A consonant that is not normally produced with lip rounding may become rounded in the presence of certain phonemes, for example, /u/, /ʊ/, or /w/. This phenomenon can be seen in the initial consonantal phoneme of "quick," "good," "zoo," and "rude." The additional articulation of lip rounding, associated with consonant production, is called **labialization**. The diacritic commonly used for a labialized phoneme is a "w" placed to the right of the normally unrounded phoneme as in [kʷwɪk], [gʷʊd], [zʷu], and [rʷud]. These transcriptions all represent regressive, or right-to-left, assimilation because the normally rounded phoneme follows the phoneme undergoing assimilation. Labialization may also occur in some cases of speech sound disorder when it is not expected to occur (not due to phonetic context).

EXERCISE 8.22

Transcribe these words, using the [ʷ] diacritic if the initial phoneme is labialized due to the phonetic environment. If the word does not have a labialized initial phoneme, leave the item blank.

Examples:

swim	[sʷwɪm]
wood	*

1. hood   _____
2. shock   _____
3. roof   _____
4. thin   _____
5. wool   _____
6. plus   _____
7. sweet   _____
8. dune   _____

*/w/ is already a labialized consonant.

More Rounded/Less Rounded [i̜] / [u̜]

One variation in vowel production, sometimes seen in disordered speech, is the production of unrounded vowels as "more rounded" and the production of rounded vowels as "less rounded." The IPA symbol for an unrounded vowel produced with "more rounding" would be [i̜]. In the case where a normally rounded vowel becomes "less rounded," the appropriate IPA symbol (i.e., [u̜]) would be used.

Ball and Müller (2005) recommend the use of existing IPA vowel symbols when transcribing vowel rounding errors. For instance, if a child produces a rounded version of /i/, it would be appropriate to use the IPA symbol /y/, which is the symbol for a rounded, high front vowel (see Figure 2.1). This phoneme is not found in English, but can be found in other languages such as German and French. Similarly, the IPA symbol for an unrounded version of the high back vowel /u/ would be /ɯ/, a vowel common in Korean. Because these IPA symbols are not common in English, you will need to refer to the IPA vowel chart in order to determine the rounded/unrounded counterparts of the English vowels.

EXERCISE 8.23

Use the appropriate IPA symbol for more or less lip rounding for each of the following vowels.

Example:

/ɪ/   [ɪ̹]

1. /e/ _____   4. /ɛ/ _____
2. /o/ _____   5. /ɔ/ _____
3. /ʊ/ _____   6. /æ/ _____

EXERCISE 8.24

Using the IPA chart (Figure 2.1) as your guide, select the appropriate IPA vowel symbol for transcription of each of the following vowel conditions.

Example:

rounded /i/   /y/

1. unrounded /o/ _____   4. unrounded /u/ _____
2. rounded /ɛ/ _____   5. rounded /e/ _____
3. rounded /ɑ/ _____   6. unrounded /ɔ/ _____

Dentalization [t̪]

Alveolar consonants sometimes may be produced with a dental, instead of an alveolar, articulation. The tongue tip makes contact with the upper front teeth (central incisors) during production. This process is termed **dentalization**. In the word "ninth," /n/ becomes dentalized in typical speech production. The alveolar /n/ has a dental articulation brought about by the final phoneme /θ/ in "ninth." It would be possible to transcribe this word as [naɱθ], given that the articulation is more forward than usual. However, when an alveolar phoneme is produced with a dental articulation, the dentalization symbol [̪] is preferred. Other words with dentalized alveolar consonants include "filth" [fɪl̪θ] and "month" [mʌn̪θ]. These examples show regressive or right-to-left assimilation. The effect of dentalization crosses word boundaries as well. For instance, in the phrase "with Terry," the /t/ becomes dentalized, that is, [wɪθt̪ɛrɪ]. Notice that the plosive /t/ is released between the teeth. This is an example of progressive or left-to-right assimilation.

Dentalization occurs in some instances of disordered speech. Some young children produce dentalized /s/ and /z/ in words, such as "shoe" [s̪u] and "zoo" [z̪u] with the tongue tip touching the upper incisors during production of /s/. This is sometimes referred to as a *frontal lisp*. Some individuals transcribe this particular speech production as a /θ/ for /s/, or a /ð/ for /z/ substitution, as in "suit" /θut/ or "zebra" /ðibrə/. It is suggested that the correct transcription for this particular production should be [s̪] or [z̪], not /θ/ or /ð/, as long as the articulation retains a sibilant quality (Hodson & Paden, 1991).

Some children with phonological disorders also produce the affricates /tʃ/ and /dʒ/ as [t̪θ] and [d̪ð], respectively, as in "rich" [rɪt̪θ] and "jam" [d̪ðæm] (Powell, 2001). In this case, the articulation for the plosive portion of the affricate is no longer alveolar, it is dental, with the tongue tip between the front teeth. Also, note the substitution of the dental fricatives /θ/ and /ð/ for the palatal fricatives /ʃ/ and /ʒ/.

Some hearing-impaired children who wear cochlear implants may produce interdental fricatives as dentalized alveolar stops, as in "thumb" [t̪ʰʌm] and "mother" [mʌd̪ɚ], and labiodental stops may be produced in place of labiodental fricatives, as in "fish" [p̪ʰɪʃ] and "vase" [b̪eɪs] (Teoh & Chin, 2009). (Try producing /p/ with a labiodental articulation [instead of bilabial] by bringing your lower lip and upper incisors together.)

EXERCISE 8.25

Transcribe the following utterances, using the diacritic [̪] when necessary. Leave the item blank if it is not necessary to use the diacritic.

1. anthem   _____

2. moth   _____

3. either   _____

4. bathroom   _____

5. math time   _____

6. wealth   _____

7. rhythm   _____

8. panther   _____

Labiodental [ɱ]

In words in which the nasal consonants /m/ or /n/ are followed by /f/, the place of articulation is altered, due to the influence of the labiodental place of articulation for /f/ (regressive assimilation). Although English does not have a labiodental nasal phoneme, other languages do. The IPA symbol for this phoneme is /ɱ/. Because English does not make use of /ɱ/ phonemically, this assimilation may be considered an allophonic variant, not a phonemic change. Words in which this labiodental nasal occurs (depending on an individual speaker's pronunciation) include "comfort" /kʌɱfɚt/, "conference" /kɑɱfrəns/, "unfair" /əɱfɛr/, "emphasis" /ɛɱfəsəs/, and "symphony" /sɪɱfənɪ/. The diacritic for dentalization also may be used to transcribe labiodental assimilation—"comfort" /kʌm̪fɚt/.

EXERCISE 8.26

Transcribe the following words using /ɱ/ where appropriate. If not appropriate, leave the item blank.

1. inferential _____
2. sphinx _____
3. Memphis _____
4. perform _____
5. unfriendly _____
6. sunflower _____
7. pharynx _____
8. kinfolk _____

Velarized [ɫ] the dark /l/

Velarization occurs when the alveolar consonant /l/ is produced in the velar region of the vocal tract. This production of /l/ is said to be *velarized* or "dark." /l/ becomes velarized in the postvocalic position of most words, as in "ball" and "eagle." The diacritic commonly used for velarization is a tilde through the middle of the phoneme, as in [bɑɫ] and [igɫ]. The velarized [ɫ] is found in all occurrences of syllabic [l̩], as in "little" [lɪɾɫ̩] and "bagel" [beɪgɫ̩]. Keep in mind that [ɫ] and [l̩] are separate allophones of /l/.

Velarized [ɫ] is sometimes found to occur at the beginning of words. This may occur as a matter of speaking style, or it may be associated with a speech sound disorder. Some hearing-impaired children produce [ɫ] at word onset as in "leave" [ɫiv] or "leg" [ɫɛg]. Word-initial [ɫ] may sound as if it is preceded by /g/ due to the velarized /l/, as in "love" [gɫʌv] (Teoh & Chin, 2009).

EXERCISE 8.27

Place an "X" next to the words that normally would *not* have a velarized /ɫ/ in their transcriptions.

1. _____ lake
2. _____ mingle
3. _____ loop
4. _____ beagle
5. _____ scalding
6. _____ liked
7. _____ hilly
8. _____ lady

The extIPA and the VoQS

In 1994, an extension to the IPA was adopted by the International Clinical Phonetics and Linguistics Association (ICPLA) as the official set of diacritics to be used in the transcription of disordered speech. This extended version of the IPA is titled the **extIPA** (pronounced /ɛkstaɪpə/) (Duckworth, Allen, Hardcastle, & Ball, 1990). The complete set of extIPA diacritics (revised to 2008) is located in Figure 8.1. You will notice that you are already familiar

extIPA SYMBOLS FOR DISORDERED SPEECH
(Revised to 2008)

CONSONANTS (other than on the IPA Chart)

	bilabial	labiodental	dentolabial	labioalv.	linguolabial	interdental	bidental	alveolar	velar	velophar.
Plosive		p̪ b̪	p̪ b̪	p̻ b̻	t̼ d̼	t̪ d̪				
Nasal			m̪	m̻	n̼	n̪				
Trill					r̼	r̪				
Fricative median		f̪ v̪	f̻ v̻	θ̼ ð̼	θ̪ ð̪	h̪ ɦ̪				fŋ
Fricative lateral+median								ɬ ɮ		
Fricative nareal	m̃							ñ	ŋ̃	
Percussive	w̪w̪						Ꞑ			
Approximant lateral					l̼	l̪				

Where symbols appear in pairs, the one to the right represents a voiced consonant. Shaded areas denote articulations judged impossible.

DIACRITICS

↔	labial spreading	s̪↔	"	strong articulation	f̬	"	denasal	m̃
͟	dentolabial	v̪	ͭ	weak articulation	v̞	͙	nasal escape	v̂
͟	interdental/bidental	n̪	\	reiterated articulation	p\p\p	ᵚ	velopharyngeal friction	s̃
=	alveolar	t̺	ᵕ	whistled articulation	s̫	↓	ingressive airflow	p↓
~	linguolabial	d̼	→	sliding articulation	θs̪	↑	egressive airflow	!↑

CONNECTED SPEECH

(.)	short pause
(..)	medium pause
(...)	long pause
f	loud speech [{f laʊd f}]
ff	louder speech [{ff laʊdɚ ff}]
p	quiet speech [{p kwaɪət p}]
pp	quieter speech [{pp kwaɪətɚ pp}]
allegro	fast speech [{allegro fast allegro}]
lento	slow speech [{lento sloʊ lento}]
crescendo, ralentando, etc. may also be used	

VOICING

	pre-voicing	˳z
	post-voicing	z˳
	partial devoicing	z̜
	initial partial devoicing	z̜
	final partial devoicing	z̜
	partial voicing	s̬
	initial partial voicing	s̬
	final partial voicing	s̬
=	unaspirated	p=
ʰ	pre-aspiration	ʰp

OTHERS

(○), (C̣), (Ṿ)	indeterminate sound, consonant, vowel	k̡	velodorsal articulation
(P̲l̲.v̲l̲s̲), (N̲)	indeterminate voiceless plosive, nasal, etc.	ᶴ	sublaminal lower alveolar percussive click
( )	silent articulation (ʃ), (m)	ꜜǃ	alveolar and sublaminal clicks (cluck-click)
(( ))	extraneous noise, e.g. ((2 sylls))	*	sound with no available symbol

FIGURE 8.1   The extended IPA. © *ICPLA 2008. Reproduced with permission.*

with some of these symbols including the symbols for denasality [͊] and nasal emission (escape) [͊]. Some of the extIPA symbols represent phonemes produced with a place of articulation not seen in typically developing speech. These include *dentolabial* (upper teeth and lower lip), *labioalveolar* (lower lip and alveolar ridge), *linguolabial* (tongue and upper lip), *interdental* (tongue tip or blade protruding between the teeth), and *bidental* (constriction formed by the upper and lower teeth). Other symbols include those for *whistled articulation* (/s/ or /z/ produced with a very narrow tongue groove that creates a whistled fricative), *nareal fricatives* (nasal phonemes produced with accompanying nasal emission due to velopharyngeal incompetency), *labial spreading* (excessive lip spreading), and for *reiterated articulation* (a repeated articulation as is seen in stuttering).

The extIPA also has several additional diacritics for indicating variations in intensity and tempo of connected speech as well as a notation system for indicating duration of pauses. As an example, normal intensity speech followed by very loud speech would be transcribed in the following manner:

$$[ðɪs ɪz nɔrməl ɪntɛnsɪtɪ spitʃ \{_{ff}fɑlod baɪ spitʃ ðæt ɪz vɛrɪ laʊd_{ff}\}]$$

Note that *braces* are used to indicate the stretch of speech that is louder. The symbol *ff* stands for *fortissimo*, an Italian term used in music to denote a passage of music that is to be played very loudly. Similarly, very soft speech would be indicated with the notation *pp*, from the Italian *pianissimo* for "very soft."

Diacritics are also provided in the extIPA to indicate variations in voicing patterns. The voicing diacritics allow for transcription of phonemes that are produced with pre-aspiration, as well as pre-, post-, or partial voicing.

Another extension to the IPA is the *Voice Quality Symbols*, or **VoQS** (Ball, Esling, & Dickson, 1995) (see Figure 8.2). This extension was developed in order to provide speech pathologists with a more in-depth system of transcribing disorders associated with voice production, such as breathiness. Breathiness occurs when the vocal folds do not make sufficient contact during voicing, allowing audible air to escape through the glottis. Causes of breathiness include growths, such as polyps or nodules, on the vocal folds. Some deaf speakers also display breathiness due to improper valving of air by the vocal folds, as air flows through the glottis from the lungs. The IPA diacritic [V̤] is used beneath specific phonemes that are produced with a breathy voice quality. If an entire utterance is breathy, it may be transcribed by using the symbol [V̤] preceding and following the breathy utterance. For example:

$$[\{V̤ \ aɪ \ hæv \ nɑdʒ̩z \ ɑn \ maɪ \ voʊkl̩ \ foldz \ V̤\}]$$

It is beyond the scope of this text to describe other conditions of the larynx that result in an alteration of voice quality. That material will be covered in coursework examining voice production (most likely at the graduate level).

Transcription of Speech Sound Disorders: Non-English Phonemes

Inspection of the IPA chart (Figure 2.1) indicates there are many consonant phonemes that do not appear in spoken English. Of the 58 pulmonic consonants listed (those produced with an egressive airstream from the lungs), only

VoQS: Voice Quality Symbols

Airstream Types

Œ	œsophageal speech	Ν	electrolarynx speech
Ю	tracheo-œsophageal speech	↓	pulmonic ingressive speech

Phonation types

V	modal voice	F	falsetto
W	whisper	C	creak
Ṿ	whispery voice (murmur)	V̰	creaky voice
Vʰ	breathy voice	C̣	whispery creak
V!	harsh voice	V!!	ventricular phonation
V̰!!	diplophonia	Ṿ!!	whispery ventricular phonation
V̱	anterior or pressed phonation	W̱	posterior whisper

Supralaryngeal Settings

L̝	raised larynx	L̞	lowered larynx
Vᶒ	labialized voice (open round)	Vʷ	labialized voice (close round)
V̬	spread-lip voice	Vᶹ	labio-dentalized voice
V̺	linguo-apicalized voice	V̻	linguo-laminalized voice
V˞	retroflex voice	V̪	dentalized voice
V̲	alveolarized voice	V̲ʲ	palatoalveolarized voice
Vʲ	palatalized voice	Vˠ	velarized voice
Vʁ	uvularized voice	Vˤ	pharyngealized voice
V̞ˤ	laryngo-pharyngealized voice	Vꟸ	faucalized voice
Ṽ	nasalized voice	Ṽ	denasalized voice
J̞	open jaw voice	J̝	close jaw voice
J̰	right offset jaw voice	J̰	left offset jaw voice
J̟	protruded jaw voice	Θ	protruded tongue voice

USE OF LABELED BRACES & NUMERALS TO MARK STRETCHES OF SPEECH
AND DEGREES AND COMBINATIONS OF VOICE QUALITY:

[ˈðɪs ɪz ˈnɔɹməl ˈvɔɪs {3V! ˈðɪs ɪz ˈveɹi ˈhɑɹʃ ˈvɔɪs 3V} ðɪs ɪz ˈnɔɹməl ˈvɔɪs wʌns ˈmɔɹ {L̝ 1V! ˈðɪs ɪz ˈlɛs ˈhɑɹʃ ˈvɔɪs wɪð ˈlovəd ˈlæɹɪŋks 1V!L̝}]

FIGURE 8.2   The VoQS. © *1994 Martin J. Ball, John Esling, Craig Dickson. Reproduced with permission.*

22 occur in English. These do not include /w/ or the affricates /tʃ/ and /dʒ/. A couple of the IPA pulmonic consonants are produced only as allophones in English, namely, the glottal stop /ʔ/ and the alveolar tap /ɾ/. The lateral alveolar fricatives /ɬ/ (voiceless) and /lʒ/ (voiced) usually occur in English only in reference to disordered speech (see the following). Although English has only

two affricates, others such as /ts/, /dz/, and /pf/ do occur in other languages. The IPA chart also lists several non-pulmonic consonants (those not requiring an airstream from the lungs in their production), none of which are found in English. Finally, of the 28 vowels listed in the IPA chart, only 12 are produced in English (not counting /ɚ/, /ɝ/, or the diphthongs). Recall that some non-English IPA vowel symbols can be used when transcribing changes in lip rounding associated with vowel production.

When transcribing disordered speech, it often becomes necessary to use some of the non-English phonemes represented in the IPA chart. This is because in some speech sound disorders, phonemes are produced with a place of articulation different from the intended target phoneme, such as substituting the voiceless velar fricative /x/ for the voiceless palatal fricative /ʃ/. Speech sound errors that require the use of non-English IPA characters in transcription generally involve changes in place of articulation of stops and fricatives. Also, some hearing-impaired speakers produce non-pulmonic implosive and ejective phonemes. Table 8.2 lists all of the non-English IPA symbols discussed in the following sections.

Glottal Stop [ʔ]

By now, you should be familiar with the use of the glottal stop in English, as in production of the word "button" /bʌʔn̩/. The glottal stop also appears in the speech of some children with phonological disorders, including those with hearing impairment (Levitt & Stromberg, 1983; Stoel-Gammon, 1983; Teoh & Chin, 2009). For instance, glottal stops may replace other stops or fricatives as in "puppy" /ʔʌʔɪ/, "sister" [ʔɪʔʊ], or "maybe" [meʔɪ]. The glottal stop also may occur at the ends of words, as in "cat" /kʰæʔ/ or "caught" [kʰɔʔ]. You must learn to listen carefully to determine whether a glottal stop is being produced. For instance, in the word "cat," you would need to determine whether the final

TABLE 8.2 Common Non-English IPA Symbols Used in Transcription of Speech Sound Disorders.

Manner of Articulation	IPA Symbol Voiceless	Voiced	Example	
Glottal Stop	[ʔ]		puppy	[ʔʌʔɪ]
Fricatives				
Bilabial	[ɸ]	[β]	fat	[ɸæʔ]
Velar	[x]	[ɣ]	game	[ɣem]
Pharyngeal	[ʕ]	[ʕ]	sheep	[ʕip]
Lateral	[ɬ]	[ɮ]	zoo	[ɮu]
Affricates				
Bilabial	[pf]	[bv]	face	[pfes]
Alveolar	[ts]	[dz]	juice	[dzus]
Velar	[kx]	[gɣ]	ghost	[gɣos]
Approximant		[ʋ]	run	[ʋʌn]
Ejectives (voiceless)	[p', t', and k']		keep	[kip']
Implosives (voiced)	[ɓ, ɗ, and ɠ]		big	[ɓɪʔ]

sound is /ʔ/, an omitted /t/ as in [kæ] or is being produced as an unreleased consonant, as in [kæt̚]. It should be noted that the presence of a glottal stop at the end of a word does not always signal the presence of a speech sound disorder. Glottal stops do occur naturally at the ends of words in some dialects of spoken English.

Cleft palate speakers also may produce glottal stops as substitutes for obstruents. In addition to possible problems with nasal emission and hypernasal resonance, cleft palate speakers may have difficulty producing stops due to decreased intraoral pressure in the oral cavity caused by the cleft. Substitution of a glottal stop assists in proper plosion with a place of articulation posterior to the cleft (so that no air escapes). Some examples include "top" [ʔɑ̃ʔʰ], "guess" [ʔɛ̃ʔ], and "comb" [ʔõm] (Trost-Cardemone, 2009). Glottal stop substitution may occur, even following surgery for the cleft, due to learned speaking habits.

Fricatives [ɸ, β, x, ɣ, ħ, ʕ, ʕ]
There are several IPA symbols for non-English fricatives that may be used in transcription of speech sound disorders. For example, *bilabial* and *velar* fricatives may be produced by some children with phonological disorders, including children with hearing loss (Louko & Edwards, 2001; Stoel-Gammon, 1983; Teoh & Chin, 2009). The bilabial fricatives [ɸ] (voiceless) and [β] (voiced) may be substituted for the labiodental fricatives /f/ and /v/, respectively. Similar to the labiodental fricatives, /f/ and /v/, the bilabial fricatives are non-strident (low intensity) and have a similar acoustic structure. Examples of bilabial fricative substitutions include "giraffe" [dəwæɸ] and "shovel" [dʌβoʊ] (Louko & Edwards, 2001).

Similarly, the velar fricatives /x/ (voiceless) and /ɣ/ (voiced) may be produced as a substitute for the velar stops /k/ and /g/. This is a substitution also seen in cleft palate speech. The velar fricatives are produced when full closure for the stops does not occur (Louko & Edwards, 2001). Some examples of velar fricative substitutions include "cat" /xæt/ or /ɣæt/, "game" /ɣem/, and "lecture" [lɛɣʒu].

In some cleft palate speakers, the fricatives /s, z, ʃ, or ʒ/ are backed and produced as pharyngeal fricatives (Trost-Cardemone & Bernthal, 1993). The IPA symbols for the pharyngeal fricatives are [ħ] (voiceless) and [ʕ] (voiced). Trust-Cardemone (2009) recommends the use of the symbol [ʕ] instead of [ħ] for the voiceless pharyngeal fricative. Some examples include "sheep" [ʕĩp] (or [ħĩp]) and "measure" [mɛ̃ʕɚ].

Lateral Fricatives [ɬ, ɮ]
Lateralization of the fricatives /s/ or /z/ occurs when the constricted airflow is diverted over the sides of the tongue, instead of being able to flow centrally. To produce a lateralized /s/, place your tongue in position for the initial phoneme in the word "let." Now, holding your tongue in place, try to produce an /s/ phoneme. Notice how the air flows over the sides of the tongue because it cannot escape anteriorly. This lateral production of /s/ or /z/ is sometimes referred to as a *lateral lisp* and is seen in some children with phonological disorders.

The IPA diacritic for a lateralized phoneme is a raised /l/, placed to the right of the indicated phoneme, as in [jɛsˡ]. There are other IPA symbols specifically used for transcription of a *lateral fricative*. The symbol [ɬ] represents a lateralized /s/, and [ɮ] represents a lateralized /z/. Examples include "yes" [jɛɫ] and "zoo" [ʐu]. Sometimes lateral fricatives are substituted for an affricate (deaffrication), as in "witch" [wɪɫ] and "jelly" [ʐɛlɪ].

The extIPA also lists two symbols for lateralized fricatives, [ls] (voiceless) and [lz] (voiced). These symbols are to be used when a fricative is produced with both a lateral *and* a central airstream.

Affricates [pf, bv, ts, dz, kx, gɣ]

Some individuals with phonological disorders may produce non-English affricates such as /pf/, /bv/ (bilabial), /ts/, /dz/ (alveolar), and /kx/, /gɣ/ (velar) (Louko & Edwards, 2001; Powell, 2001). The affricates /ts/ and /dz/ often replace /tʃ/ and /dʒ/ as in "watch" [wɑts] and "Jim" /dzɪm/. Other examples of non-English affricates include "fun" [pfʌn], "van" [bvæn], "ski" [kxi], and "go" [gɣo].

Approximant [ʋ]

Earlier in this chapter we discussed the fact that some children substitute /w/ for /r/ in a process commonly known as *gliding*. In some instances, however, the production is not truly a /w/, but somewhere between an /r/ and a /w/. What may occur in this case is the substitution of the voiced labiodental approximant [ʋ] for /r/ (Ball, 2008; Bauman-Waengler, 2012). This approximant is similar to /w/ but it is labiodental, not labiovelar; there is no constriction of the tongue in the velar region. Instead, the lower lip and teeth are used in production of this sound. Because this phoneme is an approximant, the lower lip and teeth do not touch as would be the case for the labiodental fricative /v/.

Implosives [ɓ, ɗ, ɠ] *and* Ejectives [p', t', k']

An interesting phenomenon observed in the speech of some hearing-impaired speakers is the use of non-pulmonic **ejective** and **implosive** stop consonants. Both ejectives and implosive consonants rely on a *glottalic* airstream, as opposed to a pulmonic airstream. Both implosive and ejective consonants occur in some African and Native American languages. An ejective is produced in a manner similar to a pulmonic stop consonant. However, during its production, the vocal folds close and then are *raised,* causing a decrease in the area between the closed vocal folds and the constriction in the oral cavity formed by the tongue. This results in a greater amount of intraoral pressure than would be typical of a pulmonic stop. Then, when the stop is released, there is a large burst of air due to the increased intraoral pressure. Conversely, implosives are produced by *lowering* the vocal folds, thereby increasing the area of the vocal tract and decreasing the intraoral pressure between the vocal folds and the constriction in the oral cavity. When the stop is released, air flows *into* the vocal tract (an *ingressive* airstream).

It is not completely clear why hearing-impaired individuals produce ejectives and implosives. It is believed that these behaviors develop either due to the provision of increased tactile/kinesthetic feedback (Higgins, Carney, McCleary, & Rogers, 1996) or as a result of faulty learning while developing the ability to produce voiced and voiceless stops (Monsen, 1983). The IPA symbols for the implosive and ejective stops (at the bilabial, alveolar, and velar places of articulation) are given below. The remaining implosive and ejective IPA symbols can be found in Figure 2.1.

	Implosive	Ejective
Bilabial	/ɓ/	/p'/
Dental/alveolar	/ɗ/	/t'/
Velar	/ɠ/	/k'/

Implosives and ejectives have also been known to occur in individuals who stutter and in people with phonological disorders not related to hearing impairment (Ball & Müller, 2007).

EXERCISE 8.28

Write the intended IPA symbol for each description given.

1. voiceless velar fricative   _____
2. voiceless bilabial affricate   _____
3. voiced pharyngeal fricative   _____
4. voiced bilabial fricative   _____
5. voiceless lateral fricative   _____
6. velar ejective   _____
7. labiodental approximant   _____
8. alveolar implosive   _____
9. voiced velar fricative   _____
10. labiodental nasal   _____

Complete Assignment 8-4.

Suggestions for Transcription

The complete set of combined diacritics from the revised 1996 IPA symbols, the extIPA, and from the VoQS seems extraordinarily overwhelming at first. The combined diacritic sets allow for the transcription of virtually all possible allophonic variants of English as well as most typical speech sound errors. Obviously, not all of these symbols would be used routinely in the transcription of disordered speech. This raises an interesting question. Which symbols should be used routinely when transcribing disordered speech? This is not an easy question to answer. Undoubtedly, every speech-language pathologist would have a different answer to this question. The most important consideration is the accuracy of the transcription being performed. It is not necessarily important to indicate normal allophonic variations of phonemes if they do not disrupt the production of speech. For instance, there would be no need to indicate nasalized vowels, as long as the nasalization was appropriate. If, however, a client had inappropriate nasalization of speech, the appropriate diacritic [˜] would then need to be indicated in the transcription.

When you begin transcribing both live and recorded samples of your clients, there are several factors you will need to consider so that your transcriptions will be as accurate as possible. Keep in mind that your clients' speech patterns often will be difficult to understand. This means that a good recording is necessary so that you will be able to replay the speech sample at a later time. Modern digital recorders are quite good at capturing your clients' speech. However, no matter how good the recording, certain phonemes may not always be audible during playback because some English phonemes are naturally low in intensity, especially the voiceless fricatives /f/, /θ/, and /ɸ/. This is one reason why it is extremely important for you to transcribe face-to-face during testing. Of course, wearing headphones (attached to your recorder) will aid in your transcription accuracy by reducing any background noise that might be present. Also, when you are performing a live transcription, you will be able to visually focus on the clients' articulators, especially in reference to lip rounding and tongue placement for certain phonemes. Although it is possible to make a video recording of your clients' diagnostic session, facial features may not always be clearly represented because video images provide only a two-dimensional view of the client.

Stoel-Gammon (2001, p. 15) suggests the following before beginning a transcription session:

1. Work in a quiet area.
2. Spend no more than 2 to 3 hours transcribing at any one time; take a 5- to 10-minute break every 45 minutes.
3. Before beginning, listen to an extended sample to become used to the speech patterns you will be transcribing.
4. Avoid being influenced by knowledge of the target words you are transcribing.
5. Listen to the vocalizations as many times as needed.

When listening to a recorded sample of a client's speech, it will become immediately apparent that certain speech segments will be easier to transcribe than others. Begin with the speech segments of which you are sure. You also may want to transcribe phonemes first, adding the diacritics later. Ohde and Sharf (1992, pp. 351–352) offer several beneficial suggestions to help the clinician focus on speech patterns that are particularly difficult to transcribe. Their transcription techniques include the following:

1. Count the number of syllables in each produced utterance and determine if it agrees with the number in the target utterance.
2. Identify the vowels, diphthongs, or syllabic consonants that constitute the nucleus of each syllable, using the minimal contrasts of front-back, high-low, tense-lax, and rounded-unrounded to zero in on the vowel.
3. Transcribe the syllable nuclei you are certain of, leaving space for preceding and following consonants.
4. Determine whether each vowel nucleus is initiated and terminated by a consonant or consonant cluster and if a target consonant is deleted.
5. Identify the consonants, using manner, voicing, and place feature analysis to zero in on them, and transcribe those you are certain of.
6. Decide which features of the remaining consonants you are uncertain about and how they differ from the target consonants.
7. Transcribe the consonants, using appropriate diacritics to indicate deviations from targets, if necessary.

Of course, it may not be possible for you to identify *every* phoneme that your client produces. When this happens, it may be necessary to use the appropriate symbols from the extIPA to indicate indeterminate sounds, that is sounds of which you are unsure. For instance, if you know a particular phoneme is a vowel, but you are not sure of the exact vowel, you would write V with a circle around it (i.e., Ⓥ to represent the phoneme in question). Or if you knew the phoneme was a voiceless plosive, but were not sure if it was /p, t, or k/, you would transcribe the phoneme as Pl, vls with a circle around it (i.e., Ⓟⓛ, vlꜱ).

During transcription, you should be careful about "second-guessing" or having expectations about what your client is attempting to say. In some instances, knowing what your client is saying may help you get a more accurate transcription. However, it is possible your expectations may be wrong and cause you to transcribe your client incorrectly. Louko and Edwards (2001) report a case where a child was shown a picture of "twins" and the child responded [ˈtʰoːˌwĩn]. In reality, the child was attempting to say "children," *not* "twins." Upon additional exploration, the clinician did get the child to say [tʰɪnz], proving the child's first response was not at all a production of the word "twins." Had the clinician not investigated further, her transcription of "twins" as [ˈtʰoːˌwĩn] and not [tʰɪnz] could have turned out to be problematic when determining the specific phonological errors the child was exhibiting.

Review Exercises

A. Each of the following speech productions represent one type of *syllable structure process*. Match one of the processes at the right with each transcription given.

Examples:

b	coat	/koʊ/	a. weak syllable deletion
c	kitty	/kɪkɪ/	b. final consonant deletion
			c. reduplication
			d. cluster reduction

____ 1. school	/kul/		____ 6. swing	/sɪŋ/
____ 2. candy	/kækæ/		____ 7. soap	/soʊ/
____ 3. lion	/laɪ/		____ 8. cookie	/kiki/
____ 4. mom	/mɑ/		____ 9. missed	/mɪt/
____ 5. running	/rʌn/		____ 10. water	/wɑ/

B. Each of the following transcriptions reflects an *assimilation process*. Match the type of assimilation at the right to each transcription given.

Example:

b	cup	/kʌk/	a. labial	d. prevocalic voicing
			b. velar	e. devoicing
			c. alveolar	

____ 1. pan	/tæn/		____ 6. sunny	/zʌnɪ/
____ 2. face	/veɪs/		____ 7. green	/grɪŋ/
____ 3. swim	/ɸwɪm/		____ 8. sack	/sæt/
____ 4. bad	/bæt/		____ 9. park	/kɑrk/
____ 5. numb	/mʌm/		____ 10. nag	/næk/

C. Match the appropriate *substitution process* at the right being demonstrated to the transcr
be more than one correct answer per item.

_____	1. mister	/mɪstʊ/	a. gliding
_____	2. chops	/tɑps/	b. deaffrication
_____	3. matches	/mæʃəz/	c. vocalization
_____	4. cage	/keɪʒ/	d. fronting
_____	5. shampoo	/tæmpu/	e. stopping
_____	6. reel	/wiʊ/	
_____	7. jumped	/dʌmpt/	
_____	8. little	/jɪɾoʊ/	
_____	9. press	/pwɛs/	
_____	10. yellow	/jɛwoʊ/	
_____	11. choose	/ʃuz/	
_____	12. watch	/wɑs/	

D. For each of the following words, apply the phonological process given and transcribe the resulting production.

Example:

lean final consonant deletion _____/li/_____

1. sleep cluster reduction _____
2. brag velar assimilation _____
3. jar stopping _____
4. lemon gliding _____
5. bake labial assimilation _____
6. jelly deaffrication _____
7. above weak syllable deletion _____
8. pine alveolar assimilation _____
9. came fronting _____
10. crow prevocalic voicing _____

E. Write the description for each of the following diacritics taken from the extIPA.

1. m\m\m _____ 5. θ̰ _____
2. h̬ _____ 6. s̝ _____
3. ŋ̃ _____ 7. r̃ _____
4. ḇ _____ 8. ɮ _____

F. Transcribe the following words as spoken by a 5-year-old male child who demonstrates *gliding*.

1. lobster _____ 7. dentist _____
2. nurse _____ 8. refrigerator _____
3. soldier _____ 9. telephone _____
4. astronaut _____ 10. lamp _____
5. teacher _____ 11. toothbrush _____
6. truck driver _____ 12. bathtub _____

CD #3
Track 11

13. toilet _____   20. spider _____
14. hammer _____   21. lion _____
15. alarm clock _____   22. dolphin _____
16. vacuum cleaner _____ 23. kangaroo _____
17. elephant _____   24. octopus _____
18. tiger _____   25. lawyer _____
19. squirrel _____

G. Transcribe the following words and sentences as spoken by a 7-year-old female child who demonstrates *dentalization* of alveolar fricatives.

**CD #3
Track 12**

1. cherries _____   11. octopus _____
2. celery _____   12. squirrel _____
3. cheese _____   13. snake _____
4. cereal _____   14. skunk _____
5. grapes _____   15. jeans _____
6. ice cream _____   16. sweater _____
7. peas _____   17. pajamas _____
8. pancakes _____   18. sandals _____
9. eggs _____   19. mittens _____
10. spider _____   20. slippers _____

21. We went to Ben Franklin's and looked at the toys.

_____

22. I saw some dolls that I liked.

_____

23. They traveled to Maine from Nebraska.

_____

24. We do spelling and math.

_____

25. Sometimes we play mystery games.

_____

H. Transcribe the following words as spoken by a 7-year-old female child who demonstrates both *vocalization* and *dentalization* of alveolar fricatives.

**CD #3
Track 13**

1. frog _____   11. pancakes _____
2. zebra _____   12. celery _____
3. cookies _____   13. giraffe _____
4. hamburger _____   14. lobster _____
5. skunk _____   15. rabbit _____
6. strawberries _____   16. spider _____
7. parakeet _____   17. elephant _____
8. carrots _____   18. ice cream _____
9. cereal _____   19. butter _____
10. hotdog _____   20. cherries _____

21. squirrel _____   24. potato _____

22. orange _____   25. turtle _____

23. horse _____

I. For each of the following, write the appropriate IPA symbol for the description given.

Example:

dentalized /n/ _____[n̪]_____

1. aspirated /p/ _____   6. nasalized /o/ _____

2. raised /u/ _____   7. less rounded /w/ _____

3. devoiced /r/ _____   8. unreleased /k/ _____

4. labialized /g/ _____   9. denasalized /ŋ/ _____

5. lateralized /z/ _____ 10. fronted /k/ _____

J. Select an English word in which you might find each of the following diacritics. Write the word in IPA using the appropriate transcription.

1. [t⁼] _____   6. [n̥] _____

2. [m̃] _____   7. [d̪] _____

3. [b˺] _____   8. [ɫ] _____

4. [ɛ̃] _____   9. [m̥] _____

5. [t̪] _____   10. [ʔ] _____

K. Circle the most accurate allophonic transcription for each of the following words.

1. clue   [kʰlu]   [k̥ɫu]   [k˺ɫu]
2. lymph   [lɪɱf]   [ɫɪmf]   [lɪmp˺f]
3. money   [mʌni]   [mʌ̃nɪ]   [m̥ʌnɪ]
4. coop   [k˺upʰ]   [kʰupʰ]   [kʰup⁼]
5. trial   [tʰɹ̥aɪɫ]   [t̪ʰɹaɪɫ]   [tʰɹ̥aɪɫ]
6. skunk   [sk⁼ʌŋkʰ]   [sk˺ʌŋkʰ]   [sk⁼ʌ̃ŋkʰ]
7. menthol   [mɛ̃n̪θɑɫ]   [mɛ̃nθɑl]   [mɛ̃n̪θɑɫ]
8. sweet   [swit⁼]   [sʷwit˺]   [sʷw̥itʰ]

Study Questions

1. What is the difference between an articulation disorder and a phonological disorder?
2. Define the terms *substitution, distortion, omission,* and *addition.*
3. What are the differences between syllable structure processes, assimilatory processes, and substitution processes?

4. Describe the following phonological processes:

   a. stopping

   b. fronting

   c. deaffrication

   d. gliding

   e. vocalization

   f. weak syllable deletion

   g. cluster reduction

   h. final consonant deletion

   i. reduplication

   j. labial assimilation

   k. alveolar assimilation

   l. velar assimilation

   m. prevocalic voicing

   n. devoicing

5. What is an *idiosyncratic* phonological process? Describe four such processes.

6. What is *nonlinear phonology*?

7. What is meant by the terms *nasal emission* and *denasality*?

8. When do the following stop consonant allophones generally occur in English?

   a. unreleased   b. aspirated   c. unaspirated

9. What is meant by the following terms?

   a. labialization   b. dentalization   c. velarization

10. What is the extIPA? What is the VoQS? When would these diacritic sets be employed in transcription?

11. Why is it important to become familiar with non-English IPA symbols in transcription of speech sound disorders?

12. Describe several strategies you might employ when attempting to transcribe the speech patterns of a client with a speech sound disorder.

Online Resource

American Speech-Language-Hearing Association. (1997–2014). Speech sound disorders: Articulation and phonological processes. Retrieved from *http://www.asha.org/public/speech/disorders/SpeechSoundDisorders.htm* (overview of speech sound disorders, causes, and treatment)

Assignment 8-1   Name _____

1. Match the process at the right being demonstrated with the transcriptions. Each item has only one correct answer.

____ a. lake   → /jeɪk/   ____ g. pitch   → /pɪʃ/   A. fronting

____ b. with   → /wɪt/   ____ h. dish   → /dɪs/   B. stopping

____ c. very   → /bɛrɪ/   ____ i. through → /tru/   C. deaffrication

____ d. camp   → /tæmp/   ____ j. shop   → /ʒɑp/   D. prevocalic voicing

____ e. chews → /ʃuz/   ____ k. dropped → /dwɑpt/   E. gliding

____ f. tree   → /dri/   ____ l. song   → /sɑn/

2. Match the process at the right being demonstrated with the transcriptions. Each item has only one correct answer.

____ a. tickle → /dɪkl̩/   ____ g. case → /teɪs/   A. labial assimilation

____ b. feed   → /fit/   ____ h. corn → /kɔrŋ/   B. alveolar assimilation

____ c. drop   → /drɑt/   ____ i. was   → /wʌs/   C. velar assimilation

____ d. bath   → /bæf/   ____ j. camp → /pæmp/   D. prevocalic voicing

____ e. box   → /gɔks/   ____ k. bring → /grɪŋ/   E. devoicing

____ f. pad   → /pæb/   ____ l. share → /ʒɛr/

3. For each of the following words, apply the phonological process given and transcribe the resulting production.

Example:

   lean   final consonant deletion   ____/li/____

a. cost   prevocalic voicing   _____

b. flag   final consonant deletion   _____

c. tacky   velar assimilation   _____

d. spurt   cluster reduction   _____

e. wish   fronting   _____

f. than   alveolar assimilation   _____

g. glued   gliding   _____

h. cage   devoicing   _____

i. other   stopping   _____

j. chocolate   weak syllable deletion   _____

k. badge   deaffrication   _____

l. tough   labial assimilation   _____

Assignment 8-1 (cont.)

4. Circle the transcriptions that could be examples of the process given.

   a. fronting

   leash → /lis/   pack → /pæt/

   door → /tɔr/   juice → /zus/

   b. cluster reduction

   string → /rɪŋ/   lather → /læɾɚ/

   match → /mæs/   from → /rʌm/

   c. labial assimilation

   pig → /bɪg/   drink → /brɪŋk/

   money → /mʌmɪ/   cave → /peɪv/

   d. final consonant deletion

   obey → /oʊ/   cash → /kæs/

   nest → /nɛs/   both → /boʊt/

   e. velar assimilation

   bingo → /gɪŋgoʊ/   knee → /nik/

   singer → /nɪŋɚ/   class → /glæs/

   f. stopping

   puss → /pʊt/   math → /mæt/

   Vicki → /bɪkɪ/   badge → /bæd/

   g. gliding

   trust → /twʌst/   fly → /fwaɪ/

   turn → /tʊn/   lip → /jɪp/

   h. deaffrication

   Roger → /rɑʒɚ/   catch → /kæʃ/

   sheep → /sip/   measure → /mɛzɚ/

   i. alveolar assimilation

   make → /neɪk/   then → /zɛn/

   bunny → /dʌnɪ/   sand → /tænd/

   j. vocalization

   like → /lɔk/   rain → /weɪn/

   tire → /taɪoʊ/   here → /hɪʊ/

Assignment 8-2

Name _____

CD #3
Track 14

Transcribe the following sentences, as spoken by a 7-year-old female child. This child demonstrates both gliding and vocalization.

1. I put my right shoe on my left foot.

_____

2. She'll have to wear a raincoat.

_____

3. There was a hole in the roof.

_____

4. My Grandma likes roses.

_____

5. His sandwich fell apart.

_____

6. I can't decide which I like best.

_____

7. He pushed us on the merry-go-round.

_____

8. Shannon was sick of school.

_____

9. Grandpa fell asleep on the couch.

_____

10. Jasmine hopes it'll stop raining soon.

_____

11. My shirt is in the washing machine.

_____

12. I had a seashell for show 'n' tell.

_____

Assignment 8-3

Name _____

Transcribe the following utterances, as spoken by a 4-year-old male child. This child demonstrates the idiosyncratic processes of initial consonant deletion and glottal insertion.

CD #3
Track 15

1. black _____
2. pink _____
3. red _____
4. yellow _____
5. orange _____
6. white _____
7. blue _____
8. green _____
9. apple _____

10. pear _____
11. green beans _____
12. berries _____
13. icing _____
14. cheese _____
15. hotdog _____
16. cocoon _____
17. magic _____
18. caterpillar _____

19. What is these? _____
20. big tree and lake _____
21. See worm eat big leaf. _____
22. Me see egg right there. _____
23. Worm no hungry no more. _____
24. We have that movie. _____
25. I like long necks . . . him . . . er . . .
    Joshua likes sharp tooths. _____
26. Do you color dinosaurs with me? _____

Assignment 8-4   Name _____

1. For each of the following phonemes, provide two allophones. Then transcribe two words in which those allophones may be found.

   Example:

       /p/   i) [pʰ] push [pʰʊʃ]   ii) [p˭] spin [sp˭ɪn]

   a. /l/   i)   ii)

   b. /t/   i)   ii)

   c. /k/   i)   ii)

   d. /d/   i)   ii)

   e. /r/   i)   ii)

   f. /g/   i)   ii)

   g. /z/   i)   ii)

2. Transcribe each of the following words using the devoicing diacritic [̥].

   a. sweet   _____   e. crazy   _____

   b. leave   _____   f. raise   _____

   c. plaque _____   g. fuse   _____

   d. phase   _____   h. queen   _____

3. Transcribe each of the following words using the diacritics for aspirated [ʰ] and for unaspirated [˭] where necessary.

   a. spank   _____   e. clueless   _____

   b. retain   _____   f. table   _____

   c. skewed _____   g. stared   _____

   d. peeked _____   h. supposed   _____

4. Transcribe the following words using the diacritics for dental [̪] and labiodental [ɱ] articulations, where necessary.

   a. nineteenth _____   e. breadth   _____

   b. emphatic   _____   f. although   _____

   c. infrared   _____   g. emphysema   _____

   d. enthused   _____   h. healthier   _____

Assignment 8-4 (cont.)

5. Explain the difference between the following allophones:

   Example:

   ɛ/ɛ̃   non-nasalized (oral) /ɛ/ versus nasalized /ɛ/

   a. z/ʒ
   b. pʰ/p˭
   c. l/ɬ
   d. ŋ/ŋ̃
   e. d̥/d
   f. t/t̪
   g. u/uː
   h. s/sʷ
   i. ŋ/ɱ
   j. r/r̥

6. Indicate whether the diacritic is used correctly by placing an "X" in the proper blank. If the diacritic is incorrect, explain the error.

a. plain	[plẽɪn]	_____ correct	_____ incorrect
b. licked	[l̩ɪkt]	_____ correct	_____ incorrect
c. freed	[friːd]	_____ correct	_____ incorrect
d. spread	[sp˭rɛd]	_____ correct	_____ incorrect
e. hark	[hɑrkʰ]	_____ correct	_____ incorrect
f. practice	[præk˺tɪs]	_____ correct	_____ incorrect
g. swirl	[sʷwɝl]	_____ correct	_____ incorrect
h. spry	[s̩pry]	_____ correct	_____ incorrect

7. Each of the following non-English IPA symbols may serve as a substitution for a standard English phoneme when transcribing clients with speech sound disorders. Write the articulatory description for each of the IPA symbols; then give one example of a standard English phoneme it might replace.

Example:

    [β]   voiced, bilabial fricative   /v/

1. [ʦ] _____ _____

2. [ʕ] _____ _____

3. [ɣ] _____ _____

4. [ɸ] _____ _____

5. [ɡ] _____ _____

6. [ʋ] _____ _____

7. [ʢ] _____ _____

8. [ɫ] _____ _____

9. [k'] _____ _____

10. [x] _____ _____

CHAPTER 9

Dialectal Variation

Learning Objectives

After reading this chapter you will be able to:

1. Explain the difference between formal and informal Standard American English, and General American English.
2. Describe ASHA's position concerning dialects.
3. Explain the ways in which chain shifts and mergers affect vowel production, and how they define regional dialects across the United States.
4. Describe the phonological characteristics of Southern and Eastern American English.
5. Explain the difference between a regional dialect, and a social or ethnic dialect.
6. Explain the concept of language transfer in non-native speakers of English.
7. Describe the phonological characteristics consistent with African American English.
8. Compare and contrast the vowel systems of Standard American English and Received Pronunciation.
9. Describe the phonological characteristics consistent with Spanish-Influenced English, Asian-Influenced English, and Russian, and Arabic-Influenced English.

As college freshmen, many of you moved away from home for the first time. Once you arrived at college, you immediately found yourself thrust into new surroundings. You became a little fish in a big pond, the pond made up of people from various regions of the country. You also had the opportunity to meet people with quite varied social and cultural backgrounds. For the first time in your life, you may have realized the marked dialect in the speech and language patterns of people with backgrounds different from your own. The variations in the phonological patterns of your new college acquaintances may have been subtle, in the form of a slight accent. Or perhaps the differences were not so subtle, reflecting a difference in grammatical patterns, vocabulary, and even heavier accents. Prior to this time, the primary speech and language patterns to which you were exposed were probably those of your family and friends and from the newscasters you heard on the radio or saw on TV. Your exposure to varying dialects may have been limited to TV shows that took place in the South or in New York City.

Recall that *dialect* is defined as a variation of speech or language based on geographic area, native language background, and social or ethnic group membership. The dialects of English spoken in the United States are quite variable in terms of syntax (grammatical rules), vocabulary, and phonology. The dialect you use in your daily life is the product of the region of the United States in which you grew up, your cultural background, your ethnic group membership, and also the social class to which you belong. Social class in this sense refers to type of occupation (white collar, blue collar, etc.), socioeconomic class, level of education, and in which part of town you grew up. Factors such as age and gender also play important roles in determining the language patterns you will use on a day-to-day basis. In addition, as a speaker of a language you also possess an **idiolect**, an individual, idiosyncratic speech pattern characteristic of your own personality.

Suppose you grew up in Omaha and had to travel to New York City on business. You would immediately notice a sizable variation in the pronunciation patterns of the native New Yorkers. You would probably consider the native speakers to have an accent. This judgment would be made using your own learned speaking habits as an internal yardstick or standard. Consider the fact that a New York City native would find your speech to have just as much of an accent as you do hers. Most likely, both of you would consider your own usage of English as the standard. This raises an interesting question, "Is there a standard form of American English?"

Standard American English (SAE) is a form of English that is relatively devoid of regional and social characteristics (Kretzschmar, 2008). SAE actually exists in both written and spoken forms. In the United States, there is no *one* fixed standard of English. In some countries, including Spain and France, there are academies that regulate the introduction of new words into the language as well as standardize allowable grammatical rules, especially for government publications and education. In the United States, there is no such formal academy that standardizes or regulates the rules of written and spoken English.

In the United States, SAE actually exists in two forms, **formal standard English** and **informal standard English** (Wolfram & Schilling-Estes, 2006). Formal standard English usually refers to the written form of the language; it is the English of dictionaries, grammar books, and most printed matter. As college students, you use formal standard English when writing a term paper. In spoken form, the standard may be observed in the speech of the national network newscasters who, for the most part, have limited regional accents that do not tie them to any particular geographic region. Formal standard English is the idealized form often adopted when teaching English.

In reality, most speakers in the United States do not speak formal standard English. Instead, we tend to speak some variety of informal standard English. Informal standard English is based on listener judgments of patterns of spoken English deemed to be acceptable or not. That is, societal judgment determines whether a particular speaker's dialect of English is acceptable or "standard." Informal standard English actually exists on a continuum from "standard" to "nonstandard" (Kretzschmar, 2008; Wolfram & Schilling-Estes, 2006). Two people with different language and social backgrounds might judge a third speaker differently in terms of where that person might fall on the continuum. That is, one judge may place the speaker closer to "standard" on the continuum, and the other judge might place him closer to "nonstandard." For instance, a speaker might be rated more substandard if he used sentences such as "I ain't goin' to the movies" or "We was in a hurry." An individual who is considered to be a nonstandard speaker of English is said to speak a **vernacular dialect** (Wolfram & Schilling-Estes, 2006).

An individual would be judged to be using a vernacular dialect based on the presence of stigmatizing grammatical structures in spoken language.

Formal standard English, then, at least in a spoken form, is rarely achieved by speakers of American English. Virtually every speaker of American English belongs to some dialect group defined by region, ethnic group, native language background, or social class. For this reason, it is better to think of American English as having an informal standard that exists on a continuum as opposed to one fixed, formal standard.

The term **General American English** often is used to designate a "standard" dialect that lacks any regional pronunciation, such as that associated with the South or the East. In this manner, the use of the term is somewhat synonymous with the term *Standard American English.* Wolfram and Schilling-Estes (2006) suggest that the term *General American English* be used only when comparing regional or ethnic dialects to a national standard to avoid any bias that might be inferred by use of the label "standard." If a particular dialect varies from Standard American English, it might be thought of incorrectly as being a "nonstandard" or vernacular dialect. Therefore, in this text the term *General American English* will be used only when comparing dialects to a "national standard."

EXERCISE 9.1

Which regional and social factors have influenced the particular dialect of English you speak? Do you have any particular idiosyncratic speech patterns that contribute to your idiolect?

As speech and hearing professionals, you often will be evaluating the speech and language capabilities of individuals from various regional, social, and cultural backgrounds. You will need to determine whether these individuals have a handicapping communicative problem, regardless of the particular dialect of English that they have acquired. It is important to realize that dialects of standard English should *not* be thought of as substandard versions of our language. That is, dialects should not be thought of automatically as "wrong," or in need of remediation. Instead, dialects should be considered strictly as a variety of standard English that reflects an individual's social class, ethnic group membership, or the region in which he or she grew up. In fact, dialects should be thought of as a communication *difference,* as opposed to a communication disorder, the difference being the variation in phonological rules, vocabulary, and syntax of any particular dialect.

In 2003, the American Speech-Language-Hearing Association (ASHA) published a technical report titled "American English Dialects." This report promotes the idea that "no dialectal variety of American English is a disorder or a pathological form of speech or language" (American Speech-Language-Hearing Association [ASHA], 2003). According to ASHA:

> Each dialect is adequate as a functional and effective variety of American English. Each serves a communication function as well as a social solidarity function. Each dialect maintains the communication network and the social construct of the community of speakers who use it. Furthermore, each is a symbolic representation of the geographic, historical, social, and cultural background of its speakers. (p. 45)

In some instances, speech-language pathologists (SLPs) are asked to provide an elective service known as **accent modification** in order to assist non-native English-speaking adults (those who learned English as a second language) in becoming more intelligible (easier to understand), especially in the workplace. Accent modification programs are becoming more common in university settings as the number of foreign instructors in the classroom increases. In fact, in Ohio it is mandatory that all university teaching assistants be proficient in the use of the English language. Therefore, mandatory accent modification programs have been set up in university speech and hearing clinics or in programs that teach English as a second language (ESL) to assist foreign-born instructors to improve their pronunciation of English. Keep in mind that the focus of an elective accent modification program is "to assist in the acquisition of the desired competency in the second dialect without jeopardizing the integrity of the individual's first dialect" (ASHA, 2003, p. 46).

All too often, accent modification is viewed quite narrowly as a management option similar to treatment of a speech sound disorder. It is problematic to think of accent modification merely as working on speech sound production in order to improve a client's intelligibility. Even though accent modification falls within ASHA's scope of practice for SLPs, many university training programs do not have specific coursework in that area. SLPs need to acquire additional clinical preparation if accent modification is to be successful. For instance, Sikorski (2005) states that although working with clients on the prosodic aspects of spoken language (intonation, rhythm, timing, and stress) is key in improving speech intelligibility among second-language learners of English, SLPs receive little training in this area.

Additionally, SLPs should have a thorough understanding of the client's cultural and native language background to fully understand how the native language impacts learning of English. Müller and Guendouzi (2007) suggest that for SLPs to be successful providers of accent modification, they should have training in ESL. This is because adults learning English often have difficulty not only with speech sound production, but also with English syntax and vocabulary. Working on phonology (pronunciation) in a vacuum does not address the other language issues the client may be facing that ultimately will impact language production (including phonology). Müller and Guendouzi (2007) further recommend that in order to be an effective provider of accent modification services, a speech-language pathologist should have "superior skills in the perception and analysis of speech patterns *other than their own*" (p. 119).

Several regional and ethnic dialects will be discussed in the following sections. Because this is a phonetics text, the focus will be on the *phonological* aspects of dialect. Differences in dialects related to syntax and vocabulary will not be addressed.

Regional Dialects

Several classification schemes have been used by researchers in an attempt to describe and categorize regional dialects in the United States. The regional use of certain vocabulary items have been studied to help define dialectal regions. For instance, in the eastern United States many people refer to carbonated beverages as "soda," whereas people from the Midwest generally use the term "pop," and some people from the South use the term "coke." Likewise, the terms "pail"/"bucket," "faucet"/"spigot," and "green onion"/"scallion" are used contrastively, depending on where a person lives. When using vocabulary items to demarcate regional dialects, research has shown conflicting evidence as to the actual number of dialectal regions present in the United States. Some research indicates that the United States can be divided into three separate dialectal regions—North, Midland, and South (Kurath, 1949). Another approach divides the United States into two general dialect regions, North and South (Carver, 1987). The North dialect region is divided into three layers: Upper North (including New England), Lower North, and West. The South dialect region has two layers: Upper South and Lower South. Each of these regions is further divided into additional layers, in a hierarchical arrangement.

Another approach to defining dialectal regions is to examine the *phonological patterns* of English speakers. The linguistics laboratory at the University of Pennsylvania conducted extensive telephone surveys of over 700 speakers to determine how vowel pronunciation varies across the country. This investigation, the **Telsur Project**, systematically examined speakers from 145 urban centers across the country. Several smaller cities also were included in order to provide a better representative sample of dialects across the United States. The purpose of this investigation was (1) to identify the major dialectal regions in the country using phonological data instead of vocabulary data and (2) to determine the *unique* pronunciation patterns that are found in each of the dialect regions (Labov, Ash, & Boberg, 2006). The Telsur telephone survey data confirmed the well-known fact that vowel articulation in the United States is not static; the place of articulation of American English vowels is in an active state of change. The changes in place of vowel articulation can be categorized as *chain shifts* and *mergers*.

A **chain shift** occurs when the place of articulation of one vowel changes, causing the surrounding vowels in the quadrilateral to likewise shift in production. This causes a "chain reaction" in relation to the place of articulation for other vowels. Because chain shifting affects the production of several vowels at the same time, the articulation of a single vowel is not independent of the articulation of other vowels. Instead, vowel articulation is relative; place of articulation of one vowel is determined by the place of production of other vowels. A **vowel merger** occurs when vowels with separate articulations fuse into one similar place of articulation. For example, in many regions in the United States, the vowels /ɑ/ and /ɔ/ have merged so that their production and perception is the same—that is, /ɑ/. Another example involves the merger of /ɪ/ and /ɛ/ before nasals, so that the words "pin" and "pen" both are produced and perceived as "pin."

The telephone survey data have helped identify several major dialectal regions across the United States using mostly chain shift and vowel merger data. Interestingly, three predominant dialect regions identified by the survey—the North, the South, and the Midland—are identical to the three major dialect regions that Kurath (1949) pinpointed using vocabulary items. These three dialect regions encompass most of the U.S. east of the Mississippi River, excluding the Middle Atlantic states and New England.

The data obtained from the Telsur Project has been published in a volume titled *The Atlas of North American English: Phonetics, Phonology, and Sound Change* (Labov et al., 2006). This atlas may be viewed in its entirety from the publisher's website. (See the list of online resources at the end of the chapter for the current URL.) In the next few sections, several of the dialect regions described in the atlas will be discussed, along with a brief summary of pronunciation patterns unique to each region (all data are from Labov et al., 2006). These regions include the Inland North, the South, the West, the Midland, Western Pennsylvania (W. Pa), Western New England (WNE), and Eastern New England (ENE) (see Figure 9.1).

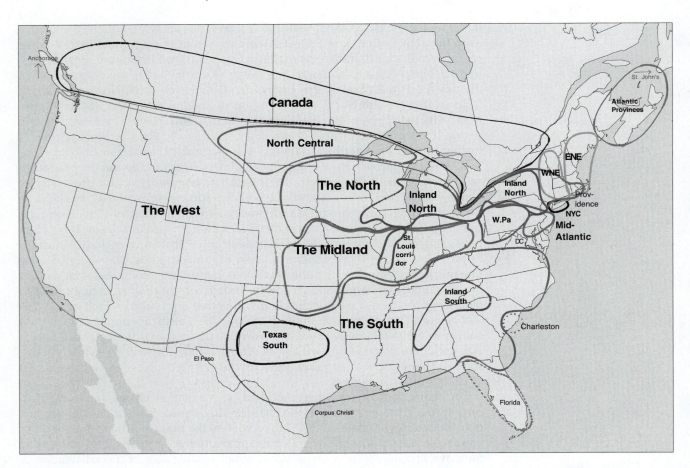

FIGURE 9.1   An overall view of North American dialects. Labov, W., Ash, S., & Boberg, C. (2006). The atlas of North American English: Phonetics, phonology and sound change. Berlin: Mouton de Gruyter.

The Inland North

The Inland North is part of a larger dialect region termed the North (see Figure 9.1). The Inland North region is comprised of New York State, Michigan, Wisconsin, and northern parts of Ohio, Indiana, and Illinois. People in the Inland North have begun to demonstrate a shift in the place of articulation of the six vowels /ɔ, ɑ, æ, ɪ, ɛ, and ʌ/ in what is known as the **Northern Cities Shift**. The Northern Cities Shift is most prominent in large urban centers such as Buffalo, Syracuse, Detroit, Chicago, and Milwaukee. A vowel quadrilateral demonstrating the Northern Cities Shift is presented in Figure 9.2. The shift reflects raising of /æ/, fronting of /ɑ/, lowering of /ɔ/, and backing of /ʌ, ɛ, and ɪ/. The shift occurs in a clockwise rotation so that the fronted production of /ɑ/ and the backed production of /ɛ/ causes them to both be produced more centrally in the oral cavity.

To clarify vowel changes associated with the shift, the vowel /æ/ is produced higher and more forward in the mouth. This causes /ɑ/ to be produced more forward in the mouth (filling in the space that was previously occupied by /æ/), so that the word "hot" /hɑt/ would be produced similar to /hæt/. As

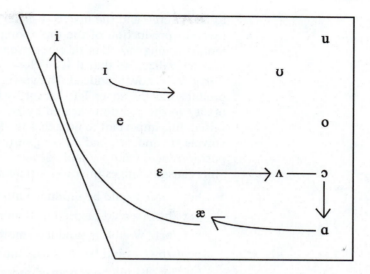

FIGURE 9.2   Vowel quadrilateral of the Northern Cities Shift (based on Labov et al., 2006).

a result, the vowel /ɔ/ is then produced lower in the mouth so that "caught" /kɔt/ would be produced more like /kɑt/. Further:

cut /kʌt/ would be produced more like /kɔt/

bet /bɛt/ would be produced more like /bʌt/

bit /bɪt/ would be produced more like /bɛt/

EXERCISE 9.2

Transcribe the following words as they would be pronounced with the Northern Cities Shift. Use the appropriate diacritics to indicate raising [˔], lowering [˕], advancement [˖], or retraction [˗] of the tongue. Refer to Figure 9.2 to help you complete this exercise.

Example:

dog	/dɔg/	[dɔ̞g]
1. lid	/lɪd/	
2. when	/wɛn/	
3. rub	/rʌb/	
4. caught	/kɑt/	
5. bag	/bæg/	

The South

The South region includes Texas, Oklahoma, a small section of northern Florida, and all of the other southeastern states (see Figure 9.1). In this region, a chain shift known as the **Southern Shift** causes the tense vowels /i/ and /e/

to be lowered and the lax vowels /æ/, /ɪ/, and /ɛ/ to be raised. The shift also involves production of the diphthong /aɪ/; it is fronted and produced as the monophthong /a/. Careful inspection of Figure 9.3 shows that /e/ is lowered and centralized so that it is in close proximity to where the fronted monophthong /a/ is now produced. The vowel /ɛ/ is raised and fronted so that it is now produced in the space left vacant by the lowering of /e/, causing the raising of /æ/ to the position vacated by /ɛ/. Concurrently, /i/ is lowered, and /ɪ/ is raised. It is important to note that the Southern Shift reflects a tensing of the lax vowels /ɪ/ and /ɛ/, and a laxing of the tense vowels /i/ and /e/ such that the positions of /i/ and /ɪ/ and /e/ and /ɛ/ are essentially reversed. The Southern Shift causes changes in vowel articulation so that:

buy /baɪ/ would be produced more like /ba/

bat /bæt/ would be produced more like /bɛt/

bet /bɛt/ would be produced more like /bet/

beet /bit/ would be produced more like /bɪt/

bit /bɪt/ would be produced more like /bit/

Fronting of the vowels /u/ and /o/ was originally part of the Southern Shift. However, fronting of these back vowels is also observed in speakers of the Midland region. As such, the shift in back vowel production is no longer a defining feature unique to the South.

Southern dialect is also marked by a second chain shift known as the **Back Upglide Shift** which can be found in the Carolinas and in Tennessee, as well as in Arkansas, Texas, Missouri, and as far north as Kansas City. This shift affects production of the vowel /ɔ/ and the diphthong /aʊ/. In this shift, the vowel /ɔ/ becomes unrounded and glides forward, becoming the diphthong /aʊ/. For example, the word "brought" /brɔt/ would be pronounced as /braʊt/. Additionally, the diphthong /aʊ/ would be fronted and produced as /æo/, or as /eo/ causing the word "crown" to be produced (and heard) as "crayon" /kræon/ or /kreon/ (Labov et al., 2006).

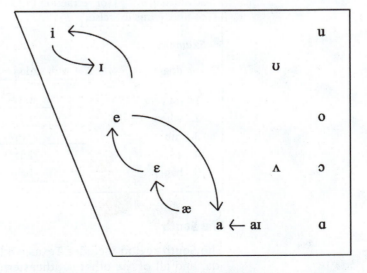

FIGURE 9.3   Vowel quadrilateral of the Southern Shift (based on Labov et al., 2006).

EXERCISE 9.3

Transcribe the following words as they would be pronounced with the Southern Shift. Use the appropriate diacritical marking for raising, lowering, or advancement to indicate the appropriate transcription as predicted by the Southern Shift. Refer to Figure 9.3 to help you complete this exercise.

Examples:

red	/rɛd/	[rɛ̞d]

1. may   /meɪ/   _____
2. lick   /lɪk/   _____
3. cat   /kæt/   _____
4. like   /laɪk/   _____
5. weed   /wid/   _____

The West

A third and somewhat different pattern of vowel articulation is currently being observed throughout a large portion of the western United States (see Figure 9.1). This is known as the **low back merger** (Labov, 1991). This change in pronunciation involves the merger of the low back vowels /ɑ/ and /ɔ/. Speakers who merge these vowels show no phonemic contrast between them during the production of words. For instance, a speaker who merges these vowels would pronounce the names "Dawn" and "Don" the same—that is, /dɑn/. In addition to the West, this merger occurs in parts of New England and also in western Pennsylvania. The Inland North, the South, the Midland, the Mid-Atlantic states, and New York City are all resistant to the low back merger, meaning that the merger is not complete in those regions; production of both /ɑ/ and /ɔ/ is still evident.

EXERCISE 9.4

Transcribe the following word pairs as you would pronounce them. Do you produce both /ɑ/ and /ɔ/ in your regional dialect of English? Or do you use the vowels /a/ or /ɒ/ (the rounded version of /ɑ/) in transcription of these words?

1. Lon   _____   lawn   _____
2. clod   _____   Claude   _____
3. caught   _____   cot   _____
4. taught   _____   tot   _____

The Midland and Western Pennsylvania

The Midland states extend westward from central Ohio and include parts of Indiana, Illinois, Iowa, Missouri, Nebraska, Kansas, and Oklahoma (see Figure 9.1). The Midland serves as a demarcation that separates the dialectal patterns of speakers from the Inland North (Northern Cities Shift) and the South (Southern Shift). That is, the Midland is resistant to the chain shifting associated with either area. The low back merger is not complete in some areas of the Midland, and some cities, notably Cincinnati and St. Louis, show their own unique dialectal patterns. According to Labov et al. (2006), "there is reason to believe that the Midland is becoming the default system of North American English" (p. 135).

Adjoining the Midland is the Western Pennsylvania dialect region which includes parts of Ohio and West Virginia. Similar to the West, the low back merger occurs in the speech patterns of individuals from western Pennsylvania. The presence of the merger helps separate Western Pennsylvania from the Midland, where the merger is still in a state of transition.

A major city in the Western Pennsylvania dialect region is Pittsburgh. The dialect spoken in Pittsburgh is often referred to as "Pittsburghese." The most defining dialectal feature unique to the Pittsburgh area is pronunciation of the diphthong /aʊ/ as the monophthong /a/ as in "downtown" /dantan/. This is known as **monophthongization** or **diphthong simplification**. Another dialectal feature associated with Pittsburgh (though it is not unique to this area) is laxing of the vowel /i/ in words such as "feel" /fɪl/ and "meal /mɪl/.

Eastern and Western New England

The Telsur data separate New England into Eastern and Western dialectal regions. This results in a separation of New Hampshire and Maine on the east from Vermont on the west. The line also divides Massachusetts and Connecticut into eastern and western portions. Western New England adjoins the Inland North region. As such, some speakers in western New England are beginning to show some evidence of the Northern Cities Shift.

The presence of the low back merger in New England separates it from the Inland North, where the merger is not complete. The low back merger is prominent in most of eastern New England and also in the northern section of western New England, notably in Vermont. The prominent dialectal feature that *separates* eastern from western New England is *vocalization* of postvocalic /r/, as in "here" /hɪə/. Vocalization of /r/ is prevalent throughout eastern New England. However, residents of western New England do not vocalize /r/, they tend to fully articulate /r/ in the postvocalic position of words.

In the next section, we will continue with a more in-depth discussion of the phonological patterns associated with both Southern and Eastern American English dialects. These two dialectal patterns are certainly the most recognized regional dialects in the United States (see Ball & Müller, 2005). In fact, some older phonetics books identified Southern and Eastern American English as two of only three regional dialects in the *entire* United States (Edwards, 1992; Gray & Wise, 1959). These older texts called the third regional dialect *General American English*. In this historic sense, General American English represented a regional dialect spoken in all areas of the country other than the East or the South. Recall in our earlier discussion of General American English that today the term has taken on somewhat of a different connotation, referring to a dialect devoid of any regional pronunciation, allowing an unbiased comparison of regional or ethnic dialects to a national "standard."

Southern American English

Southern American English is the dialect of English spoken primarily in the southern states including all or part of Alabama, Arkansas, Florida, Georgia, Kentucky, Louisiana, Mississippi, North Carolina, Oklahoma, South Carolina, Tennessee, Texas, Virginia, and West Virginia. There are some general characteristics of southern speech that are fairly typical across the southern United States. However, not all of these characteristics would necessarily apply to the same speaker due to regional variations of Southern American English across the South.

It is important to consider the fact that dialects continually change over time. According to Hartman (1985), speakers shift their speech patterns to fit a particular audience or situation, and to sound more like their peers than their parents. He also states that younger speakers often adopt broader regional pronunciations in favor of more local ones. For instance, deleting or vocalizing (derhotacizing) postvocalic /r/ has always been one noted characteristic of southern speech (e.g., pronouncing "car" as [kɑ:] or "steer" as /stɪə/). Younger southern speakers have begun to restore postvocalic /r/ in words, so much so that "r-dropping" is no longer a defining dialectal variation in the South. However, "r-dropping" continues to exist in the speech patterns of some older southern individuals. In addition to age, there appears to be a relationship between a person's educational level and production of /r/; more highly educated individuals tend to produce postvocalic /r/ in words (Hartman, 1985; Labov et al., 2006).

Examples of the more common vowel, diphthong, and consonant features associated with Southern American English are described on the next few pages. They are also summarized in Table 9.1. Keep in mind that some of these features are not necessarily limited only to speakers in the South; they may be found in other areas of the country as well.

TABLE 9.1 Common Features of Southern American English.

English Word	Southern English Transcription	Phonological Pattern
fish	/fiʃ/	tensing of vowels
egg	/eɪg/	tensing of vowels
really	/rɪlɪ/	laxing of vowels
fire	/far/	monophthongization
foil	[fɔ:l]	monophthongization
two	/tiu/	diphthongization
lettuce	/lɛɾɪs/	/ɪ/ for /ə/ substitution (i.e., ɪ/ə)
pen/pin	/pɪn/	vowel merger
Mary/merry	/mɛɾɪ/	vowel merger
Harry	/hæɾɪ/	vowel lowering
fall	/fɔl/	incomplete /ɔ/-/ɑ/ merger
terse	[tɜ:s]	derhotacization
here	/hɪə/	/r/ vocalization
far	[fɑ:]	deletion of postvocalic /r/

Source: Information from Hartman, 1985; Labov et al., 2006; Thomas, 2008.

Vowel and Consonant Characteristics

In Southern American English, diphthongs commonly are produced as monophthongs (monophthongization) by some speakers. Consistent with the Southern Shift, /aɪ/ is simplified to /a/, as in "fire" /far/ and "tired" /tard/. Also, the diphthong /ɔɪ/ is simplified to /ɔ/ and is lengthened before /l/ as in "foil" [fɔːl] and "spoil" [spɔːl]. Other vowel productions reflective of the Southern Shift include tensing of /ɪ/ before /ʃ/, as in "fish" /fiʃ/; tensing of /ɛ/ when it precedes /g/, /ʃ/, or /ʒ/, as in "leg" /leɪg/ or "treasure" /treɪʒɚ/; and laxing of /i/ when it precedes /l/, as in "really" /rɪlɪ/.

At one time, many speakers in the South (and the East) pronounced the vowel /u/ as the diphthong /ju/ (epenthesis of /j/) when it followed the alveolar consonants /t/, /d/, or /n/ as in "two" /tju/ or "new" /nju/. In time, the glide has for the most part disappeared in southern speech. In some portions of the South (mostly in North Carolina and in the southern regions of Mississippi, Alabama, and Georgia), what still occurs is the epenthesis of /i/ before /u/, resulting in a diphthong as in "too" /tiu/ or "new" /niu/ (Labov et al., 2006; Thomas, 2008). There is also a tendency for some southern speakers to substitute /ɪ/ for /ə/ in the final syllable of words such as "pigeon" /pɪdʒɪn/ and "hopeless" /hoʊplɪs/ (Thomas, 2008).

For some speakers, /ɛ/ may be raised and articulated as /ɪ/ when it precedes the nasal /n/. In this phonetic context, /ɪ/ and /ɛ/ merge so that the words "pen" and "pin" would both be produced and perceived as /pɪn/. Similarly, "sense" and "since" would both be produced and perceived as /sɪns/. In many areas of the South, the low back merger is not complete; production of /ɔ/ is found in words such as "haul," "gone," "slaughter," and "caught."

In much of the country, the three vowels /e/, /ɛ/, and /æ/ before intervocalic /r/ have merged so that the words "Mary" /merɪ/, "merry" /mɛrɪ/, and "marry" /mærɪ/ are all pronounced the same: /mɛrɪ/. In the South, /eɪ/ and /ɛ/ have merged; however, /æ/ remains distinct:

Mary and merry → /mɛrɪ/   marry → /mærɪ/

This separation of /æ/ from from the /eɪ/-/ɛ/ merger is seen in parts of Georgia, the Carolinas, and Virginia (Labov et al., 2006). When "marry" is pronounced as /mærɪ/, the rhotic diphthong is lowered from /ɛr/ to /ær/. Other examples include "carry" /kærɪ/ and "Harry" /hærɪ/. There appears to be evidence that younger southern speakers have begun to merge all three vowels into one— /ɛr/ (Thomas, 2008).

As mentioned earlier, deletion of postvocalic /r/ is not as prevalent in the South as it once was, even though some older southern speakers still delete or vocalize postvocalic /r/. In words containing the rhotic diphthong /ɑr/, /r/ may be deleted and /ɑ/ lengthened, as in "car" [kɑː] and "farmer" [fɑːmə]. In words that contain the rhotic diphthongs /ɪr/, /ɛr/, /ɔr/, and /ʊr/, /r/ may be vocalized, resulting in a substitution of the vowel /ə/ for /r/ as in "beer" /bɪə/, "door" /dɔə/ (or /doə/), "hair" /hɛə/, or "sure" /ʃʊə/. Southern speakers who vocalize postvocalic /r/ also tend to derhotacize the central vowels /ɝ/ and /ɚ/. When /ɝ/ is derhotacized, it tends to be lengthened as in "terse" [tɜːs] and "word" [wɜːd]. Examples with /ɚ/ include "others" /ʌðəz/ and "flour" /flaʊə/.

EXERCISE 9.5

Determine the phonological pattern(s) for each Southern American English pronunciation given below. Write your answer in the blank.

Example:

| ball | /bɔl/ | incomplete /ɔ/-/ɑ/merger |

1. tunes   /tiunz/   _____
2. cautious   /kɔʃɪs/   _____
3. meal   /mɪl/   _____
4. bar   [bɑ:]   _____
5. trial   /tral/   _____
6. meant   /mɪnt/   _____
7. concern   [kənsɜ:n]   _____
8. spoiled   [spɔ:ld]   _____
9. precious   /preɪʃɪs/   _____
10. tear (noun)   /tɪə/   _____

Eastern American English

What is commonly recognized as **Eastern American English** is spoken predominantly by individuals in the New England states as well as by people from parts of New York, New Jersey, and eastern Pennsylvania. The general dialectal patterns unique to the New England states were discussed previously as part of the Telsur vowel data. Because the dialectal patterns that will be introduced in the following section are observed across many areas of the East, they are quite varied. For instance, individuals from Boston may exhibit distinct phonological patterns when compared to individuals from other cities in Massachusetts and from other cities in New England. As an example, the low back merger is complete in Boston, but still has not occurred in Springfield, Massachusetts, or in Providence, Rhode Island. Similarly, some individuals in New York City demonstrate vocalization of /r/, whereas residents of neighboring cities in New York and New Jersey do not. Due to the varied nature of Eastern regional dialects, only the more common dialectal patterns will be discussed here. A summary of the major characteristics of the Eastern American English dialect is displayed in Table 9.2.

Vowel and Consonant Characteristics

Several vowel productions in Eastern American English differ from General American English. Recall that in the South, /e/ and /ɛ/ have merged so that "Mary" and "merry" are pronounced the same (i.e., /mɛrɪ/). However, in eastern Massachusetts, northern New Hampshire, and New York City, they have *not* merged; they are produced as separate vowels, distinct in production from /æ/ (Kretzschmar, 2008; Nagy & Roberts, 2008). An example of this pattern is:

    Mary → /merɪ/   ferry → /fɛrɪ/   sparrow → /spærouʊ/

TABLE 9.2 Common Features of Eastern American English.

English Word	Eastern English Transcription	Phonological Pattern
Mary, merry, marry	/meɪ, mɛɪ, mæɪ/	distinct /eɪ, ɛ, and æ/ (incomplete merger)
sparrow	/spæroʊ/	lowering of /ɛ/
half	/hɑf/ or /haf/	backing of /æ/
room	/rʊm/	laxing of /u/
horses	/hɔrsɪz/	ɪ/ə substitution
spot	/spat/	fronting of /ɑ/
smart	[sma:t]	fronting of /ɑ/; /r/ derhotacization
don, dawn	/dɑn/	low back merger (in most regions)
steer	/stɪə/	/r/ vocalization
third	[θɜːd]	derhotacization
saw	/sɔɚ/	rhotacization

Source: Information from Hartman, 1985; Labov et al., 2006; Nagy & Roberts (2008).

Some older Eastern American speakers still may substitute /ʊ/ for /u/ (vowel laxing), as in "room" /rʊm/ and "hooves" /hʊvz/. Similar to Southern American English, there is a tendency to substitute /ɪ/ for /ə/ in the final syllable of words such as "hopeless" /hoʊplɪs/. Another example of Eastern American dialect involves the substitution (backing) of either /ɑ/ or /a/ for /æ/ before the fricatives /f/, /v/, /s/, /θ/, and /ð/ or before the nasal /n/, as in "half" (/hɑf/ or /haf/) and "dance" (/dɑns/ or /dans/).

The Telsur data show that the low back merger is complete in most regions of northern New England; /ɔ/ and /ɑ/ are both pronounced as /ɑ/. However, the merger is *not* seen among speakers from the southern portion of New England, especially in Providence, Rhode Island, and in western Connecticut. The lack of the merger in western Connecticut is presumably due to the influence of neighboring New York where the distinction between /ɔ/ and /ɑ/ is still maintained (Nagy & Roberts, 2008).

A defining dialectal feature associated with New England is the fronting of /ɑ/ and /ɑr/ to /a/ and /ar/. This results in the words "mop," "spa," and "car" being pronounced as /map/, /spa/, and /kar/, respectively. Fronting of /ɑ/ and /ɑr/ is seen in most of eastern New England, except in the southeast region, in the area around Providence, Rhode Island. In western New England, only /ɑr/ is fronted, and only in Vermont; fronting of /ɑ/ is not a dialectal feature typically observed in western New England (Labov et al., 2006).

Some speakers from eastern New England not only front /ɑ/, but also derhotacize /r/ in the rhotic diphthong /ɑr/, as in "start" /stɑːt/. This production of /ɑr/ is best exemplified in the classic phrase [pɑːk jə kɑː ɪn hɑːvəd jɑːd ‖]. Speakers in both eastern New England and in the New York City metropolitan area vocalize postvocalic /r/ in the other rhotic diphthongs as well: "chair"

/tʃɛə/ "here" /hɪə/, and "tour" /tʊə/ (Hartman, 1985; Nagy & Roberts, 2008). Eastern Americans who vocalize postvocalic /r/ also tend to derhotacize the central vowels /ɝ/ and /ɚ/ as in "heard" [hɜːd] and "better" /bɛɾə/.

One last characteristic of Eastern American English involves the *rhotacization* of /ə/, resulting in /ɚ/. This occurs when a word that ends with /ə/ is followed by a word beginning with a vowel (Hartman, 1985). For example, "Cuba and Mexico" would be pronounced as /kjubɚ ænd mɛksɪkoʊ/. In addition, /ɚ/ may be found to occur in words normally ending in /ə/ or /ɔ/, as in "Linda" /lɪndɚ/, "soda" /soʊdɚ/, "idea" /aɪdiɚ/, "saw" /sɔɚ/, and "McGraw" /məʔgrɔɚ/.

EXERCISE 9.6

Determine the phonological pattern for each of the Eastern American English pronunciations given below. Write your answer in the blank.

Example:

hair	/hɛə/	/r/ vocalization
1. roof	/rʊf /	
2. laugh	/laf/	
3. murder	[mɜːdə]	
4. caught	/kɑt/	
5. can't	/kɑnt/	
6. marry	/mærɪ/	
7. pa	/pɑ/	
8. near	/nɪə/	
9. Maria	/məriɚ/	
10. dark	[dɑːk]	

Social and Ethnic Dialects

American English also has several dialects based on social class and ethnic group membership. A dialect associated with a particular social class is referred to as a **sociolect**, whereas a dialect associated with a particular ethnic group is termed an **ethnolect**. An individual's sociolect may be related to socioeconomic status, level of education, and/or vocation. It is not always easy to identify patterns of language variation or dialect based solely on social class membership or level of education. Other variables—such as age, gender, language background, and geographic region—enter into the equation. In addition, people from the same social class may have the need to adopt different dialectal patterns based on their work environment. For individuals who hold positions in which communication is important to perform their jobs (e.g., teachers, lawyers, and health-care professionals), it becomes necessary to use a variety of language that would be deemed by the public as "standard" (Wolfram & Schilling-Estes, 2006). (Recall that informal standard English is based on speaker/listener judgment.) Individuals from the same social class who are not as much "in the public eye" may adopt a more local variety of language that might be judged as being less standard.

Similarly, the social network to which a person belongs will also dictate the variety of language an individual uses. For instance, individuals whose social situations place them in a smaller social network have different communication needs than individuals whose social networks are broader and make it necessary to interact with a wider variety of individuals on a daily basis. People who belong to larger social networks would avoid the use of socially unacceptable or stigmatizing language and speech patterns in order to avoid being identified as a speaker of a vernacular (nonstandard) dialect (Wolfram & Schilling-Estes, 2006).

Ethnolects, such as African American English and Chicano English, are often identified as being associated with a particular ethnic group. According to the *Merriam-Webster* online dictionary, the word *ethnic* is defined as "of or relating to large groups of people classed according to common racial, national, tribal, religious, linguistic, or cultural origin or background" ("Ethnic," n.d.). Ethnic group membership is often related to social class, as well as language background and geographic region. Therefore, an ethnic dialect such as African American English is sometimes referred to in the literature as a social dialect (ASHA, 1983; Stockman, 2007) or even as a social *and* ethnic dialect (Pollock & Meredith, 2001). In this text, a dialect defined by association with a particular ethnic group, such as African American English, will be referred to as an *ethnic* dialect (ethnolect).

African American English

African American English (AAE) is probably the most noted dialect of English spoken in the United States. More is written about this ethnolect than any other. Not all African American people speak AAE, nor is this dialect limited solely to African Americans. *AAE* is the most recent term for this ethnolect. Previous terminology used by linguists, educators, and speech-language pathologists for this dialect have included *ebonics* (ASHA, 1983), *Black English* (Owens, 1991; Terrell & Terrell, 1993), *Vernacular Black English* (Wolfram, 1991; Wolfram & Fasold, 1974), *Black English Vernacular* (Iglesias & Anderson, 1993), and *African American Vernacular English* (Wolfram, 1994).

AAE has quite an interesting history. There are two widely believed historical accounts of its origin: the *Anglicist Hypothesis* and the *Creolist Hypothesis*. The Anglicist Hypothesis suggests that AAE can be traced back to the dialects of English spoken in Britain and brought to America by British settlers. After arriving in America, African slaves learned the regional and social varieties of English being spoken around them. Over several generations, only a vestige of their native African language remained. In this sense, their learning of English was no different than other immigrants coming to live in the United States who were learning English as a second language (Wolfram & Schilling-Estes, 2006). The Anglicist Hypothesis was popular in the 1960s and 1970s until the Creolist Hypothesis was proposed.

The Creolist Hypothesis suggests that AAE took root when Europeans traveled to Africa for reasons of business and commerce. A **pidgin** language developed between these two groups of people. A pidgin language develops when two different groups of people, with two distinct languages, attempt to communicate. The resulting pidgin language is typically characterized as having both a reduced vocabulary and grammar. The pidgin language that led to the development of AAE shared characteristics of both African and European languages. When slaves arrived in the United States, both the slaves' overseers as well as the owners of the plantations introduced new vocabulary items and grammatical structures to the pidgin. Children born to the slaves were taught this more fully developed pidgin language as their native language. Once a pidgin language is passed on to a new generation of users, the language is considered to be what is known as a **creole** language. According to the Creolist Hypothesis, AAE evolved from this creole, with characteristics of grammar and vocabulary from both African and European languages. The Creolist Hypothesis was in favor until the 1980s. Since then, research, including examination of written narratives from ex-slaves, has shown that the Anglicist Hypothesis better explains the origin of AAE.

AAE, as it is known today, has several regional variations. The form of AAE spoken in a northern city, such as Cleveland, differs from the version of AAE spoken in Atlanta. The phonological forms associated with AAE are quite variable among its speakers (Wolfram, 1994). According to Wolfram, the variability is constrained by social factors such as age, gender, and socioeconomic status, as well as by linguistic factors such as the position of sounds in words and the particular phoneme involved. Although AAE is characterized by several lexical, grammatical, and phonological features, we will focus only on the more noted phonological features common to AAE.

Consonant Characteristics

AAE can be characterized by several phonological processes that affect phoneme production, including syllable structure processes, substitution processes, and assimilation processes. The major phonological traits associated with AAE consonants and vowels are presented in the next section and summarized in Table 9.3.

Syllable Structure Processes

Deletion of stops and nasals is common in AAE. Deletion of alveolar stops usually occurs in the word-final position as in "bat" /bæ/ or "would" /wʊ/. The voiced stop /d/ also may be deleted when it is followed by the morpheme /s/ as in "needs" /niz/ or "kids" /kɪz/. When final nasals are deleted, the preceding vowel becomes nasalized as in "pin" [pĩ] or "home" [hõũ]. Also, the liquids /r/ and /l/ may be deleted in clusters, as in "through"/θu/, "wolf" /wʊf/ and "shelf" /ʃɛf/.

Another AAE syllable structure process involves the elision of the unstressed (weak) initial syllable of a word, as in "because" /kəz/ or "about" /baʊt/. Additionally, consonant clusters at the ends of words are often reduced when the final consonant is a stop. This simplification occurs when both consonants in the cluster share the same voicing pattern, that is, both voiced or both voiceless (Wolfram, 1994). Examples include "begged"/bɛg/, "desk" /dɛs/, and "ghost"

TABLE 9.3   Examples of AAE Phonology.

Word	AAE Transcription	Phonological Process
Syllable Structure Processes		
hat; bad	/hæ/; /bæ/	final stop deletion
pin; home	[pĩ]; [hõũ]	final nasal deletion with accompanying vowel nasalization
through; wolf	/θu/; /wʊf/	liquid deletion (cluster reduction)
about; tomato	/baʊt/; /meɪroʊ/	deletion of unstressed initial syllable
haste; desk	/heɪs/; /dɛs/	final cluster reduction
ghosts; desks	/goʊsəz/; /dɛsəz/	cluster reduction + plural
Substitution and Assimilation Processes		
both; mother	/boʊf/; /mʌvə/	labialization
winning; running	/wɪnɪn/; /rʌnɪn/	fronting
isn't; hasn't	/ɪdn̩t/; /hædn̩t/	stopping
hit; bag	/hɪʔ/; /bæʔ/	glottal stop substitution
more; story; chair	/moʊ/; /stoʊɪ/; /tʃɛə/	/r/ vocalization
nickel; bell	/nɪkʊ/; /bɛʊ/	/l/ vocalization
string; strong	/skrɪŋ/; /skrɑŋ/	backing
bid; bad	[bɪːt]; [bæːt]	devoicing of final stop
ask; grasp	/æks/; /græps/	metathesis
Vowel Characteristics		
pen; many	/pɪn/; /mɪnɪ/	/ɛ/-/ɪ/ merger
sister; doctor	/sɪstə/; /dɑktə/	derhotacization
tire; flour	/tar/; /flar/	diphthong simplification

Sources: Information from Pollock & Meredith, 2001; Terrell & Terrell, 1993; Wolfram, 1994; Wolfram & Fasold, 1974; Wolfram & Thomas, 2002.

/goʊs/. Words with a final cluster comprised of /s/ followed by a stop (e.g., "desk" or "ghost") will have an AAE plural form of /əz/ (Wolfram, 1994). Some examples in AAE include "desks" /dɛsəz/ and "ghosts" /goʊsəz/. This plural form is typical of General American English words ending in /s/, for example, /leɪs/ "lace" → /leɪsəz/ "laces."

Substitution and Assimilation Processes

In AAE, *stopping* occurs when voiced fricatives precede a nasal (i.e., "isn't" /ɪdn̩t/ and "even" /ibm̩/). Stopping also occurs with the interdental fricatives /ð/ and /θ/, as in "these" /diz/ and "this" /dɪs/. In addition, glottal stops may replace final stops in some instances (e.g., "bag" /bæʔ/ and "bid" /bɪʔ/).

Liquid vocalization also occurs in AAE. /r/ may be vocalized as in "story" /stoʊɪ/, "door" /doʊ/, "cheer" /tʃɪə/ and "fair" /fɛə/. Word-final /l/ may be vocalized in words such as in "nickel" /nɪkʊ/ and "bell" /bɛʊ/ (Pollock & Meredith, 2001).

There are several other consonant substitutions observed in speakers of AAE: (1) the interdental fricatives /θ/ and /ð/ may be *labialized* and produced as /f/ and /v/, respectively, both in medial and word-final positions, as in "Ruth" /ruf/ and "brother" /brʌvə/; (2) /ŋ/ may be *fronted* to /n/ in words containing "ing" as in "hanging" /hæŋɪn/; and (3) /t/ in word-initial /str/ consonant clusters may be *backed* to /k/, as in "string" /skrɪŋ/ (Wolfram & Thomas, 2002).

One assimilation process characteristic of AAE phonology is the *devoicing* of final voiced stops (e.g., "rag" [ræːk] or "bad" [bæːt]). Note that the longer vowel length associated with voiced stops is maintained in this condition (Wolfram, 1994). Also, final clusters comprised of /s/ + stop may be reversed in certain words (metathesis), as in "ask" /æks/.

Vowel Characteristics

Similar to some speakers of Southern American English, the vowels /ɝ/ and /ɚ/ may become derhotacized, as in "third" [θɜːd] or "mother" /mʌvə/. Also, in AAE some speakers merge /ɪ/ and /ɛ/ so that "many" and "Benny" would be produced and perceived as /mɪnɪ/ and /bɪnɪ/, respectively. Finally, diphthongs are sometimes monophthongized in AAE, as in "tire" /tar/. Recall that this is a characteristic also observed in some southern speakers.

EXERCISE 9.7

Examine each of the words below. Then look at the AAE phonological pattern that should be applied to each word. Provide the appropriate transcription in the blank.

Example:

	east	cluster reduction	/is/
1.	ran	nasal deletion	
2.	with	labialization	
3.	Carol	/r/ deletion	
4.	weeds	stop deletion	
5.	wasn't	stopping	
6.	yelling	fronting	
7.	brother	derhotacization	
8.	behind	deletion of unstressed initial syllable	
9.	Denny	vowel merger	
10.	pickle	liquid vocalization	

Learning English as a Second Language

The demographic profile of the population of the United States has changed markedly over the last 50 years. The national origins quota system was eliminated when President Lyndon Johnson signed into law the Immigration Act of 1965. Since that time, there has been a steady increase in the number of immigrants coming to the United States from other countries (especially from countries in the Eastern hemisphere).

It is estimated that almost 40 million residents of the United States were foreign-born in 2011. According to the U.S. Census Bureau, a foreign-born individual is someone who is not a U.S. citizen at birth. A U.S. citizen is anyone who is born in the United States, Puerto Rico, Guam, American Samoa, the U.S. Virgin Islands, and the Commonwealth of the Northern Mariana Islands. The foreign-born population currently accounts for nearly 13 percent of the total U.S. population, the largest percentage of foreign-born individuals living in the country since 1920 (Grieco et al., 2012b). The total foreign-born population in the United States has increased by over 30 million since 1960, when the number of foreign-born individuals accounted for only 5.4 percent of the population (Grieco et al., 2012a). One-third of the increase in the foreign-born population (10 million) occurred between 2000 and 2010.

In 2010, the largest number of foreign-born residents came from Latin America (21.2 million, or 53 percent), with the largest percentage of that group coming from Mexico (55 percent). Individuals from Asia accounted for 29 percent of the foreign-born population, whereas individuals from Europe accounted for only 12 percent (Grieco et al., 2012a). It is interesting to contrast these statistics with census data from 1960, which indicated the largest number of foreign-born residents were from Europe (75 percent). In 1960, only 14 percent of the U.S. foreign-born population was made up of individuals from Asia and Latin America, compared to 82 percent in 2010. Since 2008, the Asian foreign-born population has increased at a greater rate than individuals coming from Latin America and the Caribbean (Walters & Trevelyan, 2011). According to the 2010 U.S. census, more than 50% of the foreign-born population lived in New York, Texas, Florida, and California, with over 25% of the foreign-born population living in California alone (Grieco et al., 2012b).

There are over 300 languages spoken in the United States other than English. In 1980, 23.1 million people (age 5 or older) spoke a non-English language in the home. By 2011, that number jumped to 59.5 million people. This reflects an overwhelming increase of 158 percent, especially when one considers that the U.S. population increased at a rate of only 38 percent during the same time (Ryan, 2013). Other than English, Spanish is the most spoken language in the United States. (English and Spanish are both Indo-European languages.) Of the nearly 60 million people who currently speak a language other than English, 37 million (62 percent) speak Spanish, 18 percent speak another Indo-European language, 15 percent speak an Asian language, and 4 percent speak some other language. Next to Spanish, Chinese is the most spoken language in the home (2.8 million speakers), followed by Tagalog (Filipino; 1.6 million), Vietnamese (1.4 million), French (1.3 million), Korean (1.1 million), and German (1 million) (Ryan, 2013). (Tagalog [pronounced /təˈɡɑloɡ/] and Filipino are often used synonymously to refer to the national language of the Philippines. Both Filipino and English are considered official languages.)

During the last decade, the number of Spanish, Vietnamese, Russian, and Hindi speakers in the United States has increased dramatically, as have several African languages including Yoruba, Swahili, Amharic, and Ibo. Conversely, the number of Italian, German, Polish, Yiddish, and Greek speakers has declined (Ryan, 2013).

Approximately 44 percent of the residents of California, 37 percent of the residents of New Mexico, and 35 percent of the residents of Texas speak a non-English language. In addition, Arizona, Florida, Hawaii, Nevada, New York, and New Jersey each report that more than 25 percent of their residents speak a second language. Close to one-half of all U.S. residents who speak a second language live in California, Texas, or New York. Twenty-five percent of all people who speak a second language live in California alone. Not surprisingly, New York City and Los Angeles are the two cities with the largest number of individuals who speak a second language at home, numbering more than 6 million apiece (Ryan, 2013).

For someone learning a second language, the phonology of the person's native language (L_1), will influence the pronunciation of the second (target) language (L_2). The influence of one's native language on the learning of a new language is termed **language transfer**. Language transfer is the incorporation of L_1 language features (including phonology) into the L_2 as the second language is being learned.

Due to the influence of L_1 on L_2 as a new language is being learned, there often will be a mismatch between the two phonological systems. According to Yavaş (2006), this mismatch can take several forms, causing the L_2 learner to be perceived as having a "foreign accent." The first example of a phonological mismatch is the lack of a phoneme in the native (L_1) language that does exist in L_2. For example, the voiceless plosive /p/ is absent in Arabic. Arabic speakers learning English will typically substitute /b/ for /p/ (i.e., /bɑrtɪ/ for "party") because these two phonemes differ only in voicing, but share place and manner specifications. A second divergence in phonological systems occurs when phonemes in the L_2 exist only as allophones in the L_1. For instance, in Korean, /s/, /z/, and /ʃ/ are all allophones of /s/; they do not exist as separate phonemes. A third divergence occurs when a phoneme common to both L_1 and L_2 are pronounced differently. For instance, in some Asian languages, initial voiceless stops are unaspirated, whereas in English, they are aspirated. A fourth mismatch occurs when the allowable syllable structures of L_1 and L_2 differ. In Mandarin Chinese, the only final sounds allowed are /n/ and /ŋ/. A Mandarin speaker of English may then delete the final consonant in a word if the final sound is not /n/ or /ŋ/ (i.e., /fu/ for "food"). Another example involves production of the consonant clusters /sk/, /st/, and /sp/ by Spanish speakers learning English. These clusters do not occur in the initial position of Spanish words as they do in English. Either /ə/ or /ɛ/ is added prior to the cluster, splitting its components so that each element of the cluster will appear in two separate syllables, for example, /əspat/ or /ɛspat/ for "spot" or /əskul/ or /ɛskul/ for "school." Finally, suprasegmental differences between L_1 and L_2 often cause mismatches in pronunciation.

In addition to language transfer issues, the dialect of an individual's L_1 will have an impact on the pronunciation of the target language (L_2). As an example, a native, Spanish-speaking person originally from Mexico City would have a different English accent than would a native Spanish speaker originally from Chihuahua. This is because the dialects of Spanish spoken in those two Mexican cities vary. Additionally, the accent of an English second-language learner may reflect regional variations of English depending on where the person lives in the United States.

As practicing clinicians, you need to have a heightened awareness of the dialects and language practices of second-language learners, especially if you choose to work with children. You will need to learn what is considered to be normal phonological development and what is not, depending on an individual's L_1. The children you will be serving will have varied language backgrounds. That is, some will come from homes where only the L_2 is spoken, some will come from homes where only the L_1 is spoken, and others may rely more on one language than the other, or they may be completely bilingual.

An individual who is attempting to master English as a second language is said to be an **English Language Learner (ELL)**. This term, adopted by the National Council of Teachers of English (NCTE), is similar to the term *Limited English Proficiency (LEP)* still in use by the U.S. Department of Education in reference to children who do not meet state standards in relation to English mastery. The term *ELL* underscores learning rather than focusing on deficiencies (National Council of Teachers of English [NCTE], 2008).

As English develops, the ELL child may display a dialectal variation of English due to language transfer, factors associated with the child's environment and to familial language practice. If the child's language and speech performance are related to dialectal variation and not a communication disorder, therapeutic treatment is not necessarily indicated. Of course, it is possible for ELL children to have communication deficits associated with hearing loss, cleft palate, fluency disorders, language disorders, or phonological disorders (not due to language transfer). In any of these instances, treatment might be warranted.

Spanish-Influenced English

In 2010, the Hispanic population in the United States numbered 50.5 million, or 16 percent of the total population (Humes, Jones, & Ramirez, 2011). Since the previous census in 2000, the Hispanic population in the United States increased by 15.2 million (an increase of 43 percent), accounting for greater than one-half of the increase in the U.S. population during that same time (Ennis, Rios-Vargas, & Albert, 2011). Fifty-five percent of the Hispanic population lives in California, Texas, and Florida. The Hispanic population continues to be the largest minority group in the United States.

According to the U.S. Census Bureau, the term *Hispanic* or *Latino* refers to an individual of Cuban, Mexican, Puerto Rican, or South or Central American descent, or someone from another Spanish culture or origin, regardless of race (Ennis et al., 2011). The five races listed in the 2010 census included *White, Black or African American, American Indian or Alaska Native, Asian,* and *Native Hawaiian or Other Pacific Islander.* An additional category "some other race" was listed for individuals who were "unable to identify" with any of the five given race groupings (Humes et al., 2011). Greater than 50 percent of Hispanic census respondents indicated their race as White, and about one-third indicated their race as "some other race." During the 2010 census, only 6 percent of Hispanics identified themselves as belonging to more than one race (Humes et al., 2011).

Almost two-thirds of the Hispanic population in the United States comes from Mexico (63 percent), followed by Puerto Rico (9.2 percent), and Cuba (3.5 percent). Approximately 27 percent of census respondents indicated their place of origin as "other Hispanic or Latino," which included individuals from the Dominican Republic and from countries in Central American or South America (Ennis et al., 2011).

Many Hispanic children in the United States are born into families in which Spanish is the primary language spoken, both by parents and by other family members. Recall that Spanish is spoken in 62 percent of the homes in the United States in which a second language is spoken. The extent to which a Hispanic child becomes masterful in the use of the English language depends on (1) the age when the child was first exposed to English, (2) the degree of acceptance of English by the immediate family members, (3) the degree of exposure to English in the child's daily environment, and (4) whether the child's family is monolingual or bilingual (Perez, 1994; Reed, 1994).

In relation to bilingualism, the family members may be fluent in both Spanish and English. However, not all bilingual individuals are skilled in both languages. Some bilingual individuals are more fluent in one language than the other. In some cases, there may be limited skill in both languages.

Phonological Characteristics of Spanish-Influenced English

Because some Hispanic children may be considered ELL when they enter school, speech-language pathologists should understand how Spanish may influence the further development of English. Otherwise, it would not be possible to tell whether a child's particular speech patterns were related to Spanish-Influenced English (SIE) or were reflective of a speech sound disorder.

The phonemic system of Spanish varies from that of English, both in terms of vowels and consonants. There are several consonants that are shared by both Spanish and English. These include the stops /p, /t/, /k/, /b/, /d/, and /g/, the nasals /m/ and /n/, the fricatives /f/ and /s/, the affricate /tʃ/, and the approximants /w/, /l/, and /j/ (Iglesias & Goldstein, 1998). Spanish has several phonemes that are not found in English. These include the voiceless, velar fricative /x/, the voiced palatal nasal /ɲ/, and the trilled /r/ (Bleile & Goldstein, 1996). (Recall that the English approximant /r/ is not trilled and is officially represented by the IPA symbol /ɹ/.) Spanish also contains the voiced fricatives /β/ (bilabial) and /ɣ/ (velar), which are actually allophones of /b/ and /g/, respectively (Goldstein, 2001). In addition, English contains sounds that do not occur in Spanish. These include the aspirated stops [pʰ, tʰ, and kʰ]; the nasal /ŋ/, the obstruents /v, s, ʃ, θ, tʃ, and dʒ/; and the liquid /ɹ/. Some of these phonemes, however, exist in some Spanish dialects (Goldstein, 2001), and some exist as allophones (e.g., /ŋ/).

The differences in the English and Spanish consonant systems, and their effect on Spanish Influenced English, can be categorized in terms of syllable structure, substitution, and assimilation processes (Perez, 1994). Examples of SIE consonant production are summarized in Table 9.4.

Syllable Structure Processes
As mentioned earlier, the consonant clusters /sk/, /st/, or /sp/ do not occur in the initial position of words in Spanish. Therefore, a common SIE production involves the epenthesis of /ə/ to the initial portion of the cluster, creating two syllables, as in /əspat/ "spot." Unstressed syllables are sometimes deleted as in "explain" /spleɪn/. Final consonant clusters may be reduced as in "rest" /rɛs/ and "hold" /hol/. Another syllable structure process involves final consonant deletion (e.g., "date" /deɪ/).

Substitution and Assimilation Processes
The voiceless interdental fricative /θ/ does not exist in Spanish. Because of this, /θ/ is stopped and produced as /t/ as in "think" /tɪŋk/. Also, /t/ may be dentalized as in "tea" [t̪i]. The voiced fricative /v/ also is not a phoneme found in Spanish. Therefore, it is sometimes stopped as and produced as /b/ as in the word "vine" /baɪn/. It may also be produced by substituting a voiced bilabial fricative /β/ as in /βaɪn/ (fronting). Affrication may occur in production of both glides and fricatives as in "you" /dʒu/ and "sheep" /tʃip/. Similarly,

TABLE 9.4   Common Spanish-Influenced English Consonant Productions.

English Word	SIE Transcription	Phonological Pattern
Syllable Structure Processes		
stand	/əstand/ or /ɛstand/	epenthesis of /ə or ɛ/preceding initial /s/ + stop clusters
explain	/spleɪn/	unstressed syllable deletion
rest	/rɛs/	final consonant cluster reduction
hold	/hol/	final consonant cluster reduction
date	/deɪ/	final consonant deletion
Substitution and Assimilation Processes		
think	/tɪŋk/	stopping
vase	/bes/	stopping
tea	[t̪i]	dentalization
vine	/βaɪn/	fronting
you	/dʒu/	affrication of a glide
sheep	/tʃip/	affrication of a fricative
choose	/ʃuz/	deaffrication
zoo	/su/	devoicing (initial)
was	/wʌs/	devoicing (final)

Sources: Information from Goldstein, 2001; Perez, 1994.

deaffrication may occur as in "cheap" /ʃip/. Devoicing of consonants (an assimilation process) occurs in words such as "zebra" /sibrə/ and "has" /hæs/.

Vowel Characteristics
In English, there are 14 vowels (excluding the diphthongs). Spanish, on the other hand, has only 5 vowels: /i, e, a, o, and u/ (Iglesias & Goldstein, 1998; Perez, 1994). Therefore, knowledge of Spanish (L$_1$) may influence the production of English (L$_2$) vowels. Some vowel productions in SIE are predictable from a transfer point of view. That is, English words that contain vowels not typical of Spanish may be produced by substituting one of the five Spanish vowels located in close proximity to the English vowel in the vowel quadrilateral. Examples include a/ʌ, as in /sam/ for "some", and /i/ for /ɪ/, as in /sit/ for "sit." There are other vowel productions in SIE that are not predictable from a transfer view of speech sound production. In most cases, the substitution is for a vowel that shares a similar place of production. Examples include æ/ɛ, as in /mæn/ for "men" and ʊ/u as in /rʊm/ for "room" (Perez, 1994). More examples of SIE vowel productions are given in Table 9.5.

TABLE 9.5 Common Spanish-Influenced English Vowel Productions.

English Word	SIE Transcription	Vowel Substitution
lid	/lid/	i/ɪ
need	/nɪd/	ɪ/i
late	/lɛt/	ɛ/eɪ
tennis	/teɪnɪs/	eɪ/ɛ
dead	/dæd/	æ/ɛ
bag	/bɑg/ or /bɛg/	ɑ or ɛ/æ
look	/luk/	u/ʊ
pool	/pʊl/	ʊ/u
bug	/bɑg/ or /bɑg/	ɑ or a/ʌ
word	/wɛrd/	ɛr/ɝ
boat	/bot/	diphthong simplification

Source: Information from Goldstein, 2001; Perez, 1994.

EXERCISE 9.8

Determine the phonological pattern being demonstrated in each of the following SIE pronunciations. Write your answer in the blank.

Examples:

need	/nɪd/	ɪ/i substitution
juice	/tʃus/	devoicing

1.	last	/læs/	final consonant deletion
2.	much	/mɑtʃ/	_____
3.	check	/ʃɛk/	_____
4.	yes	/dʒɛs/	_____
5.	spoiled	/ɛspɔɪld/	_____
6.	them	/dɛm/	_____
7.	Cher	/tʃɛr/	_____
8.	voice	/bɔɪs/	_____
9.	mood	/mut/	_____
10.	wound	/wun/	_____

Asian-Influenced English I: East Asian Languages

The 2010 U.S. census indicates that 17.3 million residents are Asian (5.6 percent of the entire population). This reflects an increase of 43 percent from the previous census in 2000. Of the 17.3 million Asians in the United States, 11.5 million are foreign-born. Of all racial groups in the country, the Asian population has shown the greatest growth during the last decade. Thirty-two percent of all Asians live in California. An additional 25 percent of the Asian population lives in New York, Texas, Hawaii, and New Jersey (Gryn & Gambino, 2012; Hoeffel, Rastogi, Kim, & Shakid, 2012).

Approximately 9 million people living in the United States speak an Asian language at home; this reflects an increase of approximately 2.4 million since 2000 (Ryan, 2013). Recall that Asian languages are spoken in 15 percent of homes where more than one language is spoken. The five most common Asian languages spoken in the United States are Chinese, Tagalog (Filipino), Vietnamese, Korean, and Japanese (Ryan, 2013). (For the remainder of the chapter, the term *Filipino* will be used to refer to speakers of Tagalog.)

China, Korea, and Japan are located in East Asia, whereas the Philippines and Vietnam are located in Southeast Asia. The languages spoken in these countries come from different language families, and as such, are quite diverse. However, for purposes of discussion, they will be referred to collectively as East Asian languages. The phonological systems of East Asian languages are quite dissimilar from each other and from English phonology. It is not surprising that language transfer issues are apparent when East Asians learn English as a second language.

Some East Asian languages, such as Chinese and Vietnamese, are *tone languages*. In a tone language, a word's meaning may differ when pronounced with a varying tone or intonation pattern. For instance, in Mandarin (a dialect of Chinese), the syllable /ba/ may mean "eight," "to pull," "handle," "to give up," or "okay," depending on the intonation produced as the word is articulated (Cheng, 1994). In a tone language, intonation is considered to be phonemic because each tone will convey a different meaning to the listener. As you know, in English, tone is not phonemic. Instead, tone generally indicates the speaker's mood or intent or signals whether the utterance is a statement or a question.

Syllable Structure Processes

In Vietnamese and Chinese, most words are monosyllabic. In Chinese, each printed character is only one syllable in length. Therefore, when a Chinese person is learning English, there is a tendency to pronounce multisyllabic words syllable by syllable, in a telegraphic manner (Cheng, 2001). In Chinese and Vietnamese, consonant clusters do not exist. Instead, Vietnamese has vowel clusters, diphthongs, and triphthongs (Hwa-Froelich, Hodson, & Edwards, 2002). In Korean, consonant clusters do not exist in initial or final positions of words (Cheng, 1987a). Therefore, when producing an English word containing a consonant cluster, it may be simplified by deleting the last consonant of the cluster, or a vowel may be inserted within the cluster. Some examples from Chinese include "train" /təreɪn/ and "three" /təri/ (Shen, 1962). Both Japanese and Filipino speakers also insert vowels into consonant clusters in certain phonetic contexts. For instance, in Filipino, the clusters /sp/, /st/, or /sk/ do not occur at the beginning of a word, similar to Spanish. Therefore, Filipino speakers insert a vowel either prior to, or within the cluster as in "start" /istɑrt/ or "square" /iskuwir/ (Tayao, 2008).

It is quite common in English for words and syllables to have a coda; 21 English consonants may occur at the end of a word. In Japanese, the only final consonant is /n/. In Mandarin, there are only 2 final consonants, /n/ and /ŋ/. Cantonese (another dialect of Chinese), has 7 final consonants, /m, n, ŋ, p, t, k, and ʔ/, and Vietnamese has 6, including /p, t, k, m, n, and ŋ/ (Cheng, 1987b, 2001).

Chinese, Japanese, and Vietnamese speakers often delete the final consonants of English words because it is not common for syllables and words to have a coda in their native languages. On the other hand, Japanese speakers will sometimes add a vowel to the end of a syllable or word in an attempt to create an open syllable, such as "desk" /dɛskɚ/ (Cheng, 2001). In other cases, substitutions for missing consonants are produced as a general result of language transfer between the particular East Asian language (L_1) being spoken and English (L_2).

Substitution Processes

Table 9.6 provides a summary of some of the more common English consonant substitutions (as a result of language transfer) as spoken by Cantonese Chinese, Vietnamese, Korean, Japanese, and Filipino speakers. In the following paragraphs, consonant substitutions due to language transfer will be discussed in terms of basic similarities between the languages. As you read, continually refer to Table 9.6 in order to examine the full set of substitutions in more detail.

The interdental fricatives /θ/ and /ð/ do not occur in Filipino, and are stopped and produced as /t/ and /d/, respectively by Filipino English speakers. Note in Table 9.6 that stopping of /θ/ and /ð/ is common among all five groups of East Asian speakers of English.

TABLE 9.6 Consonant Substitutions of Chinese (Cantonese), Vietnamese, Korean, Japanese, and Filipino Speakers of English.

Intended Phoneme		Observed Phoneme				
		Cantonese	**Vietnamese**	**Korean**	**Japanese**	**Filipino**
Fricatives	θ	s, t, f	s, t	t	t, s, z	t, s
	ð	d, z	d, z	d	d, z, θ, t, s	d
	ʃ	s	s	s	s, tʃ, t	s, ts
	ʒ		z, dʒ	z	dʒ	s, ds
	f		p	p	h	p
	v	f, w	j, b, p	p, b	b, f, w	b
	s		ʃ	ʃ	ʃ	
	z	s	s, ʃ	s, ts, dz	dz, dʒ, s, ts	s
Affricates	tʃ		s, ʃ	t		t, s, ts
	dʒ		z, ʒ, d	tʃ	ʒ	ds
Stops	p	pʼ	pʼ, p⁼, b, f	pʼ, b		p⁼
	t	tʼ	tʼ, t⁼	tʼ, d	tʃ	t⁼
	k	kʼ	kʼ, k⁼	kʼ, g		k⁼
	b	pʼ	p		p	
	d	tʼ	t		dʒ, t	
	g	kʼ	k			
Liquids	r	l		l	l	
	l	n	n	r	r	

Sources: Information from Bada, 2001; Ball & Müller, 2005; Bautista, 2008; Cheng, 1987a, 1987b; Hwa-Froelich, et al., 2002; Shen, 1962; Tayao, 2008; Yavaş, 2006.

Cantonese, Vietnamese, Japanese, and Filipino speakers also may substitute /s/ or /z/ for the two interdental fricatives. The labiodental fricatives /f/ and /v/ are stopped and produced as /p/ and /b/ by Vietnamese, Korean, Japanese, and Filipino speakers. Japanese speakers substitute /h/ for /f/ and Chinese, and Japanese speakers substitute either /f/ or /w/ for /v/ (all labial sounds).

The alveolar fricative /s/ is backed and produced as /ʃ/ by Vietnamese, Korean, and Japanese speakers, whereas /z/ is devoiced and produced as /s/ by English speakers of all the language depicted in Table 9.6. Other substitutions for /z/ include affrication to /ts/, /dz/, or /dʒ/ (Korean and Japanese). The palatal fricative /ʃ/ is fronted and produced as /s/ by all speakers. Japanese speakers may affricate or stop /ʃ/ substituting /tʃ/ and /t/, respectively. Some Filipino speakers affricate /ʃ/, resulting in /ts/. Substitutions for /ʒ/ include /z/ (fronting) and /dʒ/ (affrication) by Vietnamese, Korean and Japanese speakers, and /s/ (fronting and devoicing) or /ds/ (affrication) by Filipino speakers.

The voiceless affricate /tʃ/ is deaffricated and produced as /s/ or /ʃ/ by Vietnamese speakers, and as /t/, /s/, or /ts/ by Filipino and Korean speakers. The voiced affricate /dʒ/ is also deaffricated and produced as /ʒ/ by Vietnamese and Japanese speakers. Vietnamese speakers also may substitute /z/ or /d/ for /dʒ/, whereas Korean speakers devoice /dʒ/, and Filipino speakers substitute ds/dʒ.

In relation to stop consonants, Cantonese, Vietnamese and Korean speakers all produce final voiceless stops as unreleased consonants (i.e., [p˺], [t˺], and [k˺]). Unreleased voiceless stops may be perceived by English speakers as voiced; for example, [p˺]would be perceived as /b/ (Ball & Müller, 2005). In addition, Cantonese speakers produce all final *voiced* stops as their unreleased voiceless cognates (i.e., [k˺] for /g/). Further, Vietnamese and Filipino speakers produce all initial voiceless stops as unaspirated consonants (i.e., [p⁼], [t⁼], and [k⁼]). Unaspirated stops at the beginning of a word also may cause English listeners to perceive the consonant as being voiced (Hwa-Froelich et al., 2002). Some other stop consonant substitutions include voicing of voiceless stops (Korean) and devoicing of voiced stops (Vietnamese and Japanese).

The liquids /r/ and /l/ are often not differentiated in Cantonese, Korean, and Japanese, resulting in r/l and l/r substitutions. Also, /n/ is substituted for /l/ in both Cantonese and Vietnamese.

L_2 English vowel production is challenging as well due to the differences between English and East Asian vowel systems. Both Japanese and Filipino have only five vowels. Transfer becomes an issue when attempting to produce all of the English vowels with such a small set of L_1 vowels. None of the vowel systems in Chinese, Vietnamese, Korean, Japanese, or Filipino maintain a tense/lax vowel distinction, as in English. For instance, in Korean the vowel system is composed of /i, e, ɛ, a, u, o, and ʌ/ as well as other vowels not typical of English (Handbook of the International Phonetic Association, 1999). Note the absence of /ɪ, ɛ, and ʊ/, the lax counterparts of /i, e, and u/. Korean speakers therefore may substitute tense for lax vowels when pronouncing English words, as in "sit" /sit/ or "book" /buk/.

EXERCISE 9.9

The transcription of each of the following words indicates an English production that is the result of language transfer associated with one of the East Asian languages given in Table 9.6. For each transcription given, list the languages where such a substitution *might be possible*.

Word	Transcription	East Asian Language(s)
Example:		
rice	/laɪs/	Cantonese, Korean, Japanese
1. think	/tɪŋk/	
2. shoes	/tsuz/	
3. vine	/faɪn/	
4. badge	/pæz/	
5. this	/zɪs/	
6. from	/hrəm/	
7. pay	[p⁼eɪ]	
8. seas	/ʃiz/	
9. check	[tɛk˺]	
10. leap	[nip˺]	

Asian-Influenced English II: Asian Indian English

The Asian Indian population has grown by 68 percent since the 2000 U.S. census, displaying faster growth than any other Asian group (Hoeffel et al., 2012). Of the 11.5 million Asian foreign-born living in the United States, nearly 2 million (16 percent) are from India, ranking second only to China (Gryn & Gambino, 2012). As a result, there has been a great increase in the number of Asian Indian English speakers across the country during the last decade. For this reason, it is of interest to more closely examine the growing number of Asian Indians learning English as a second language.

India is located in southern Asia. The majority of the 122 languages spoken in India belong to one of two language families, Dravidian and Indo-Aryan (part of the Indo-European language family). During the last decade, English speakers of Punjabi, Bengali, and Marathi (Indo-Aryan languages) have increased by 86 percent, whereas English speakers of Malayalam, Telugu, and Tamil (Dravidian languages) have increased by 115 percent. English speakers of Hindi (also Indo-Aryan), the official language of the Union Government of India, have increased by 105 percent (Ryan, 2013). According to the Constitution of India, each of its 29 states has the legal authority to adopt its own *state language* for purposes of communication and for conducting official business not only within each state, but also between each state and the Union Government. India currently has over 20 state languages, including English.

The majority of Asian Indians learn English as a second language. The English-speaking ability of foreign-born Asian Indians is quite variable. Some individuals may not have had excessive training in English before coming to the United States. The level of English instruction in India's schools is variable depending on whether a child is enrolled in a government (public) or private school. Children who are enrolled in private schools generally begin English instruction at an earlier age than children in government schools. Although 26 percent of children enrolled in private schools are given instruction exclusively in English, only 2 percent of children in government schools receive exclusive English instruction (Desai, Dubey, Vanneman, & Banerji, 2008). Instruction at the university level is variable as well. Most universities adopt English as the primary medium of instruction. On the other hand, some universities use the state language as the primary medium of instruction. In these institutions, students are offered English only as a secondary subject. Even in university English classes, the primary medium of instruction still might be in the official language of the university, resulting in limited English proficiency.

Regardless of educational background, language transfer issues related to the speaker's L$_1$ have a large impact on spoken English (L$_2$). Pronunciation is affected not only by regional dialect but also by the pronunciation patterns taught by the second-language learners' teachers who often are non-native English speakers as well (Gargesh, 2008).

British and American Influence on Indian English

Prior to 1947, India was under British rule. Since that time, Indian English pronunciation (as well as the spelling of certain words) continues to be heavily influenced by British English. Standard British English pronunciation is often referred to as **received pronunciation (RP)**. The term *received* in this sense means an acceptable form of English based on social judgment (Cruttenden, 2008). Standard RP originally emerged during the 16th century as a regional dialect in southern England, especially in the area around London. This dialect was used for purposes of commerce and politics, and became the spoken English of the ruling class and of the Court. RP ultimately became more associated with prestige and social status than regional pronunciation (Cruttenden, 2008). Certain changes in English production came about as RP developed over time. For example, "r-dropping" of postvocalic /r/ became part of RP during the 18th century (Wells, 1982a). Prior to that time, postvocalic /r/ was fully articulated in spoken English.

The use of RP has continued to evolve over the years. Regional versions of RP have emerged that display more of a variety of pronunciations, similar to Informal Standard American English. At one time, the British Broadcasting Corporation (BBC) required that all newscasters use RP so that they did not display any regional pronunciations that might be difficult to understand or that might offend the listening audience. For a time, RP was also called "BBC English." More recently, BBC newscasters have begun to exhibit some of their own individual regional pronunciations. Today, there is actually a stigma attached to use of RP in its original intended prestige form because it has become synonymous with elevated social status.

When comparing RP and Standard American English, consonant production is virtually identical. What sets the two dialects apart is differences in vowel production. This is especially true of back vowels and diphthong production. RP has an additional back vowel /ɒ/ (low back rounded) that occurs in British production of the words "lot" and "cough." This vowel is distinct from the back vowels /ɔ/ and /ɑ/ which are both evident in RP; they have not merged as they have in many regions of the United States. Therefore, pronunciation of the words "palm" /pɑm/, "thought" /θɔt/, and "lot" /lɒt/ are all produced with different vowels. Do not be alarmed if the vowels in these three words sound alike to you! In terms of diphthongs, /oʊ/ is pronounced as /əʊ/, as in "goat"/gəʊt/. Whereas /r/ is dropped in production of the rhotic diphthongs /ɑr/ and /ɔr/, as in "car" [kɑ:] and "for" [fɔ:], /ə/ replaces /r/ (vocalization) in the other rhotic diphthongs /ɪr/, /ɛr/, and /ʊr/. Examples include "beer" /bɪə/, "fair" /fɛə/, and "pure" /pjʊə/. In stressed syllables, /ɝ/ is derhotacized and produced as /ɜ/, as in "heard" /hɜd/. Table 9.7 displays in more detail differences between the RP and Standard English vowel systems (Wells, 1982a); similarities between the two are not shown.

TABLE 9.7 Differences in the Standard English and Received Pronunciation Vowel Systems (all back vowel comparisons shown).

Key Word	Standard American English	Received Pronunciation
dance	/dæns/	/dɑns/
road	/roʊd/	/rəʊd/
palm	/pɑm/	/pɑm/
thought	/θɔt/ (or /θɑt/)	/θɔt/
lot	/lɑt/	/lɒt/
earth	/ɝθ/	/ɜθ/
near	/nɪr/	/nɪə/
fair	/fɛr/	/fɛə/
cure	/kjʊr/	/kjʊə/
fourth	/fɔrθ/	[fɔ:θ]
cart	/kɑrt/	[kɑ:t]

Source: Information from Wells, 1982a.

EXERCISE 9.10

Using Table 9.7 as your guide, transcribe each of the following words using the appropriate RP vowel(s).

1. merged _____   4. appear _____
2. chance _____   5. repair _____
3. ghostly _____ 6. north star _____

In India, RP was originally considered the standard of pronunciation when teaching English to first- or second-language learners. This was to ensure that speakers would be intelligible to speakers of English in other regions or in other countries. Teaching standard RP to second-language learners, although an ideal, has not met with much success. In actual practice, RP is not the form of pronunciation adopted by many Asian Indian English speakers, including many teachers of English. Over time, **Educated Indian English** (also known as **Educated Indian Pronunciation**) has emerged as a preferred method of pronunciation adopted by educators in India (Nihalani, Tongue, Hosali, & Crowther, 2004; Sailaja, 2009). Educated Indian English has kept the basic phonological concepts of RP but has allowed for incorporation of regional variations, especially for English sounds that are difficult to produce. Proponents of Educated Indian English believe that what is important in becoming intelligible speakers of English is not so much perfection in phoneme production, but the ability to use the proper suprasegmental aspects of English. Educated Indian English allows then for variability in phoneme production as long as regional variations "do not damage the overall phonological (i.e., sound) system of the language" (Nihalani et al., 2004, p. 205).

American English pronunciation and culture also has begun to have a strong influence on Indian English pronunciation. American movies and TV shows have gained widespread popularity in India. Many U.S.-based companies have established a major presence in India. These companies train employees to modify their accents to approximate American English pronunciation patterns. American restaurant and fast-food chains have become popular in India as well, adding to the proliferation of American English in India (N. Radhakrishnan, personal communication, May 2, 2014).

Speaking English continues to be a mark of social status in India. Learning English in private schools and in universities (where English is the primary mode of instruction) is a measure of prestige, as is eating in English-speaking restaurants and watching movies with English dialogue. The use of *Hinglish*, a hybrid language that mixes English words and phrases with Hindi (as well as other Asian Indian languages) continues to grow not only in conversational settings, but in music and in the popular press.

Consonant Characteristics of Asian Indian English

Even with its many variations due to regional differences, differences in educational background, and influence of British or American pronunciation, Asian Indian English can be characterized by several common phonological processes that affect consonant production, including substitution, assimilation, and syllable structure processes. In addition, some Indian English pronunciation is based on the spelling of certain words. The major pronunciation patterns associated with Indian English consonants are presented in the next section and are also summarized in Table 9.8.

Substitution and Assimilation Processes

Indian English speakers do not aspirate the voiceless stops /p/, /t/, and /k/ at the beginning of stressed syllables. For example, "pen" would be produced as [pɛn] instead of [pʰɛn]. Even though many Indian languages have aspirated voiceless stops in syllable-initial position, they are produced with greater aspiration than the aspiration associated with American or British English. Because of this, English voiceless stops are *perceived* by Indian English speakers as having no aspiration and therefore are produced without aspiration.

The plosives /t/ and /d/ may be produced in Indian English as *retroflex* stops, and not alveolar in reference to place of production. The phonetic

TABLE 9.8 Asian Indian English Pronunciation.

English Word	Asian Indian English	Phonological Process
Substitution and Assimilation Processes		
pen	[pˀɛn]	unaspirated
dog	/ɖɒg/	retroflex
river	[rɪbʰər]	stopping; aspiration
vine	/ʋaɪn/ or /waɪn/	gliding
this	[d̪ɪs]; [d̪ʰɪs]	dentalization; dentalization and aspiration
sheet	/sit/	fronting
Sue	/ʃu/	backing
dose	[ɖo:dʒ]	affrication; retroflex /ɖ/
measure	/mɛzɚ/; /mɛʃɚ/	fronting; fronting and devoicing
wall	/wɔl/ or /wɔɭ/	l/ɫ; or l/ɫ
bring	/brɪŋg/	regressive assimilation
candy	/kæɳɖi/	retroflex /ɳ/ due to regressive assimilation
Syllable Structure Processes		
spot; school	/səpat/ or /ɪskul/	epenthesis of /ə/ or /ɪ/
works; desk	/ʋɚs/; /dɛs/	cluster simplification
legal	/ligəl/	epenthesis of /ə/ instead of syllabic /l/
old; every	/wolɖ/; /jɛʋri/	epenthesis of a glide
yet; won't	/ɛʈ/; /onʈ/	glide deletion
Pronunciation Based on Spelling		
walked	/wɒkd/	d/t with past-tense "-ed" spelling
keys	/kis/	s/z with plural "-s" spelling
innate	[ɪnne:ʈ]	epenthesis of consonant with geminate
which; ghost	/wfɪɪtʃ/; [gfio:st]	pronunciation of both letters in "wh" and "gh"

Sources: Information from Gargesh, 2008; Nihalani et al., 2004; Wells, 1982b.

symbols for retroflex /t/ and /d/ are /ʈ/ and /ɖ/, respectively. Retroflex consonants are characterized as having a distinct place of production. Recall that the only other retroflex consonant in English is seen in some individuals' productions of /r/ (postalveolar). To produce a retroflex stop, the tongue tip is curled up and back so that the underside of the tongue tip comes in contact with the rear portion of the alveolar ridge near the anterior portion of the palate. Refer to the IPA chart (Figure 2.1) to see how the retroflex consonants are displayed. Examples in Indian English include /ʈɪp/ "tip" and /ɖɒg/ "dog." Due to regressive assimilation, /n/ can be produced as a retroflex consonant when it occurs prior to a retroflex stop, so that the word "candy" is produced as /kænɖɪ/. Another example of regressive assimilation involves production of the velar nasal /ŋ/. It is produced as an allophone of /n/ when it precedes a velar consonant as in "bring" /brɪŋg/ or "hang" /hæŋg/ (Gargesh, 2008). Note that that final /g/ is still produced. In General American English, /g/ is in free variation in these words and either pronunciation would be deemed acceptable even though in most cases, the final /g/ would not be pronounced.

In some regions of India, the labiodental fricatives /f/ and /v/ are stopped and aspirated so that "fine" becomes [pʰaɪn] and "river" becomes [rɪbʰər]. Also, there is no distinction between /v/ and the labiovelar glide /w/. /w/ is often substituted for /v/ as in "veggie" /wɛdʒɪ/. In addition, Indian English speakers may substitute the labiodental approximant /ʋ/ for either /v/ or /w/. Recall that this phoneme is produced without the lower teeth contacting the lower lip. An Indian English production of the word "vine" would be /ʋaɪn/, but would most likely sound like /waɪn/ to a speaker of Standard English.

The interdental fricatives /θ/ and /ð/ do not exist in Indian languages. Instead, they are stopped and dentalized. This is directly related to language transfer because dentalized stops are phonemic in Indian languages. This results in productions of "thick" and "this" as [t̪ɪk] and [d̪ɪs], respectively. In some parts of India, /θ/ and /ð/ in words might be produced as aspirated dentalized stops, as in [t̪ʰɪk] and [d̪ʰɪs].

The sibilant consonants /s, z, ʃ, and ʒ/ have varying productions among Indian English speakers. In some regions of India, /s/ is backed and produced as /ʃ/ as in "Sue" /ʃu/. Conversely, the opposite occurs in some areas so that /ʃ/ is fronted and pronounced as /s/ as in "shoe" /su/. Also, /z/ may be affricated and produced as /dʒ/ as in "doze" /ɖoːdʒ/ and "crazy" /kredʒi/. The palatal fricative /ʒ/ does not exist in most Indian languages. Therefore it is replaced by either /dʒ/, /z/, or /ʃ/ as in "measure" /mɛdʒɚ/, /mɛzɚ/, or /mɛʃɚ/ (Gargesh, 2008; Nihalani et al., 2004; Wells, 1982b).

In reference to liquids, Indian English speakers produce light /l/ at the beginning of words, as in "lip" [lɪp]. However, dark /l/ is not always produced. For example, speakers of Hindi may produce "wall" as [wɔl] instead of [wɔɫ]. On the other hand, speakers of Malayalam and Kannada may produce a retroflex lateral /l/ (transcribed as /ɭ/) instead of dark [ɫ]- "wall" /wɔɭ/ (S. Karthikeyan, personal communication, May 19, 2014). Production of /r/ is variable in Indian English. Many speakers produce postvocalic /ɹ/ as a palatal liquid approximant as in Standard English, while others produce it as an alveolar trill /r/. In some dialects where a strong RP influence exists, or where teaching method still promotes RP, /ɹ/ is vocalized in rhotic diphthongs and in the postvocalic position of words.

Syllable Structure Processes
Consonant clusters are often simplified in Indian English. Similar to Spanish-Influenced English, the consonant clusters /sp/, /st/, or /sk/ do not occur in the initial position of words in many Indian languages. In some regions of India, speakers add /i/ or /ɪ/ to the initial portion of the cluster (epenthesis), creating two syllables, as in "spot" /ispat/ or "school" /ɪskul/. In other regions, speakers will insert /ə/ *into* the cluster: "spot" /səpɔt/ or "school" /səkul/ (Gargesh, 2008; Wells, 1982b). Word-final clusters also are simplified, for example, "desk" /ɖɛs/ and "works" /ʋɚs/. Also, syllabic consonants do not exist in in Indian English. Syllabic /l̩/ and /n̩/ are replaced with the sequence

of /əl/ or /ən/ as in "legal" /ligəl/ or "written" /rɪʈən/ (Wells, 1982b). (Note the replacement of the glottal stop with the retroflex /ʈ/ in "written" /rɪʔn̩/.)

Some Indian English speakers display epenthesis of the glides /j/ or /w/ before a vowel in some words (e.g., "okay" /wokeɪ/ and "every" /jɛʋri/). The glide chosen is dependent on the place of articulation of the following vowel. If it is a back vowel, /w/ is appended. If it is a front vowel, /j/ is appended. Furthermore, some speakers omit the glide when the following vowel is mid or high as long as the vowel is similar in tongue advancement—"yet" /ɛt/ (front) and "won't" /ont/ (back) (Wells, 1982b).

Pronunciation Based on Spelling

In Indian English, the way a word is spelled often may influence its production. For example, the past tense of verbs ending with "-ed" will be pronounced with /d/ even when the preceding phoneme is voiceless. Some examples of this include "walked" /wɑkd/ and "laced" /leɪsd/. Similarly, the plural form of nouns ending with "-s" will be pronounced with /s/ regardless of the voicing of the preceding phoneme, as in "keys" /kis/ and "dogs" /dɒgs/. Another pronunciation based on spelling involves *geminates* (double consonants) in words like "innate" and "fully." Some Indian English speakers will lengthen the consonant accordingly as /ɪnneʈ/ and /fʊlli/, respectively (Gargesh, 2008). Also, both consonants may be pronounced in words that begin with "wh," as in "which" /wɦɪɪtʃ/ or /ʋɦɪɪtʃ/. (The phoneme /ɦ/ is a *voiced* glottal fricative, the cognate of the voiceless glottal fricative /h/.) Similarly, in words that begin with "gh" as in "ghost," the "h" is pronounced as in [gɦio:st] (Wells, 1982b).

Vowel Characteristics

For the most part, vowel pronunciation in Indian English parallels vowel pronunciation of RP. In Indian English, /ɔ/ may be produced as either /a/ or /ɒ/. Similar to RP, the vowel /æ/ may be produced as either /a/ or /ɑ/, in words such as "bath" /baʈ/ or "dance" /dɑns/. The diphthongs /eɪ/ and /oʊ/ are produced as lengthened monophthongs, as in "day" [d̪e:] and "coat" [ko:ʈ]. Schwa /ə/ does exist in Indian English; however, /ʌ/ does not. Therefore, schwa appears in stressed syllables, unlike both RP and Standard English. Some examples include "other" [əd̪ɚ] and "mud" /məd̪/.

Suprasegmental Aspects

Recall that Educated Indian English stresses the importance of appropriate prosody in order to maximize the intelligibility of spoken English. The correct use of prosody provides a particular challenge for Indians who are learning English as a second language because the suprasegmental aspects of Standard American English (L₂) are quite different from Asian Indian languages (L₁). Standard English duration, rhythm, and intonation often are not maintained by Indian L₂ learners of English. Similarly, pauses may be taken in places where they might be unexpected. Additionally, sentence stress may be assigned to words that might not usually receive sentence stress based on the speakers' intent. Incorrect production of these prosodic cues often lead to breakdowns in communication because a listener will not be familiar with the prosodic cues provided by the speaker.

Duration of vowels and consonants is often affected not only by context of the utterance, but also by the intent and emotion the speaker wishes to convey. For instance, vowels may be prolonged when producing adjectives such as "tall," "big," "long," and so on. When wishing to express emotion and emphasis, plosives may be produced with excessive intraoral pressure, resulting in a louder release burst and greater aspiration. Also, past-tense "-ed" is sometimes overemphasized as in "walked" /wɔkdu/.

Recall that in Standard English, falling intonation contours are generally used when asking a "wh" question, such as "What is your name?" Some Asian Indian speakers might ask this question with a *rising* contour when they are addressing someone they have just met (so that the highest pitch would be on the word "name"). Also, announcements in public places (such as airports) are often made with a rising intonation contour instead of a falling contour (typical of most Standard English statements). For example, the statement "The plane is delayed due to the weather" would be pronounced with a pitch rise on the last word of the sentence, "weather." A native English speaker might assume that more information is going to be provided following the utterance due to the rise in the intonation contour (see Sailaja, 2009).

Remember that yes/no questions are typically produced with a rising intonation contour, as in "Are you going to the party?" Some Indian English speakers produce yes/no questions in the form of a statement, with "ah" as a tag question (similar to "huh?") at the end of the sentence, as in "You are going to the party, ah?" In this manner, the intonation falls throughout the utterance "You are going to the party," with a rise in pitch only during production of the tag question "ah" (V. Ramachandra, personal communication, May 19, 2014).

Often, the word (lexical) stress patterns of Asian Indians is quite dissimilar from the stress patterns of Standard English speakers. The speaker's L$_1$ can account for some of these differences (Gargesh, 2008). There are several rules that attempt to predict the word stress patterns used by Indian speakers of English. According to these rules, stress is often determined by the phonetic makeup of each syllable (i.e., the specific grouping of consonants and vowels in each syllable). However, word stress patterns are not always predictable from these rules. Furthermore, stress patterns can be tied to a speaker's idiolect (Wells, 1982b). Incorrect word stress often leads to problems in intelligibility because the resulting word may often appear unrecognizable. Some examples of Asian Indian English stress patterns in bisyllabic and multisyllabic words follow. Be sure to pay particular attention to the primary stress marks in each word; secondary stress marks also are indicated.

audiology	[ˌɒdɪəˈlɒdʒi]	contents	[kənˈtɛnts]
Kentucky	[ˈkænʈɪki]	adolescent	[əˈdɒləsənt]
perimeter	[ˈpɛrɪˌmitɚ]	sentence	[sɪnˈtæns]
biology	[ˌbaɪoˈlɒdʒi]	academics	[əˈkædəmɪks]

Asian Indian English speakers also confuse the stress patterns in English words that are spelled the same, but have different stress depending on whether the word is a noun or a verb. Some examples include "RECord" (noun), pronounced as the verb [rɪˈkɔːrd], and "PROject" (noun), pronounced as the verb [proˈdʒɛkt] (Wells, 1982b). In these two examples, both nouns are pronounced as (what would normally be perceived as) verbs due to the shift in word stress to the second syllable. It is easy to see how the mismatch between the word and the stress pattern could possibly lead to confusions in conversation.

EXERCISE 9.11

Fill in the blank with the Asian English phonological process being demonstrated. For some items there will be more than one answer.

Example:

		Phonological Process
pen	[p⁼ɛn]	unaspirated stop

1. shawl — /sɒl/ — _____
2. skin — /ɪskɪn/ — _____
3. bottle — /bɒtəl/ — _____
4. yes — /ɛs/ — _____
5. vase — /ʋes/ — _____
6. pleasure — /plɛzɚ/ — _____
7. sing — /sɪŋg/ — _____
8. them — /d̪ʰɛm/ — _____
9. don't — /doɳt/ — _____
10. doll — /ɖɔl̪/ — _____

Russian- and Arabic-Influenced English

The number of Russian and Arabic speakers in the United States continues to grow. Between 2000 and 2011, the number of Russian speakers in the country increased by 28 percent, whereas the number of Arabic speakers increased by 55 percent. Russian and Arabic are among the top 10 non-English languages spoken in the country, Arabic ranking eighth and Russian ranking ninth (Ryan, 2013).

Arabic is an Afroasiatic language, while Russian is a member of the Indo-European family of languages. Both Arabic and Russian have very different phonemic systems when compared to English, even though Russian (a Balto-Slavic language) and English (a Germanic language) are both Indo-European languages. Each language will be examined separately to help explain some of the mismatches between Arabic and Russian (L_1) and American English (L_2).

Russian-Influenced English

Russian has only five vowels, /i, e, a, u, and o/, and only one true diphthong, /aʊ/ (Berger, 1952). For this reason, Russian speakers learning English have difficulty with vowel production. In unstressed syllables, the five vowels are reduced to three: /i, a, and ə/, and similar to East Asian languages, lax vowels are tensed as in the following substitutions: i/ɪ, e/ɛ or æ, u/ʊ, and o/ɔ. The vowel /a/ may be produced as a substitute for /æ, a, and ʌ/ (Yavaş, 2006). See Table 9.9 for a summary of Russian-Influenced English pronunciations.

TABLE 9.9 Common Russian-Influenced English Vowel and Consonant Productions.

English Word	Russian-Influenced English Transcription	Substitution
Vowel Articulations		
sit	/sit/	i/ɪ
book	/buk/	u/ʊ
hat	/hat/	a/æ
caught	/kot/	o/ɔ
men	/men/	e/ɛ
Consonant Articulations		
pool	[p⁼ul]	unaspirated stop
tame	/ţem/	dentalization
mood, bags	/mut/, /baks/	devoicing
this, thin	/dis/, /tin/	stopping
laughing	/lafɪŋk/	epenthesis
quota	/kvotə/	frication
vodka	/wodkə/	gliding
ham	/xam/	fronting
run (/ɹʌn/)	/ran/	r/ɹ substitution

Sources: Information from Berger, 1952; Power, 2014b; Yavaş, 2006.

The Russian consonant system also varies significantly when compared to English. For example, voiceless stop consonants in Russian tend to be unaspirated. Therefore, English words that begin with a voiceless stop may be unaspirated when spoken by a Russian individual learning English. An unaspirated voiceless stop at the beginning of a word will tend to sound voiced. For example, "came" [k⁼eɪm] will sound like "game" [geɪm] (Baker, 1982; Berger, 1952). Also, alveolar phonemes may be produced as dentalized consonants: [ţ, ḓ, and ṉ] (Yavaş, 2006).

There are several consonants in English that do not exist in Russian: /ð, θ, dʒ, w, and r/; /ŋ/ exists only as an allophone of /n/. Because of phonological mismatch (transfer) between languages:

1. The interdental fricatives /ð/ and /θ/ are often stopped, as in "them" /dɛm/ and "thin" /tɪn/.
2. The affricate /dʒ/ may be devoiced and produced as /tʃ/, as in "jam" /tʃam/.
3. The glide /w/ may be produced as /v/ (frication), as in "when" /vɛn/.
4. The approximant /ɹ / is pronounced as a trill, that is, /r/.
5. The velar nasal /ŋ/ is produced *as an allophone of* /n/ only when it occurs before a velar stop.

Therefore, in words where /ŋ/ does not precede a velar stop, one is added (epenthesis), as in "running" /ranɪŋk/. In this context, the added velar is also devoiced: /rʌnɪŋg/→ /rʌnɪŋk/ (Yavaş, 2006).

Additionally, some Russian speakers front the production of the voiceless glottal /h/ and produce it as a voiceless velar fricative /x/ as in "hot" /xɑt/. Also, /v/ is produced either as the voiced bilabial fricative /β/, /w/, or /vw/ (Berger, 1952). For example, "vodka" could be produced as /βɔdkə/, /wɔdkə/, or /vwɔdkə/.

In Russian, voiced obstruents do not occur in word-final positions resulting in devoicing of the final phoneme, such as "lag" /lak/ (Baker, 1982; Berger, 1952). Also, clusters made up of voiced stops and fricatives do not occur together in the final position of a word. Therefore, the word "bags" would be pronounced as /bæks/ (/g/ and /z/ both being produced as their voiceless cognates /k/ and /s/). Finally, voiceless and voiced phonemes do not occur together at word boundaries (Berger, 1952). For example, "hit the ball," would be produced as /hɪdðəbal/. Note the effect of regressive assimilation in this case.

EXERCISE 9.12

Fill in the blank with the correct phonological process being demonstrated. For some items there will be more than one answer.

Example:

			Phonological Process
__X__	pack	[p⁼ak]	unaspirated stop, a/æ substitution
____	1. foot	/fut/	_____
____	2. very	/wɛri/	_____
____	3. badge	/batʃ/	_____
____	4. swim	/svɪm/	_____
____	5. those	/dos/	_____
____	6. eating	/itɪ̩ŋk/	_____
____	7. rugs	/raks/	_____
____	8. kiss	/xis/	_____

Arabic-Influenced English

Arabic has only three vowels—/i/, /a/, and /u/ (all tense)—which occur in both short and long forms. The vowels /ɪ/ and /e/ may be produced as /i/, the vowels /æ/, /ɑ/, and /ʌ/ produced as /a/, and /ʊ/ is produced as /u/; the vowel /ɛ/ may be produced as either /a/ or /i/ (Ball & Müller, 2005; Yavaş, 2006). Note that tense vowels often substitute for lax vowels. The only diphthongs in Arabic are /eɪ/ and /aʊ/.

Several English obstruents do not exist in Arabic: /p, v, ʒ, and tʃ/ (Altaha, 1995; *Handbook of the International Phonetic Association*, 1999). Some of the obstruents do exist in some dialects of Arabic, however. Due to phonological transfer:

1. /p/ is voiced and produced as /b/, as in "peel" /bil/.
2. /v/ is devoiced and produced as /f/, as in "vote" /fot/.
3. /tʃ/ and /ʒ/ are often produced as /ʃ/ as in "choose" /ʃuz/ (deaffrication) and "measure" /mɛʃɚ/ (devoicing).

As in Russian, /ŋ/ exists as an allophone of /n/ before velar stops (Yavaş, 2006). Therefore, in words where /ŋ/ does not precede a velar stop, /g/ is added, as in "running" /ranɪŋg/ (epenthesis). Also, the English liquid /ɹ/ does not exist and is produced as the alveolar trill /r/. Phonemes of Arabic not found in English include the voiceless uvular plosive /q/, the velar fricatives /x/ (voiceless) and /ɣ/ (voiced), the voiceless pharyngeal fricative /ħ/, and several pharyngealized consonants including /tˤ, dˤ, sˤ, ðˤ, lˤ, and ʕˤ/ (*Handbook of the International Phonetic Association*, 1999).

In Arabic, it is not possible to have a cluster of two or three consonants at the beginning of a word. For this reason, vowels are added in production of clusters, as in /sikrim/ for "scream" and /sitrit/ for "street" (Altaha, 1995).

Arabic speakers learning English will sometimes pronounce silent letters because Arabic's alphabet is phonemic, as in "knot" /knat/, "could" /kuld/, and "lamb" /læmb/. Other difficulties that arise from English spelling intrusions include problems pronouncing words with the letter "c" as in "city" /kiti/ or "soccer" /sasɚ/. In a similar manner, because the letter "g" can be pronounced as either /dʒ/ or /g/, Arabic speakers may produce "gear" as /dʒir/ and "origin" as /arigin/. Also, the spelling "dg" may be pronounced as two separate phonemes, as in /badgit/ for "budget" (Altaha, 1995). Refer to Table 9.10 for a summary of Arabic-Influenced English productions.

TABLE 9.10 Common Arabic-Influenced English Vowel and Consonant Productions.

English Word	Arabic-Influenced English Transcription	Phonological Pattern
Vowel Articulations		
bit	/bit/	i/ɪ
cup	/kap/	a/ʌ
cap	/kap/	a/æ
set	/sit/ or /sat/	i or a/ɛ
look	/luk/	u/ʊ
Consonant Articulations		
put	/but/	voicing
love	/laf/	devoicing
lesion	/liʃən/	devoicing
watch	/waʃ/	deaffrication
reed (/ɹid/)	/rid/	r/ɹ (producing a trilled /r/)
wing	/wɪŋg/	epenthesis
scream	/sikrim/	epenthesis

Sources: Information from Altaha, 1995; Baker, 1982; Ball & Müller, 2005; Power 2014a; Yavaş, 2006.

EXERCISE 9.13

Indicate with an "X" the productions that are consistent with the phonological patterns associated with Arabic-Influenced English. Fill in the blank with the correct description of the pattern. For some items there will be more than one phonological pattern being demonstrated.

Example:

Phonological Process

| X | luck | /luk/ | u/ʊ substitution (vowel tensing) |

___	1. azure	/aʃɚ/	_____
___	2. Paul	/bal/	_____
___	3. hat	/xæt/	_____
___	4. check	/ʃɛk/	_____
___	5. did	/did/	_____
___	6. vase	/fes/	_____
___	7. hearing	/hiriŋg/	_____
___	8. win	/vin/	_____

Review Exercises

A. Transcribe each of the following words as if they were pronounced by a Southern American English Speaker.

1. steal _____
2. steer _____
3. ferry _____
4. dew _____
5. mesh _____
6. fought _____
7. coil _____
8. treasure _____
9. lines _____
10. when _____

B. Provide English orthography for each of the following Southern American English pronunciations.

1. /lɪmɪn/ _____
2. /spoət/ _____
3. /preɪʃɪʃ/ _____
4. /pjuə/ _____
5. /wiʃ/ _____
6. /wɔtʃ/ _____
7. /hɪl/ _____
8. [wɜːðɪ] _____
9. /tʃɛə/ _____
10. /stiu/ _____
11. [kɑːt] _____
12. /kærɪ/ _____

C. Transcribe each of the following words as if they were pronounced by an Eastern American English speaker. All of these words involve some form of /r/ vocalization or derhotacization.

1. beware _____
2. start _____
3. hanger _____
4. severe _____
5. clergy _____
6. store _____
7. squirt _____
8. glare _____
9. doctor _____
10. carbon _____

D. Provide English orthography for each of the following Eastern American English pronunciations.

1. /kɑnt/ _____   6. /ɛksploə/ _____
2. /brʊm/ _____   7. [tʃaːɾə] _____
3. /mærou/ _____   8. /ladʒɪst/ _____
4. /baθ/ _____   9. /dɪmɑnd/ _____
5. /pærɪt/ _____   10. /kənspaɪə/ _____

E. Examine each of the words below. Then look at the AAE phonological pattern that should be applied to each word. Provide the appropriate transcription in the blank.

Example:

east	cluster reduction	/is/ _____
1. moth	labialization	_____
2. because	deletion of unstressed initial syllable	_____
3. then	/ɛ/-/ɪ/ merger	_____
4. can	nasal deletion	_____
5. Harold	/l/ vocalization	_____
6. them	stopping	_____
7. mind	monophthongization	_____
8. wastes	cluster reduction + plural	_____
9. eleven	stopping	_____
10. straight	backing	_____

F. Indicate with an "X" the productions that are consistent with the phonological patterns associated with AAE. Write the phonological pattern being demonstrated in the blank.

Example:

east	/is/	cluster reduction
1. bread	/brɛ/	_____
2. broom	/brʊm/	_____
3. suppose	/pouz/	_____
4. raced	/reɪs/	_____
5. cat	/kæʔ/	_____
6. Ben	/bɪn/	_____
7. light	/lat/	_____
8. hold	/houd/	_____
9. cola	/koulɚ/	_____
10. washing	/waʃɪn/	_____
11. carry	/kærɪ/	_____
12. men	/mɛ̃ː/	_____

G. For these Spanish-Influenced English words, write the description of the phonological pattern being displayed in the blank.

    Examples:

late	/lɛt/	ɛ/eɪ substitution
zebra	/sibrə/	devoicing

    1. bath   /bæt/   _____

    2. been   /bin/   _____

    3. chore   /ʃɔr/   _____

    4. oven   /avən/   _____

    5. young   /dʒɑŋ/   _____

    6. told   /tol/   _____

    7. cushion   /kuʃən/   _____

    8. Tom   /t̪ɑm/   _____

    9. shallow   /tʃælou/   _____

    10. vine   /baɪn/   _____

    11. them   /dɛm/   _____

    12. stood   /əstʊd/   _____

H. Examine the phonological pattern in the Asian-Influenced English pronunciation of each word. From Table 9.6, determine the Asian language(s) in which the given pattern may occur. Write your answer in the blank.

    Example:

them	/zɛm/	Vietnamese, Japanese, Mandarin, and Cantonese

    1. like   /raɪk/   _____

    2. very   /wɛrɪ/   _____

    3. vine   /baɪn/   _____

    4. shine   /saɪn/   _____

    5. joke   /tʃouk/   _____

    6. put   [p˭ʊt]   _____

    7. thank   /fæŋk/   _____

    8. chant   /tsænt/   _____

    9. zoo   /dzu/   _____

    10. talk   /tʃɑk/   _____

I. Using Tables 9.9 and 9.10, determine whether the phonological process given is indicative of either Russian-Influenced English, Arabic-Influenced English, or both. Mark the appropriate blank with an "X." Then give the name of the process being demonstrated.

Example:

		Russian	Arabic	Both	Phonological Process
lesion	/liʃən/	___	X	___	devoicing
1. pass	/bæs/	___	___	___	
2. very	/wɛri/	___	___	___	
3. they	/deɪ/	___	___	___	
4. good	/gud/	___	___	___	
5. funny	/fani/	___	___	___	
6. happy	/xæpi/	___	___	___	
7. dogs	/daks/	___	___	___	
8. school	/sikul/	___	___	___	
9. yes mom	/jɛzmɑm/	___	___	___	
10. eating	/itɪŋg/	___	___	___	
11. roof (/ɹuf/)	/ruf/	___	___	___	
12. should	/ʃuld/	___	___	___	

J. Eastern American English Transcription Practice.

CD #3
Track 16

Transcribe each of the following sentences as spoken by a female from New York City.

1. Ma, I gotta go to the store with Paul today.

_____

2. What are you talking about? Forget about it already.

_____

3. Carly, why do you have to ruin everything?

_____

4. I have a dentist appointment at 6:30.

_____

5. Robert needs to go to the barber; his hair is too long.

_____

6. I walked over to the mall yesterday afternoon to get a new pair of shoes.

_____

7. My dog likes to run all around the yard and bark.

_____

8. When I was playing basketball, I ran all over the court.

_____

9. I gotta go food shopping. I need watermelon, corn, and soda.

_____

10. My friend Mary is a weirdo. She don't want to leave me alone.

_____

K. Eastern American English Transcription Practice.

Transcribe each of the following sentences as spoken by a female from Massachusetts.

1. Park the car in the garage.

_____

CD #3
Track 17

2. I am going to the market in Boston.

_____

3. I love to shop Harvard Square.

_____

4. Have you guys been to the Cape or Martha's Vineyard for the summer?

_____

5. Don't forget to bring your pocketbook.

_____

6. Donna loves to drink tonic.

_____

7. Can you wear your dungarees and sneakers?

_____

8. Get a fork for that huge helping of pasta and gravy.

_____

9. Go ahead and give Mommy some jimmies for her banana split.

_____

10. John Miller is a decent human being.

_____

L. Southern American English Transcription Practice.

Transcribe each of the following sentences as spoken by a female from Tennessee.

1. She's driving to Louisiana tomorrow morning.

_____

CD #3
Track 18

2. I'm going to boil a dozen eggs for Easter.

_____

3. Last night, I was talking to my friend Mary Lynn.

_____

4. I am fixing to have to buy some tires for my car.

_____

5. I am looking for my blue ballpoint pen.

_____

6. You better cover that broiling pan with aluminum foil.

_____

7. Wait a minute, Larry. I need another minute to make up my mind.

_____

8. I left the chicken out on the counter and it spoiled.

_____

9. The University of Tennessee is in Knoxville.

_____

10. Hurricanes and tornadoes are both large damaging windstorms.

_____

M. African American English Transcription Practice.

Transcribe each of the following sentences as spoken by a female from Ohio.

1. The boy needs more money.

_____

**CD #3
Track 19**

2. We fixin' to go to the store.

_____

3. He be playing ball at the park.

_____

4. There four new kids in my class.

_____

5. My sister and brother was at that concert.

_____

6. My family go to church every Sunday.

_____

7. Your momma car in the middle of the street.

_____

8. She found five quarters in her purse.

_____

9. Kwanzaa got her hair done.

_____

10. The students helped themselves to breakfast.

_____

N. Spanish-Influenced English Transcription Practice.

Transcribe each of the following sentences as spoken by a female from Spain.

1. Please put the flowers in the vase.

_____

**CD #3
Track 20**

2. It was a very special occasion.

_____

3. You should quit yelling at your mother.

_____

4. I was not sure I would be able to help.

_____

5. My favorite teacher's name is Mister Jones.

_____

6. Don't let your dog play in my yard.

_____

7. Why don't you put these clothes in the garage?

_____

8. Yesterday, I went to the zoo with Doug.

_____

9. Shelley put the potato chips on the lower shelf.

_____

10. I was very excited about winning the football game.

_____

O. Asian-Influenced English Transcription Practice.

Transcribe each of the following sentences as spoken by a female from Japan.

1. I have one younger brother in my family.

_____

**CD #3
Track 21**

2. I would like a grilled cheese sandwich for lunch, please.

_____

3. It is supposed to rain heavily for much of the week.

_____

4. The river is heavily polluted.

_____

5. My sister Kyoko will be 23 years old next Thursday.

_____

6. Would you like to go shopping with me after I get off work?

_____

7. Would your other brother help me lift this? It's heavy.

_____

8. Thank you very much for the beautiful flowers.

_____

9. I have a hard time distinguishing between the singular and plural forms.

_____

10. The only connecting flight is through Portland, Oregon.

_____

P. Asian-Influenced English Transcription Practice.

**CD #3
Track 22**

Transcribe each of the following sentences as spoken by a male from Hong Kong. This male speaks the Cantonese dialect of Chinese.

1. Typing email helps me think in English.

2. I went to the zoo to see the new panda bears.

3. What do you think of the new television show?

4. I have two or three friends who are going to the soccer game.

5. Usually, she is not so forgetful.

6. I bet you that I will win the race.

7. My girlfriend sent me flowers last week for my birthday.

8. There are several people I need to get to know.

9. The layout of this city is not very convenient.

10. I plan to go to Purdue for my master's degree.

Q. Asian Indian English Transcription Practice.

**CD #3
Track 23**

Transcribe each of the following sentences as spoken by a female from New Delhi, India.

1. My Auntie is going to study audiology at the University of Kentucky.

2. I need to pay my tuition in the Bursar's office.

3. They need your help immediately.

4. My father planted herbs around the perimeter of my garden.

5. The contents of the potion include calcium and potassium.

6. I put vinegar and oil on my tomato and lettuce salad.

7. I just got a box of chocolate-covered caramels.

8. My adolescent cousin brother excelled at academics.

_____

9. She should schedule an appointment with the biology department.

_____

10. Please rewrite the last sentence of the paragraph.

_____

R. Russian-Influenced English Transcription Practice.

Transcribe each of the following sentences as spoken by a male from Russia.

1. I would like a vodka and tonic, please.

_____

CD #3
Track 24

2. Put the books over there on the table.

_____

3. It was difficult for me to learn the correct pronunciation.

_____

4. I have been living in the United States since last August.

_____

5. He has many problems with his vocabulary.

_____

6. The Russian economy depends on the current price of oil.

_____

7. My younger brother Alexander is studying metallurgy at Moscow State University.

_____

8. The author of the book was a famous writer.

_____

9. I had several visitors from Virginia last month.

_____

10. How many other people needed to take the class?

_____

S. Arabic-Influenced English Transcription Practice.

Transcribe each of the following sentences as spoken by a male from Saudi Arabia.

1. Please use that word in a sentence.

_____

CD #3
Track 25

2. I need sugar substitute for my coffee.

_____

3. Dr. Cooper told me to make a copy of my homework assignment.

_____

4. Their friend Robin got married to Victor, my next-door neighbor.

_____

5. I was depressed because we have had so much bad weather.

_____

6. Pete got a prison sentence because he hit the policeman.

_____

7. My favorite cotton shirt shrunk in the laundry.

_____

8. Penny visited her fiancé on Friday.

_____

9. I need to study English phonology to improve my pronunciation.

_____

10. I grew a beard so that I would appear older.

_____

Complete Assignment 9-1.

Study Questions

1. What is a dialect? What is the difference between a regional dialect and an ethnic dialect?
2. What is ASHA's position on *accent modification*?
3. Contrast the terms *Standard American English* and *General American English*.
4. What is chain shifting? How is chain shifting affecting English vowel production? Which areas of the country are associated with chain shifting?
5. Which features of Southern American English and Eastern American English are similar?
6. In which areas of the country does /r/ vocalization and derhotacization of vowels affect pronunciation?
7. What is African American English (AAE)? What are the two theories used to explain its origin?
8. Describe several vowel and consonant features of AAE that differ from General American English.
9. What is meant by the term *language transfer*? How does transfer affect phoneme acquisition by an individual learning English as a second language?
10. How does language transfer affect phoneme production in Spanish-Influenced English?
11. Describe some general characteristics of Asian languages that add to the difficulty of learning English as a second language.
12. How do the Russian and Arabic phonological systems differ from General American English?

Online Resources

American Speech-Language-Hearing Association. (n.d.). Second language acquisition. Retrieved from *http://www.asha.org/public/speech/development/second.htm* (overview of issues involving second-language acquisition)

The David Pakman Show. (2013). American English is changing fast. Retrieved from *http://www.youtube.com/watch?v=aL0--f89Qds* (interview with William Labov on *Dialect Diversity in America*)

International Dialects of English Archive. (2014). Maintained by Paul Meier. Retrieved from *http://www.dialectsarchive.com*
(online archive of dialect and accent recordings; designed for the performing arts)

Labov, W., Ash, S., & Boberg, C. (2008). *The atlas of North American English: Phonetics, phonology, and sound change.* De Gruyter Mouton [e-book]. Retrieved from *http://www.degruyter.com/view/product/178229*
(open-access version of *The Atlas of North American English*; complete description of the major dialects of North American English as determined by the Telsur telephone survey; to access the table of contents, click on the "Read Content" link in the upper left-hand corner of the web page)

Power, T. (n.d.). English language learning and teaching. Retrieved from *http://www.tedpower.co.uk/phono.html*
(L_2 English pronunciation instruction for L_1 speakers from 20 other countries)

Sailaja, P. (2009). *Dialects of English: Indian English* [audio files]. Retrieved from *http://www.lel.ed.ac.uk/dialects/india.html*
(audio samples of Indian English)

The Speech Accent Archive. (n.d.). George Mason University. Retrieved from *http://accent.gmu.edu/*
(audio samples of non-native speakers of English from around the world)

Assignment 9-1

Name _____

CD #3
Track 26

"The Grandfather Passage" (Darley, Aronson, & Brown, 1975) will be spoken by several individuals who demonstrate different dialects of American English. Transcribe the passage carefully for each speaker, using phonemic (broad) transcription. (In some instances, it may be necessary to use narrow transcription.) In addition to the phonological patterns produced by these speakers, pay attention to the suprasegmental patterns displayed.

You wish to know all about my grandfather. Well, he is nearly 93 years old, yet he still thinks as swiftly as ever. He dresses himself in an old black frock coat, usually several buttons missing. A long beard clings to his chin, giving those who observe him a pronounced feeling of the utmost respect. When he speaks, his voice is just a bit cracked and quivers a bit. Twice each day he plays skillfully and with zest upon a small organ. Except in the winter when the snow or ice prevents, he slowly takes a short walk in the open air each day. We have often urged him to walk more and smoke less, but he always answers, "Banana oil!" Grandfather likes to be modern in his language.

1. African American English (Ohio)

CD #3
Track 27

_____

_____

_____

_____

_____

_____

_____

_____

2. Eastern American English (Massachusetts)

CD #3
Track 28

_____

_____

_____

_____

_____

_____

_____

_____

Assignment 9-1 (cont.)

**CD #3
Track 29**

3. Cantonese-Influenced English

_____
_____
_____
_____
_____
_____
_____
_____

**CD #3
Track 30**

4. Spanish-Influenced English

_____
_____
_____
_____
_____
_____
_____
_____
_____

**CD #3
Track 31**

5. Southern American English (Tennessee)

_____
_____
_____
_____
_____
_____
_____
_____
_____

Assignment 9-1 (cont.)

**CD #3
Track 32**

6. Japanese-Influenced English

_____

_____

_____

_____

_____

_____

_____

_____

**CD #3
Track 33**

7. Eastern American English (New York City)

_____

_____

_____

_____

_____

_____

_____

_____

_____

**CD #3
Track 34**

8. Russian-Influenced English

_____

_____

_____

_____

_____

_____

_____

_____

Assignment 9-1 (cont.)

CD #3
Track 35

9. Arabic-Influenced English

_____
_____
_____
_____
_____
_____
_____
_____
_____

CD #3
Track 36

10. Asian Indian English

_____
_____
_____
_____
_____
_____
_____
_____
_____

References

Altaha, F. M. (1995). Pronunciation errors made by Saudi University students learning English: Analysis and remedy. *I.T.L Review of Applied Linguistics,109–110*, 110–123.

American Speech-Language-Hearing Association. (1983). Social dialects. *ASHA, 25*(9), 23–27.

American Speech-Language-Hearing Association. (2003). *Technical report: American English dialects. ASHA Supplement 23,* 45–46.

Bada, E. (2001). Native language influence on the production of English sounds by Japanese learners. *The Reading Matrix, 1*(2). Retrieved from http://www.readingmatrix.com /articles/bada/article.pdf

Baker, A. (1982). *Introducing English pronunciation: A teacher's guide to tree or three? and ship or sheep?* Cambridge, UK: Cambridge University Press.

Ball, M., & Müller, N. (2005). *Phonetics for communication disorders.* Mahwah, NJ: Erlbaum.

Ball, M. J. (2008). Transcribing disordered speech: By target or by production? *Clinical Linguistics & Phonetics, 22,* 864–870.

Ball, M. J., Esling, J., & Dickson, J. (1995). The VoQS system for the transcription of voice quality. *Journal of the International Phonetics Association, 25*(2), 71–80.

Ball, M. J., & Müller, N. (2007). Non-pulmonic-egressive speech in clinical data: A brief review. *Clinical Linguistics & Phonetics, 21,* 869–874.

Bauman-Waengler, J. (2012). *Articulatory and phonological impairments: A clinical focus* (4th ed.). Boston, MA: Pearson.

Bautista, M. L. S. (2008). A lectal description of the phonological features of Philippine English. In K. Bolton & M. L. S. Bautista (Eds.), *Philippine English: Linguistic and literary perspectives* (pp. 157–174). Hong Kong: Hong Kong University Press.

Berger, M. D. (1952). *The American English pronunciation of Russian immigrants.* Unpublished doctoral dissertation, Columbia University, New York, NY.

Bleile, K., & Goldstein, B. (1996). Dialect. In K. Bleile, *Articulation and phonological disorders: A book of exercises* (pp. 73–82). San Diego, CA: Singular.

Boone, D., & McFarlane, S. (1994). *The voice and voice therapy* (5th ed.). Boston, MA: Allyn & Bacon.

Borden, G., Harris, K., & Raphael, L. (1994). *Speech science primer* (3rd ed.). Baltimore, MD: Williams & Wilkins.

Calvert, D. (1986). *Descriptive phonetics.* New York, NY: Thieme.

Carrell, J., & Tiffany, W. (1960). *Phonetics: Theory and application to speech improvement.* New York, NY: McGraw-Hill.

Carver, C. (1987). *American regional dialects: A word geography.* Ann Arbor: University of Michigan Press.

Cheng, L. (1987a). *Assessing Asian language performance*. Rockville, MD: Aspen.

Cheng, L. (1987b). Cross-cultural and linguistic considerations in working with Asian populations. *ASHA, 29*(6), 33–38.

Cheng, L. (1994). Asian/Pacific students and the learning of English. In J. Bernthal & N. Bankson (Eds.), *Child phonology: Characteristics, assessment and intervention with special populations* (pp. 255–274). New York, NY: Thieme.

Cheng, L. (2001). Transcription of English influenced by selected Asian languages. *Communication Disorders Quarterly, 23*(1), 40–46.

Chomsky, N., & Halle, M. (1968). *The sound pattern of English*. Cambridge, MA: MIT Press.

Cruttenden, A. (2008). *Gimson's pronunciation of English* (7th ed.). London, UK: Hodder Education.

Crystal, D. (1987). *The Cambridge encyclopedia of language*. Cambridge, UK: Cambridge University Press.

Daniloff, R., Schuckers, G., & Feth, L. (1980). *The physiology of speech and hearing*. Upper Saddle River, NJ: Prentice Hall.

Darley, F., Aronson, F., & Brown, J. (1975). *Motor speech disorders*. Philadelphia, PA: W.B. Saunders.

Desai, S., Dubey, A., Vanneman, R., & Banerji, R. (2008). Private schooling in India: A new educational landscape. *India Policy Forum, 5*(1), 1–58.

Duckworth, M., Allen, G., Hardcastle, W., & Ball, M. (1990). Extensions to the International Phonetic Alphabet for the transcription of atypical speech. *Clinical Linguistics and Phonetics, 4*(4), 273–280.

Edwards, H. (1992). *Applied phonetics*. San Diego, CA: Singular.

Elbert, M., & Gierut, J. (1986). *Handbook of clinical phonology: Approaches to assessment and treatment*. San Diego, CA: College Hill Press.

Ennis, S. R., Rios-Vargas, M., & Albert, N. G. (2011). *The Hispanic population: 2010*. 2010 Census Briefs, C2101BR-04. Retrieved from the U.S. Census Bureau website: http://www.census.gov/prod/cen2010/briefs/c2010br-04.pdf

Erber, N. (1983). Speech perception and speech development in hearing-impaired children. In I. Hochberg, H. Levitt, & M. Osberger (Eds.), *Speech of the hearing impaired: Research, training and personnel preparation* (pp. 131–145). Baltimore, MD: University Park Press.

Ethnic. (n.d.). In *Merriam-Webster's online dictionary*. Retrieved from http://www.merriam-webster.com/dictionary/ethnic

Fletcher, H. (1953). *Speech and hearing in communication*. Princeton, NJ: Van Nostrand.

Fudge, E. (1984). *English word-stress*. London, UK: Allen & Unwin.

Gargesh, R. (2008). Indian English: Phonology. In R. Mesthrie (Ed.), *Varieties of English 4: Africa, South, and Southeast Asia* (pp. 231–243). Berlin: De Gruyter Mouton.

Goldstein, B. (2001). Transcription of Spanish and Spanish-Influenced English. *Communication Disorders Quarterly, 23*(1), 54–60.

Gray, G., & Wise, C. (1959). *The bases of speech* (3rd ed.). New York, NY: Harper and Row.

Grieco, E. M., Acosta, Y. D., de la Cruz, G. P., Gambino, C., Gryn, T., Larsen, L. J., . . . Walters, N. P. (2012a). *The foreign-born population in the United States: 2010*. American Community Survey Reports, ACS-19. Retrieved from the U.S. Census Bureau website: http://www.census.gov/prod/2012pubs/acs-19.pdf

Grieco, E. M., Trevelyan, E., Larsen, L., Acosta, Y. D., Gambino, C., de la Cruz, P., . . . Walters, N. P. (2012b). *The size, place of birth, and geographic distribution of the foreign-born population in the United States: 1960 to 2010*. Population Division Working Paper No. 96. Retrieved from the U.S. Census Bureau website: http://www.census.gov/population/foreign/files/WorkingPaper96.pdf

Grunwell, P. (1987). *Clinical phonology* (2nd ed.). Baltimore, MD: Williams & Wilkins.

Grunwell, P., & Harding, A. (1996). A note on describing types of nasality. *Clinical Linguistics and Phonetics, 10*, 157–161.

Gryn, T., & Gambino, C. (2012). *The foreign-born from Asia: 2011*. American Community Survey Briefs, ACSBR/11-06. Retrieved from the U.S. Census Bureau website: http://www.census.gov/prod/2012pubs/acsbr11-06.pdf

Handbook of the International Phonetic Association. (1999). Cambridge, UK: Cambridge University Press.

Hartman, J. (1985). Guide to pronunciation. In F. Cassidy (Ed.), *Dictionary of American regional English: Volume I, introduction and A–C* (pp. xli–lx). Cambridge, MA: Belknap Press.

Higgins, M. B., Carney, A. E., McCleary, E., & Rogers, S. (1996). Negative intraoral air pressures of deaf children with cochlear implants: Physiology, phonology, and treatment. *Journal of Speech and Hearing Research, 39,* 957–967.

Hodson, B. W., & Paden, E. P. (1991). *Targeting intelligible speech: A phonological approach to remediation* (2nd ed.). Austin, TX: Pro-Ed.

Hoeffel, E. M., Rastogi, S., Kim, M. O., and Shahid, H. (2012). *The Asian population: 2010.* 2010 Census Briefs, C2010BR-11. Retrieved from the U.S. Census Bureau website: http://www.census.gov/prod/cen2010/briefs/c2010br-11.pdf

Humes, K. R., Jones, N. A., & Ramirez, R. R. (2011). *Overview of race and Hispanic origin.* 2010 Census Briefs, C2010BR-02. Retrieved from the U.S. Census Bureau website: http://www.census.gov/prod/cen2010/briefs/c2010br-02.pdf

Hwa-Froelich. D., Hodson, B. W., & Edwards, H. E. (2002). Characteristics of Vietnamese phonology. *American Journal of Speech-Language Pathology, 11,* 264–273.

Iglesias, A., & Anderson, N. (1993). Dialectal variation. In J. Bernthal & N. Bankson (Eds.), *Articulation and phonological disorders* (3rd ed., pp. 147–161). Upper Saddle River, NJ: Prentice Hall.

Iglesias, A., & Goldstein, B. (1998). Language and dialectal variations. In J. Bernthal & N. Bankson (Eds.), *Articulation and phonological disorders* (4th ed., pp. 148–171). Boston, MA: Allyn & Bacon.

Ingram, D. (1976). *Phonological disability in children.* London, UK: Edward Arnold.

Jones, D. (1963). *The pronunciation of English.* Cambridge, UK: Cambridge University Press.

Jones, D. (1967). *An outline of English phonetics.* Cambridge, UK: W. Heffner.

Kent, R. (1997). *The speech sciences.* San Diego, CA: Singular.

Kent, R., & Read, C. (2002). *Acoustic analysis of speech* (2nd ed.). Boston, MA: Cengage.

Kretzschmar, W. (2008). Standard American English pronunciation. In E. W. Schneider (Ed.), *Varieties of English 2: The Americas and the Caribbean* (pp. 37–51). Berlin: De Gruyter Mouton.

Kurath, H. (1949). *Word geography of the eastern United States.* Ann Arbor: University of Michigan Press.

Labov, W. (1991). The three dialects of English. In P. Eckert (Ed.), *New ways of analyzing sound change* (pp. 1–44). San Diego, CA: Academic Press.

Labov, W., Ash, S., & Boberg, C. (2006). *The atlas of North American English: Phonetics, phonology and sound change.* Berlin: De Gruyter Mouton.

Ladefoged, P., & Johnson, K. (2011). *A course in phonetics* (6th ed.). Boston, MA: Wadsworth.

Lehiste, I. (1970). *Suprasegmentals.* Cambridge, MA: MIT Press.

Levitt, H., & Stromberg, L. (1983). Segmental characteristics of the speech of hearing-impaired children: Factors affecting intelligibility. In I. Hochberg, H. Levitt, & M. J. Osberger (Eds.), *Speech of the hearing impaired: Research, training, and personnel preparation* (pp. 53–73). Baltimore. MD: University Park Press.

Louko, L. J., & Edwards, M. L. (2001). Issues in collecting and transcribing speech samples. *Topics in Language Disorders, 21*(4), 1–11.

Lowe, R. (1996). *Workbook for the identification of phonological processes.* Austin, TX: Pro-Ed.

MacKay, I. (1987). *Phonetics: The science of speech production* (2nd ed.). Boston, MA: College Hill Press.

Monsen, R. B. (1983). General effects of deafness on phonation and articulation. In I. Hochberg, H. Levitt, & M. J. Osberger (Eds.), *Speech of the hearing impaired: Research, training, and personnel preparation* (pp. 23–34). Baltimore, MD: University Park Press.

Müller, N., & Guendouzi, J. A. (2007). Accent modification. In S. McLeod (Ed.), *The international guide to speech acquisition* (pp. 114–121). Clifton Park, NJ: Thomson Delmar Learning.

Nagy, N., & Roberts, J. (2008). New England: Phonology. In E. W. Schneider (Ed.), *Varieties of English 2: The Americas and the Caribbean* (pp. 52–66). Berlin: De Gruyter Mouton.

National Council of Teachers of English. (2008). *English language learners: A policy research brief.* Retrieved from http://www.ncte.org/library/NCTEFiles/Resources/PolicyResearch/ELLResearchBrief.pdf

Nihalani, P., Tongue, R. K., Hosali, P., & Crowther, J. (2004). *Indian and British English: A handbook of usage and pronunciation* (2nd ed.). New Delhi, India: Oxford University Press.

Ohde, R., & Sharf, D. (1992). Phonetic analysis of normal and abnormal speech. New York, NY: Merrill.

Owens, R. (1991). *Language disorders: A functional approach to assessment and intervention* (2nd ed.). Boston, MA: Allyn & Bacon.

Perez, E. (1994). Phonological differences among speakers of Spanish-Influenced English. In J. Bernthal & N. Bankson (Eds.), *Child phonology: Characteristics, assessment and intervention with special populations* (pp. 245–254). New York, NY: Thieme.

Peterson, G. E., & Barney, H. L. (1952). Control methods used in a study of the vowels. *Journal of the Acoustical Society of America, 24,* 175–184.

Pickett, J. M. (1999). *The acoustics of speech communication.* Boston, MA: Pearson.

Pike, K. L. (1945). *The intonation of American English.* Ann Arbor: University of Michigan Press.

Pollock, K. E., & Meredith, L. H. (2001). Phonetic transcription of African American Vernacular English. *Communication Disorders Quarterly, 23*(1), 47–53.

Poole, I. (1934). Genetic development of articulation of consonant sounds in speech. *Elementary English Review, 11,* 159–161.

Powell, T. W. (2001). Phonetic transcription of disordered speech. *Topics in Language Disorders, 21*(4), 52–72.

Power, T. (2014a). *Ted Power: English language learning and teaching.* Arabic language backgrounds. Retrieved from http://www.tedpower.co.uk/l1arabic.html

Power, T. (2014b). *Ted Power: English language learning and teaching.* Russian language backgrounds. Retrieved from http://www.tedpower.co.uk/l1russian.html

Prather, E. D., Hedrick, D. L., & Kern, C. A. (1975). Articulation development in children aged two to four years. *Journal of Speech and Hearing Disorders, 40,* 179–191.

Pullum, G. K., & Ladusaw, W. A. (1996). *Phonetic symbol guide* (2nd ed.). Chicago: University of Chicago Press.

Reed, V. (1994). *An introduction to children with language disorders* (2nd ed.). New York, NY: Merrill.

Ryan, C. (2013). *Language use in the United States: 2011.* American Community Survey Reports, ACS-22. Retrieved from the U.S. Census Bureau website: http://www.census.gov/prod/2013pubs/acs-22.pdf

Sailaja, P. (2009). *Dialects of English: Indian English.* Edinburgh, UK: Edinburgh University Press.

Sander, E. (1972). When are speech sounds learned? *Journal of Speech and Hearing Disorders, 37,* 55–63.

Shen, Y. (1962). *English phonetics: (Especially for teachers of English as a foreign language).* Ann Arbor: University of Michigan Press.

Shriberg, L., & Kent, R. (2013). *Clinical phonetics* (4th ed.). Boston, MA: Pearson.

Sikorski, L. (2005). Foreign accents: Suggested competencies for improving communicative pronunciation. *Seminars in Speech and Language, 26*(2), 126–130.

Singh, S., & Singh, K. (2006). *Phonetics: Principles and practices* (3rd ed.). San Diego, CA: Plural.

Smit, A. (1993). Phonologic error distributions in the Iowa-Nebraska Articulation Norms Project: Word-initial consonant clusters. *Journal of Speech and Hearing Research, 36,* 931–947.

Smit, A., Hand, L., Freilinger, J., Bernthal, J., & Bird, A. (1990). The Iowa Articulation Norms Project and its Nebraska replication. *Journal of Speech and Hearing Disorders, 55,* 779–798.

Stampe, D. (1969). *The acquisition of phonetic representation.* Paper presented at the Fifth Regional Meeting of the Chicago Linguistic Society, Chicago, IL.

Stockman, I. J. (2007). African American English speech acquisition. In S. McLeod (Ed.), *The international guide to speech acquisition* (pp. 148–160). Clifton Park, NY: Thomson Delmar Learning.

Stoel-Gammon, C. (1983). The acquisition of segmental phonology by normal and hearing-impaired children. In I. Hochberg, H. Levitt, & M. J. Osberger (Eds.), *Speech of the hearing-impaired: Research, training, and personnel preparation* (pp. 267–280). Baltimore, MD: University Park Press.

Stoel-Gammon, C. (2001). Transcribing the speech of young children. *Topics in Language Disorders, 21*(4), 12–21.

Stoel-Gammon, C., & Dunn, C. (1985). *Normal and disordered phonology in children.* Austin, TX: Pro-Ed.

Tayao, M. L. G. (2008). Philippine English: Phonology. In R. Mesthrie (Ed.), *Varieties of English 4: Africa, South, and Southeast Asia* (pp. 292–306). Berlin: De Gruyter Mouton.

Templin, M. C. (1957). *Certain language skills in children.* Minneapolis: University of Minnesota Press.

Teoh, A. P., & Chin, S. B. (2009). Transcribing the speech of children with cochlear implants: Clinical application of narrow phonetic transcriptions. *American Journal of Speech-Language Pathology, 18,* 388–401.

Terrell, S., & Terrell, F. (1993). African American cultures. In D. Battle (Ed.), *Communication disorders in multicultural populations* (pp. 3–37). Boston, MA: Andover Medical.

Thomas, E. (2008). Rural southern white accents. In E. W. Schneider (Ed.), *Varieties of English 2: The Americas and the Caribbean* (pp. 87–114). Berlin: De Gruyter Mouton.

Trost-Cardamone, J. E. (2009). Articulation and phonologic assessment procedures and treatment decisions. In K. T. Moller & L. E. Glaze (Eds.), *Cleft lip and palate: Interdisciplinary issues and treatment* (3rd ed., pp. 377–413). Austin, TX: Pro-Ed.

Trost-Cardamone, J. E., & Bernthal, J. E. (1993). Articulation assessment procedures and treatment decisions. In K. T. Moller & C. D. Starr (Eds.), *Cleft palate: Interdisciplinary issues and treatment* (pp. 307–336). Austin, TX: Pro-Ed.

Walters, N. P., & Trevelyan, E. N. (2011). *The newly arrived foreign-born population of the United States: 2010.* American Community Survey Briefs, ACSBR/10-16. Retrieved from the U.S. Census Bureau website: http://www.census.gov/prod/2011pubs/acsbr10-16.pdf

Wellman, B., Case, M., Mengert, E., & Bradbury, D. (1931). *Speech sounds of young children.* (University of Iowa Studies in Child Welfare, 5.) Iowa City: University of Iowa Press.

Wells, J. C. (1982a). *Accents of English 1: An introduction.* Cambridge, UK: Cambridge University Press.

Wells, J. C. (1982b). *Accents of English 3: Beyond the British Isles.* Cambridge, UK: Cambridge University Press.

Wolfram, W. (1991). *Dialects and American English.* Upper Saddle River, NJ: Prentice Hall.

Wolfram, W. (1994). The phonology of a sociocultural variety: The case of African American Vernacular English. In J. Bernthal & N. Bankson (Eds.), *Child phonology: Characteristics, assessment and intervention with special populations* (pp. 227–244). New York, NY: Thieme.

Wolfram, W., & Fasold, R. W. (1974). *The study of social dialects in American English.* Upper Saddle River, NJ: Prentice Hall.

Wolfram, W., & Schilling-Estes, N. (2006). *American English: Dialects and variation* (2nd ed.). Malden, MA: Blackwell.

Wolfram, W., & Thomas, E. R. (2002). *The development of African American English.* Malden, MA: Blackwell.

Yavaş, M. (2006). *Applied English phonology.* Malden, MA: Blackwell.

Answers to Questions

Chapter 1

Chapter Exercises

1.1 1. are you → ya; going to → gonna
2. can't you → cantcha; see her → see 'er
3. did you → ja

1.2 1. ə   2. θ   3. ʊ   4. ŋ   5. ɹ

Chapter 2

Chapter Exercises

2.1 __4__ lazy   __4__ smooth   __3__ cough

__5__ spilled   __6__ driven   __1__ oh

__3__ comb   __2__ why   __5__ raisin

__4__ thrill   __3__ judge   __3__ away

2.2 1. measure   2. rag   3. though   4. wood   5. was

2.3 Possible answers include:
1. deduct   4. scrutinize   7. dishonest   10. magnetize
2. protection   5. laborious   8. indecent
3. potential   6. greatly   9. later

2.4 __1__ caution   __2__ running   __2__ lived   __3__ relistened

__2__ warmly   __1__ finger   __2__ talker   __1__ kangaroo

__3__ prorated   __2__ clarinetist __2__ sharply   __2__ swarming

2.5   1. lend   ɛ   4. should   ʊ
      2. man   æ   5. rude   u
      3. flick   ɪ   6. week   i

2.6   1. ram   m   4. sung   ŋ
      2. laugh   f   5. bath   θ
      3. wish   ʃ   6. leave   v

2.7   1. ʃ   5. ʊ   9. dʒ
      2. ð   6. f   10. k
      3. tʃ   7. t   11. ʒ
      4. ɪ   8. ŋ   12. ɚ

2.8   Sample minimal pairs include:

      1. lame, came   4. wood, hood   7. toad, toes   10. rug, rush
      2. rate, sate   5. coil, toil   8. well, wedge
      3. doll, hall   6. harm, hard   9. cheat, cheese

2.9   X 1. kale, mail   X 6. find, fanned
      X 2. blog, blot   ___ 7. daughter, slaughter
      ___ 3. smart, smarts   X 8. twitch, switch
      ___ 4. rinse, sins   ___ 9. rings, brings
      ___ 5. bird, burned   X 10. limes, rhymes

2.11 ouch   **crab**   **hoe**   oats   elm   **your**
      re act   **car go**   **be ware**   a **tone**   **cour** age   eat ing

2.12 shrine   scold   plea   produce   schism   **away**
      elope   selfish   **auto**   biceps   flight   truce

2.13 through   spa   **rough**   bough   row   spray
      law **ful**   **fun** ny   cre **ate**   **in verse**   **can** dy   replay

2.14 O pliant   C comply   O coerced   C minutes
      O decree   C encase   C flatly   O preface

2.15 C pliant   O comply   C coerced   C minutes
      O decree   C encase   O flatly   C preface

2.16 1. shampoo   4. Marie
      2. careful   5. injure
      3. okay

2.17 propose   **contest**   **protest**   congress   **research**
      project   consume   **compress**   reasoned   **confines**

2.18 decoy   **mirage**   **pastel**   puzzle   **regret**   **platoon**
      stipend   thesis   **undo**   reason   falter   **Maureen**
      timid   planted   **derail**   virtue   **restricts**   peon
      transcend   **parade**   circus   **suspend**   movie   shoulder
      lucid   **cajole**   **devoid**   **cassette**   **provide**   merchant

2.19 **pondering**   **edited**   **consequent**   **misery**   **calendar**   **ebony**
plentiful   **asterisk**   pharyngeal   persona   distinctive   example
surrounded   December   **caribou**   **underling**   Barbados   lasagna
terrified   hydrangea   **telephoned**   contended   perfected   **India**
musical   **skeletal**   courageous   umbrella   **Philistine**   perusal

2.20 **stupendous**   pliable   **creative**   carefully   elevate   magical
corporal   answering   spectacle   **presumption**   **placenta**   **bananas**
plantation   clarinet   murderer   predisposed   **decorum**   horribly
heroic   violin   integer   **discover**   clavicle   **majestic**
daffodil   **subscription**   expertise   **immoral**   muscular   **Hawaii**

2.21   1, 3   phonemic
   2, 4   allophonic
   2, 4   impressionistic

Review Exercises

A. 1. bread   4   4. news   3   7. **fluid**   5   10. tomb   3
   2. coughs   4   5. **plot**   4   8. **spew**   4   11. walked   4
   3. throw   3   6. stroke   5   9. **fat**   3   12. **last**   4

B. 1. clueless   2   6. rewrite   2
   2. tomato   1   7. winterized   3
   3. pumpkin   1   8. edits   2
   4. likable   2   9. thoughtlessness   3
   5. cheddar   1   10. coexisting   3

C. 1. puss   6. flew
   2. dogs   7. limb
   3. league   8. wheeze
   4. pant   9. giraffe
   5. beau   10. cloth

D. 1. ten   6. name
   2. less   7. nip
   3. stop   8. nab
   4. tan   9. cat
   5. dean   10. newt

E. 1. chef   6. song
   2. cut   7. gnaw
   3. think   8. chore
   4. came   9. goat
   5. please   10. their

F. Possible answers include:
   1. slit, skit   6. fun, fine
   2. band, canned   7. sought, caught
   3. sink, think   8. hid, herd
   4. win, chin   9. shook, book
   5. paid, page   10. rib, rube

G. 1. **maybe, baby**   6. **bribe, tribe**
    2. plaid, prod   7. smart, dart
    3. **looks, lacks**   8. **shout, pout**
    4. mail, mailed   9. window, minnow
    5. **prance, prince**   10. **lumpy, bumpy**

H. 1. mar<u>bl</u>e ___C___   6. <u>a</u>wesome ___O___
    2. <u>pr</u>evious ___O___   7. mis<u>tak</u>e ___C___
    3. pa<u>tr</u>on ___C___   8. luck<u>y</u> ___O___
    4. <u>tr</u>ifle ___O___   9. profi<u>t</u> ___C___
    5. <u>so</u>dium ___O___   10. <u>sy</u>stem ___C___

I.

	Onset Yes	Onset No	Coda Yes	Coda No
1. mentions	X		X	
2. icon		X		X
3. camper	X		X	
4. instinct		X	X	
5. able		X		X
6. lotion	X			X
7. charming	X		X	
8. asterisk		X	X	
9. Japan	X			X
10. aloof		X		X

J. __1__ 1. loser   __2__ 6. provoke   __1__ 11. plastic
    __2__ 2. unsure   __1__ 7. stagnant   __2__ 12. divorce
    __1__ 3. anxious   __2__ 8. beside   __1__ 13. western
    __2__ 4. disturb   __2__ 9. germane   __1__ 14. language
    __1__ 5. Grecian   __2__ 10. gourmet   __2__ 15. defer

K. __2__ 1. provincial   __1__ 6. hypocrite   __3__ 11. picturesque
    __1__ 2. sorceress   __3__ 7. indisposed   __1__ 12. relegate
    __1__ 3. indigent   __2__ 8. uncertain   __2__ 13. foundation
    __2__ 4. commander   __2__ 9. magenta   __2__ 14. contagious
    __3__ 5. arabesque   __1__ 10. platypus   __1__ 15. constable

L. __3__ 1. problematic   __3__ 6. correlation   __3__ 11. protozoan
    __1__ 2. mercenary   __1__ 7. catamaran   __1__ 12. contradiction
    __2__ 3. statistical   __2__ 8. continuant   __1__ 13. protoplasm
    __1__ 4. ecosystem   __1__ 9. allegory   __1__ 14. Argentina
    __2__ 5. gregarious   __2__ 10. carnivorous __2__ 15. obstructionist

Chapter 3

Chapter Exercises

3.1 Possible answers include:
    voiced   /r/, /l/, /d/
    voiceless   /p/, /t/, /h/

3.2 The phoneme /b/ is produced by closing the lips.
    The phoneme /w/ is produced by rounding the lips; the lips do not close.

3.3 __X__ choose   __X__ way   _____ car

    _____ lamb   __X__ road   __X__ look

    _____ this   __X__ heard   _____ mess

3.4 The phoneme in the word <u>th</u>ink is voiceless: /θ/
    The phoneme in the word <u>th</u>at is voiced: /ð/

3.5 1. soft palate or velum   5. (hard) palate
    2. alveolar ridge   6. glottis
    3. tongue   7. teeth
    4. lips

Review Exercises

A. 1. b   2. c   3. d   4. a

B. 1. fundamental frequency   4. diaphragm
   2. mandible   5. subglottal
   3. a. in front of   6. habitual
      b. below   7. blade; apex
      c. above   8. front; back
      d. to the rear   9. timbre

C. 1. c   5. c   9. a
   2. a   6. d   10. d
   3. b   7. c
   4. b   8. b

D. 1. T   5. T   9. F
   2. F   6. F   10. T
   3. F   7. T
   4. T   8. T

E. 1. b   5. b   9. e
   2. d   6. c   10. a
   3. a   7. b
   4. d   8. d

Chapter 4

Preliminary Exercise 1

U	1.	R	6.
R	2.	U	7.
R	3.	U	8.
U	4.	U	9.
R	5.	R	10.

Preliminary Exercise 2

T	1.	T	5.
L	2.	T	6.
L	3.	L	7.
L	4.	T	8.

Chapter Exercises

4.1—The Vowel /i/

A.

paper	train	**Cleveland**	**seaside**
please	picture	trip	trail
tribal	**machine**	labor	**trees**
settle	**screen**	**Toledo**	lip
nice	foreign	**Levi**	**jeans**

B.

/ist/	/flip/	**/min/**	**/hid/**
/iv/	/hig/	/lim/	/wins/
/rift/	/if/	**/trit/**	**/lik/**

C.

/lip/	leap	/it/	eat	/brizd/	breezed
/pip/	peep	/hip/	heap	/spik/	speak
/mit/	meat, meet	/sip/	seep	/klin/	clean
/rid/	reed, read	/did/	deed	/krist/	creased

D.

___	dream	drip	X	east	eaves
X	seek	wheel	___	chief	vein
___	same	land	___	base	lease
X	creek	steam	___	need	pain
X	bean	heed	X	creed	cream

4.2—The Vowel /ɪ/

B. peace   friend   enthrall   **bitter**
   mythical   **silver**   woman   **tryst**
   click   **ingest**   **build**   **fear**
   thread   **pink**   **bowling**   tried
   pride   **clear**   **sporty**   **synchronize**

C. /vɪl/   **/sɪst/**   **/fɪld/**   **/wɪns/**
   /izɪ/   /klip/   **/spid/**   /hik/
   /hɪr/   /ɪl/   /sɪg/   **/pɪgɪ/**

D. /stip/   steep   /pɪk/   pick
   /pliz/   please   /kɪst/   kissed
   /mɪt/   mitt   /bik/   beak
   /dɪd/   did   /pɪp/   pip
   /fɪr/   fear   /mɪstɪ/   misty
   /rilɪ/   really   /ɪndid/   indeed

E. X feel   teach   X win   king
       lip   thread   X mint   inch
    X been   drink   X deed   flea
       vent   list   X dish   ill
       tied   pig   X kick   mill

F. 1. ___ flirt   5. _X_ smeared   9. ___ stirred
   2. _X_ peerless   6. ___ worried   10. ___ stared
   3. ___ bird   7. _X_ steered   11. _X_ earring
   4. ___ shrill   8. ___ harder   12. ___ cursor

4.3—The Vowel /e/ - /eɪ/

B. **trail**   **rage**   wheel   **palatial**
   vice   **razor**   manage   green
   transit   machine   **whale**   **potato**
   lazy   bread   football   temperate
   dale   **tackle**   **daily**   bright

C. **/freɪd/**   /pɪln/   /trips/   **/spid/**
   /kreɪt/   /deɪs/   **/blid/**   **/treɪ/**
   /neɪp/   **/biz/**   /dɪnt/   /feɪlm/
   /deɪlɪ/   **/deɪm/**   /fril/   /streɪp/

D. /bleɪz/   blaze   /pleɪket/   placate

   /pleɪd/   played   /rimeɪn/   remain

   /beɪn/   bane   /ɪnmeɪt/   inmate

   /iveɪd/   evade   /ribet/   rebate

   /krɪmp/   crimp   /steɪnd/   stained

   /rikt/   reeked   /deɪzɪ/   daisy

E. **O** crayon   **C** unmade

   O prepay   **O** stay

   C baking   **O** tailor

   O masonry   **C** betrayed

F. ___ braid hid   **X** state rain

   ___ feed hate   ___ fist flea

   X lane aim   **X** cringe hid

   X fill kissed   ___ deal will

   ___ treat sling   **X** wheel meat

G. **eɪ** neighbor   **e** Crayola

   eɪ crate   **eɪ** basin

   e donate   **eɪ** stay

   eɪ hooray   **e** prostrate

   eɪ saber   **e** incubate

4.4—The Vowel /ɛ/

B. pimple   trip   **ensure**   tryst
   syrup   **caring**   women   **contend**
   pencil   butter   build   **pretzel**
   thing   **thread**   **prepare**   tried
   jeep   pistol   **unscented** **remember**

C. **/mɛrɪ/**   /hint/   /split/   /ɪstɛr/
   /slɛpt/ **/fɛr/**   /ɪrk/   **/meɪd/**
   /sɪsɪ/   /kleɪ/   **/wɛl/**   **/krip/**

D. /reɪk/   rake   /stɛr/   stare

/fɪz/   fizz   /treɪl/   trail

/smɛl/   smell   /pritɛnd/   pretend

/sid/   seed   /hɛvɪ/   heavy

/kreɪn/   crane   /friz/   freeze

/breɪzd/   braised   /blɛst/   blessed

E.
X	fill	fear		X	step	edge
X	made	cage		___	bread	breathe
___	wind	best		___	flit	red
___	trade	peel		X	sill	kit
X	rid	sing		X	care	meant

F.
C	1. trail		O	6. spree
O	2. repay		C	7. arouse
C	3. strike		C	8. rough
O	4. plea		O	9. undo
C	5. late		O	10. chow

G.
1. **X** share   6. **X** careful

2. ___ early   7. **X** sparrow

3. ___ dearly   8. ___ third

4. **X** compare   9. ___ corridor

5. ___ fluoride   10. ___ certain

4.5—The Vowel /æ/

B.
straddle	**practice**	**lapse**	**revamp**
pale	**panther**	**repast**	straight
Lester	pacific	**pacify**	farmer
baseball	**hanged**	**chances**	cards
jazz	pistol	tamed	**bombastic**

C.
/klæd/	/prid/	/strɪv/	/wæd/
/slæpt/	**/bɪrd/**	/bæz/	**/trækt/**
/web/	/steɪp/	**/sprɪg/**	/læzɪ/

D. /klæn/   clan   /spɪr/   spear
    /sprɪnt/   sprint   /hɛrɪ/   hairy, Harry
    /rɛk/   wreck   /pækt/   packed
    /teɪstɪ/   tasty   /dræg/   drag
    /præns/   prance   /bɛrɪ/   berry
    /læft/   laughed   /tinz/   teens

E. ___   badge   rage   X   hair   bend
    ___   seed   shade   X   lick   beer
    ___   cab   blonde   ___ beak   bless
    X   tray   whale   ___ trap   bake
    X   crank   shag   X   lapse   crag

4.6—The Vowel /u/

A. **ghoul**   oboe   **crew**   plural
    butter   stuck   **Lucifer**   must
    should   luck   lusty   shook
    fuchsia   look   molding   **stupor**
    loosely   **glue**   blouse   **choose**

B. /ust/   **/krud/**   /prus/   **/tul/**
    /suv/   /tug/   /pus/   **/wund/**
    /pul/   /rup/   **/lus/**   /slug/

C. /spun/   spoon   /sup/   soup
    /tun/   tune   /lud/   lewd
    /rut/   root   /stru/   strew
    /mud/   mood   /flu/   flew, flue, flu
    /klu/   clue   /grum/   groom
    /ruf/   roof   /snut/   snoot

D. ___ 1. could   showed   ___ 6. brood   hood
    X   2. suit   loon   X   7. stood   could
    ___ 3. lute   book   ___ 8. hoops   poor
    X   4. crew   scoot   X   9. feud   moose
    X   5. push   foot   ___ 10. muse   cook

E. ___ 1. oozing   ___ 4. ruined   ___ 7. Pluto   ___ 10. spooky
    X   2. cute   ___ 5. sloop   X   8. useful
    X   3. huge   X   6. fuming   X   9. viewing

4.7—The Vowel /ʊ/

B.

hole	**wooden**	snooze	stunned
shut	punched	luscious	spook
hood	**couldn't**	**pulled**	**shook**
flushed	**mistook**	beauty	person
rudely	**cooker**	brood	**stood**

C.

/buk/	/stʊ/	**/rul/**	/sul/
/lʊv/	**/lum/**	**/rʊk/**	**/frut/**
/trups/	/stʊr/	**/buts/**	/slʊg/

D.

/pʊs/	puss	/tʊr/	tour
/tru/	true	/hʊk/	hook
/stʊd/	stood	/lum/	loom
/dum/	doom	/fluk/	fluke
/gru/	grew	/prun/	prune
/gʊd/	good	/krʊk/	crook

E.

___	1.	loot	foot	___	6.	what	look
X	2.	tune	mute	X	7.	nook	stood
X	3.	coupe	soon	___	8.	rust	rook
___	4.	flood	cute	X	9.	goof	cruise
X	5.	would	soot	___	10.	mutt	look

4.8—The Vowel /o/ - /oʊ/

B.

mope	aloof	root	**toll**
noose	**slowed**	pond	push
soda	lost	**loaded**	**lasso**
nosy	book	sugar	**remote**
dole	**spoke**	doily	**wholly**

C.

/toʊ/	**/boʊn/**	**/stup/**	/prʊb/
/bʊt/	**/floʊd/**	**/boʊd/**	**/krud/**
/stub/	**/stud/**	/flʊk/	**/woʊnt/**

D.

/moʊld/	mold	/tupeɪ/	toupee
/kupt/	cooped	/bruzd/	bruised
/boʊnɪ/	bony	/bændeɪd/	Band-Aid
/ivoʊk/	evoke	/kʊkɪ/	cookie
/stoʊd/	stowed	/koʊɛd/	coed
/doʊpɪ/	dopey	/rizum/	resume

E. __o__ Romania   __ou__ snowman   __ou__ bowling

    __ou__ corroded   __o__ location   __ou__ though

    __ou__ stolen   __ou__ jello   __o__ notation

    __ou__ magnolia   __o__ coagulate   __o__ potential

4.9—The Vowel /ɔ/

A. /**bɔt**/   /drʊm/   /stɔn/   /**brɔn**/
    /**koʊt**/   /grɔn/   /**tɔk**/   /**pʊl**/
    /**lups**/   /**fɔrt**/   /**flum**/   /ɔrn/

B. /spɔrt/   sport   /sprɔl/   sprawl

    /kʊd/   could   /stʊd/   stood

    /proʊb/   probe   /frɔt/   fraught

    /pruv/   prove   /kɔrps/   corpse

    /stɔrd/   stored   /hʊkt/   hooked

    /ɔfʊl/   awful   /doʊnet/   donate

C. 1. _____ farm   4. __X__ storm   7. _____ lured

    2. _____ third   5. _____ worm   8. _____ worth

    3. __X__ horrid   6. __X__ thorn   9. _____ spar

4.10—The Vowel /ɑ/

B. /wond/   /tɔb/   /**hɑrm**/   /**blɑb**/
    /**koʊd**/   /sɔt/   /blɑd/   /**ɑrmɪ**/
    /**frɔd**/   /pʊnt/   /**ɑd**/   /**kɑd**/

C. /frɑst/   frost   /zɑr/   czar

    /lʊkt/   looked   /prund/   pruned

    /bɔrd/   board, bored   /blɔnd/   blonde

    /kroʊm/   chrome   /ɑnsɛt/   onset

    /wɑnt/   want   /krɔdæd/   crawdad

    /stɑrvd/   starved   /ɑrdvɑrk/   aardvark

D. 1. _____ war   7. _____ orchard

    2. _____ cleared   8. __X__ March

    3. _____ quartz   9. _____ poorly

    4. _____ flare   10. __X__ smarter

    5. __X__ starred   11. __X__ carbon

    6. _____ dirt   12. _____ spore

4.11—The Vowel /ə/

A. rowing · **lasagna** · **wooded** · **Laverne** · **decision**
injure · poorly · ruled · **control** · glamour
motion · holding · **untamed** · **opera** · puppy
fuchsia · laundry · **petunia** · cockroach · **lotion**

B. /sətɪn/ · **/drɑmə/** · **/səpoʊz/**
/zəbrɑ/ · /ləpʊr/ · /rəpik/
/əbeɪt/ · **/bəlun/** · **/brəzɪl/**
/əluf/ · /rədæn/ · /əndu/

C.
/pinət/	peanut	/kənteɪn/	contain
/əkrɑs/	across	/lɛmən/	lemon
/vəlɔr/	velour	/bətɑn/	baton
/səpɔrt/	support	/əwɔrd/	award
/kɔfɪn/	coffin	/eɪprəl/	April
/plətun/	platoon	/kəsɛt/	cassette

4.12—The Vowel /ʌ/

B. awful · **custard** · pushy · cologne · charades
blunder · laborious · cushion · **abundant** · mundane
laundry · **Sunday** · **hundred** · plural · wander
Hoover · lawyer · **trumpet** · shouldn't · conducive

C.
1. hooked	/hʌkt/	X	6. rookie	/rʌkɪ/	X
2. bond	/bʊnd/	X	7. mistook	/mɪstʊk/	___
3. bluff	/blʌf/	___	8. lucky	/lʌkɪ/	X
4. hood	/hud/	X	9. rubbing	/rʊbɪŋ/	X
5. cluck	/klʌk/	___	10. crooked	/krɔkəd/	X

D. /klʊstɪ/ · **/rizən/** · **/mʌstɪ/**
/əpʌft/ · /krɑmd/ · /əndʌn/
/dʊkɪ/ · **/pʊlɪ/** · **/plʌmət/**
/sʌntæn/ · /vɪstʌ/ · **/plæzə/**

E.
/pɛrəs/	Paris	/robʌst/	robust
/hʌnɪ/	honey	/sʌdən/	sudden
/əlɑt/	allot; a lot	/kəbus/	caboose
/kənvɪns/	convince	/tʌndrə/	tundra
/gɑrdəd/	guarded	/kəlæps/	collapse
/flʌbd/	flubbed	/bəfun/	buffoon

F. lumber /ʌ/   suspend /ə/
  abort /ə/   suppose /ə/
  shaken /ə/   induct /ʌ/
  contain /ə/   serpent /ə/
  thunder /ʌ/   rusty /ʌ/

G. _____ 1. nuts could   _____ 6. crook fund

    _____ 2. foot stoop   __X__ 7. blood crust

    __X__ 3. done rubbed   __X__ 8. runs floods

    __X__ 4. crumb rust   __X__ 9. loom food

    __X__ 5. cook should   _____ 10. rush look

4.13—The Vowel /ɚ/

B. **clover**   rebel   barley   dearly
  fearless   endear   **perjure** **fester**
  carbon   torment **harbor** electric
  tremor   written   poorly   breezy
  laundered **perhaps** torpedo **surprise**

C. /kʌnvɚt/   /pɚteɪn/   **/pɚsɛnt/** /lɛpɚd/
  /rabɚ/   /tɚoʊd/   **/drimɚ/** /fɚəst/
  /sɚvɛs/   /ɚɛdɪ/   /ʌnfɛr/   **/hɪndɚ/**

D. /drɛsɚ/   dresser   /kəntɔrt/ contort

  /kæmrə/ camera   /pɚɑnə/   piranha

  /rʌbɚ/   rubber   /pɚu/   Peru

  /mɑrbəl/ marble   /sɪmɚ/   simmer

  /tɚeɪn/   terrain   /kɛrosin/ kerosene

  /flʌstɚd/ flustered   /əweɪtəd/ awaited

4.14—The Vowel /ɝ/

B. forward   pretend   January   barren
  disturbed **turban** **stirrup** morale
  terrible   arid   steered   persistent
  conversion warship distort   choir
  muster   **wordy**   **conserve** fearless

C. /kʌstɚd/   /lɝdɪ/   **/kərɪr/** /vɝsəz/
  /pɝsən/   **/hɝdəd/** **/fɝmɚ/** /dɝsənt/
  /plædɝ/   **/fɔrən/** /ɝbɔrt/ **/kɝsɚ/**

D. /smɝkt/ smirked   /kənvɚt/ convert

    /ovɝt/ overt   /wɪspɚ/ whisper

    /kɛrət/ carrot   /bɝbən/ bourbon

    /sʌbɚb/ suburb   /skwɝts/ squirts

    /supɝb/ superb   /səhɛrə/ Sahara

E. erasure   /ɚ/   ermine   /ɝ/
    surprise /ɚ/   color   /ɚ/
    furnace   /ɝ/   infer   /ɝ/
    curtail   /ɚ/   terror   /ɚ/
    immerse   /ɝ/   duster   /ɚ/

F. _____ 1. herd   cheered   _____ 6. hair   queer
    _____ 2. cord   word   X   7. birch lurk
    _____ 3. lured   stored   X   8. hoard lord
      X   4. ark   smart   _____ 9. pear   heard
      X   5. fears   cheer   _____ 10. term peered

G.   ɝ   1. myrth   ɪr 11. appearance
     ɛr 2. flared   ɛr 12. Carol
     ɪr 3. cirrus   ɝ   13. furtive
     ɛr 4. serenade   ɛr 14. larynx
     ɝ   5. Merlin   ɪr 15. experience
     ɛr 6. cherub   ɝ   16. disturbing
     ɔr 7. portion   ɪr 17. clearance
     ɑr 8. farming   ɝ   18. nervous
     ɛr 9. sparrow   ɝ, ʊr 19. furious
     ɝ 10. nervous   ɛr 20. clairvoyant

4.15—The Diphthong /aɪ/

B. power   spacious   machine   replaced
    slice   delicious   **formica**   traded
    contrite **spider**   maybe   **piped**
    lever   **Cairo**   **cider**   **supplied**
    rivalry razor   piano   spigot

C. /fraɪdeɪ/   /braɪmɚ/   /taɪfraɪn/   /rəvaɪz/
    /məbaɪ/   /naɪlɔn/   /prədaɪt/   /traɪdɛnt/
    /traɪd/   /laɪɚ/   /haɪəst/   /straɪpt/

D. /sɚpraɪz/ surprise   /klaɪmæks/ climax

/kəlaɪd/ collide   /preɪlin/ praline

/treɪlɚ/ trailer   /baɪsɛps/ biceps

/praɪmeɪt/ primate   /waɪɚd/ wired

/vaɪrəs/ virus   /taɪred/ tirade

/deɪlaɪt/ daylight   /daɪmənd/ diamond

4.16—The Diphthong /ɔɪ/

B.
repay	**hoisted**	**voiceless**	reward
loiter	crowded	fiery	tiled
straight	feisty	**coy**	**cloying**
crime	**broiler**	stoic	**destroy**
goiter	razor	**avoid**	supplied

C.
/kwaɪət/	/sprɔɪdɪn/	/dɔɪəz/	/plɔɪdənt/
/mɝdɚ/	**/blaɪndlɪ/**	/ənstraɪt/	**/taɪpsɛt/**
/pɔɪzən/	**/vɔɪdəd/**	**/rikɔɪld/**	/taɪwɑn/

D. /ɔɪlɪ/ oily   /ændrɔɪd/ android

/maɪstroʊ/ maestro   /laɪvlɪ/ lively

/taɪfɔɪd/ typhoid   /ɪnvɔɪs/ invoice

/parbɔɪl/ parboil   /ɔɪstɚ/ oyster

/haɪndsaɪt/ hindsight   /haɪɔɪd/ hyoid

/baɪaʊt/ buyout   /deɪlaɪt/ daylight

4.17—The Diphthong /aʊ/

B.
toilet	**dowdy**	**frown**	**bounty**
mousy	**allowed**	loaded	probate
beauty	explode	soils	**proud**
astound	toil	**chowder**	crowbar
hello	toad	chastise	scrolled

C.
/taɪɚd/	**/laʊzɪ/**	**/aɪvrɪ/**	**/hoʊmbɔɪ/**
/rɪbaʊ/	/blaʊkɚ/	/rɔɪdɪ/	/kaʊtaʊ/
/waʊntɪd/	/roʊgbɪ/	/paʊzɚ/	**/aʊɚlɪ/**

D. /bɔɪfrɛnd/ boyfriend   /roʊboʊt/ rowboat

/klɑndaɪk/ Klondike   /pispaɪp/ peace pipe

/daʊntaʊn/ downtown   /sɚaʊnd/ surround

/sloʊɚ/ slower   /doʊnʌt/ doughnut

/faʊndəd/ founded   /klaɪənt/ client

/vaɪzɚ/ visor   /braʊzɚ/ browser

Review Exercises

A.

ʊ	high	back	yes	lax
ɝ	mid	central	yes	tense
ə	mid	central	no	lax
o	high-mid	back	yes	tense
u	high	back	yes	tense
ɛ	low-mid	front	no	lax
ɚ	mid	central	yes	lax
ʌ	low-mid	back-central	no	lax
e	high-mid	front	no	tense
ɪ	high	front	no	lax
ɑ	low	back	no	tense
ɔ	low-mid	back	yes	tense
æ	low	front	no	lax

B.
1. æ, bad
2. ʌ, sun
3. ɛ, slept
4. u, soup
5. ɔ, cord
6. ʊ, foot
7. ɪ, fizz
8. ɑ, park
9. ɝ, word
10. oʊ, crows

C.
1. Sunday	L	T		6. concern	L	T
2. bashful	L	L		7. regroup	T	T
3. laundry	T	L		8. obese	T	T
4. confused	L	T		9. layette	T	L
5. fender	L	L		10. abrupt	L	L

D.
1. foolish	R	U		6. Pluto	R	R
2. curfew	R	R		7. person	R	U
3. decade	U	U		8. pursuit	R	R
4. collate	R	U		9. rugby	U	U
5. football	R	U/R*		10. lower	R	U

*Depending on pronunciation (i.e., /ɑ/ or /ɔ/).

E.   /eɪ/ 1. straight   /ɛ/ /ɪ/ 11. empty
     /i/   2. bees   /eɪ/ /ɪ/ 12. rabies
     /ɛ/   3. bread   /ɪ/ /ɛ/ 13. instead
     /æ/   4. can   /æ/ /i/ 14. stampede
     /ɪ/   5. filled   /eɪ/ /e/ 15. vacate
     /ɪ/   6. bring   /i/ /ɪ/ 16. pleasing
     /æ/   7. lapse   /æ/ /ɪ/ 17. transit
     /æ/   8. sang   /i/ /æ/ 18. beer can
     /ɛ/   9. fair   /ɪ/ /æ/ 19. implant
     /i/ 10. mean   /ɛr/ /ɪ/ 20. barely

F.   /oʊ/ 1. moat   /ɔ/ /ʊ/ 11. awful
     /ʊ/   2. push   /ɔr/ /ɑ/ 12. Clorox
     /ɑ/   3. laud   /oʊ/ /oʊ/ 13. loco
     /ɑ/   4. locks   /oʊ/ /oʊ/ 14. oboe
     /u/   5. crude   /ɑ/ /oʊ/ 15. taco
     /oʊ/ 6. chose   /ɑ/ /ɑr/ 16. monarch
     /ɑ/   7. raw   /ɑ/ /ɔr/ 17. popcorn
     /ʊr/ 8. lure   /u/ /ʊ/ 18. truthful
     /ɔr/ 9. sword   /ɑ/ /u/ 19. costume
     /ɑr/ 10. card   /u/ /ɑ/ 20. crouton

G.   /ɝ/ /ə/(ɪ) 1. certain   /ɝ/ /ə/   11. purpose
     /ʌ/ /ə/   2. rusted   /ʌ/ /ə/(ɪ) 12. sudden
     /ɚ/ /ɝ/   3. perturb   /ʌ/ /ɚ/   13. luster
     /ə/ /ɝ/   4. assert   /ɝ/ /ə/   14. purchase
     /ʌ/ /ɚ/   5. upper   /ɝ/ /ɚ/   15. sherbet
     /ɝ/ /ɚ/   6. merger   /ʌ/ /ɚ/   16. mother
     /ʌ/ /ɚ/   7. clutter   /ə/ /ɝ/   17. converge
     /ɝ/ /ə/   8. verbal   /ɝ/ /ɚ/   18. herder
     /ə/ /ɝ/   9. traverse   /ɝ/ /ə/   19. worded
     /ɝ/ /ɚ/   10. learner   /ʌ/ /ɚ/   20. mustard

H.
1.	word	/wɝd/	
2.	lard	/lɔrd/	/ɑr/
3.	carp	/kɝp/	/ɑr/
4.	war	/wɑr/	/ɔr/
5.	mere	/mɪr/	
6.	wide	/weɪd/	/aɪ/
7.	curd	/kʊrd/	/ɝ/
8.	stay	/steɪ/	
9.	pray	/praɪ/	/eɪ/
10.	crow	/kraʊ/	/oʊ/
11.	coin	/kɔɪn/	
12.	pride	/praɪd/	
13.	firm	/fɪrm/	/ɝ/
14.	tour	/tʊr/	
15.	fair	/fɛr/	

16.	maestro	/maɪstroʊ/	
17.	flour	/floʊɚ/	/aʊ/
18.	pouring	/pɔrɪŋ/	
19.	liar	/laɪɚ/	
20.	appear	/əpɛr/	/ɪr/
21.	tighter	/taɪtɝ/	/ɚ/
22.	parrot	/pɝət/	/ɛr/
23.	corner	/kɔrnɚ/	
24.	oyster	/ɔɪstɛr/	/ɚ/
25.	squarely	/skwɛrlɪ/	
26.	silence	/sɪləns/	/aɪ/
27.	smarter	/smɔrtɚ/	/ɑr/
28.	avoid	/əvaɪd/	/ɔɪ/
29.	prowess	/proəs/	/aʊ/
30.	license	/leɪsəns/	/aɪ/

I.
1. p___ pier (peer), pour (poor), pore, par, pear (pair), purr

2. r___ rear, roar, rare

3. d___t dart, dirt

4. w___d weird, ward, word

5. k___d cord, card, cared, curd

J.
1. ___d id, aid, Ed, add, oohed, owed, awed, odd

2. ___n in, an (Ann), own, on, urn (earn)

3. l___st least, list, laced, lest, last, lost, lust

4. sk___n skin, skein, scan, scone

5. st___d steed, stayed (staid), stead, stewed, stood, stowed, stirred, stud

6. b___rd beard, bared, board (bored), bard, bird

7. t___nt tint, taint, tent, taunt

8. s___t seat, sit, sate, set, sat, suit, soot, sought, sot

9. r___t writ, rate, ret, rat, root, wrought, rote, rot, rut

10. r___bd ribbed, robed, robbed, rubbed

11. sp___t spit, spate, spat, spot, spurt

12. w___d weed, wade, wed, wooed, wood (would), wad, word

K.   1. customs
      2. abound
      3. toward
      4. slender
      5. carefree
      6. vacant
      7. bunted
      8. cloudy
      9. stapler
     10. contort

     11. sirens
     12. cloistered
     13. Ohio
     14. radio
     15. corrosive
     16. platonic
     17. resonate
     18. digress
     19. siphoned
     20. Arkansas

     21. wonderful
     22. calendar
     23. remorseful
     24. stupendous
     25. laxative
     26. sincerely
     27. colander
     28. Raisinettes
     29. baritone
     30. December

     31. Mexico
     32. quagmire
     33. orderly
     34. herbicide
     35. repulsive
     36. character
     37. sassafras
     38. xylophone
     39. quarterback
     40. embarrassed

L.   /ɛ/ /ɪ/   1. epic
      /æ/ /ɚ/   2. faster
      /ʌ/ /ɚ/   3. wonder
      /ɑ/ /ɛ/   4. octet
      /ʊ/ /ə/   5. woolen
      /i/ /oʊ/ 6. depot
      /oʊ/ /ɚ/   7. soldier
      /ɪ/ /ɪ/   8. itchy
      /ɝ/ /ɪ/   9. worship
      /æ/ /ə/ 10. palace
      /ɛr/ /ɪ/ 11. barely
      /eɪ/ /ə/ 12. nation
      /i/ /ə/ 13. genius
      /ʌ/ /ɚ/ 14. cupboard
      /ɑr/ /u/ 15. cartoon
      /æ/ /ɪ/ 16. nasty
      /ɪr/ /ə/ 17. fearless
      /ʌ/ /ɚ/ 18. number
      /æ/ /ə/ 19. sanction
      /oʊ/ /ə/ 20. ocean

      /ɪ/ /ɪ/ 21. inkling
      /ɛr/ /æ/ 22. Fairbanks
      /ɑr/ /u/ 23. car pool
      /ə/ /i/ 24. machine
      /æ/ /ə/ 25. Athens
      /ɑ/ /ə/ 26. autumn
      /i/ /ə/ 27. rebus
      /ɔr/ /ɛ/ 28. torment
      /ʌ/ /ɚ/ 29. utter
      /ʊ/ /ə/ 30. bushel
      /ɔr/ /ɚ/ 31. corner
      /ɑ/ /ɪ/ 32. quandary
      /æ/ /ɚ/ 33. aster
      /oʊ/ /u/ 34. phone booth
      /ɝ/ /ə/ 35. turban
      /i/ /eɪ/ 36. key case
      /ɔr/ /ɚ/ 37. boarder
      /ɛr/ /ɪ/ 38. blaring
      /æ/ /ə/ 39. strangle
      /ɔ/ /ə/ 40. awesome

M. /ɔɪ/ /ɚ/   1. broiler   /ɛ/   /ɚ/   16. gender

    /ɑʊ/ /æ/   2. mousetrap   /aɪ/ /ə/   17. China

    /ɔr/ /ɑ/   3. boardwalk   /ɔ/   /ɪ/   18. jaundiced

    /oʊ/ /ɚ/   4. closure   /ɝ/   /ɔɪ/ 19. turquoise

    /aɪ/ /ɑ/   5. nylons   /ɪ/   /ɔɪ/ 20. invoice

    /ɛr/ /ɔɪ/ 6. steroid   /aɪ/ /æ/   21. financed

    /ɑr/ /ʌ/   7. starstruck   /ɝ/   /ə/   22. merchant

    /ə/   /i/   8. regime   /o/   /eɪ/ 23. proclaim

    /æ/   /ʊ/   9. bashful   /oʊ/ /e/   24. probate

    /ɝ/   /ɚ/   10. perjure   /ə/   /aɪ/ 25. July

    /ɪr/ /ɪ/   11. spearmint   /ɑr/ /ə/   26. martian

    /aɪ/ /ʌ/   12. lightbulb   /u/   /ɚ/   27. future

    /i/   /ɔɪ/ 13. destroy   /ɑ/   /ɛ/   28. prospect

    /æ/   /ə/(ɪ) 14. banquet   /ɑ/   /ə/   29. product

    /aɪ/ /ɔr/ 15. eyesore   /o/   /u/   30. tofu

Chapter 5

Preliminary Exercise 1

    a   1. seem   b   6. oily

    c   2. trade   a   7. hotdog

    b   3. away   b   8. hasten

    a   4. cruise   b   9. open

    c   5. oaf   c   10. football

Preliminary Exercise 2

    f   1. /r/   b   4. /f/

    a   2. /d/   d   5. /n/

    e   3. /w/   c   6. /tʃ/

Preliminary Exercise 3

    ___   1. me, we   ___   6. shoot, suit

    X   2. seal, zeal   ___   7. flame, blame

    ___   3. plan, clan   X   8. dram, tram

    ___   4. lice, rice   ___   9. yes, chess

    X   5. grain, crane   X   10. vender, fender

Chapter Exercises

5.1—The Stop Consonants

A.   ___ 1. wish   ___ 6. runs   ___ 11. church   X 16. think

         X 2. spring   X 7. whisper   X 12. tomb   ___ 17. rummage

         ___ 3. loom   X 8. question   X 13. logical   ___ 18. realm

         X 4. brush   X 9. system   ___ 14. jeans   X 19. guess

         X 5. window   ___ 10. phase   X 15. Stephen   X 20. fox

B.

1.	*Contains a high front vowel*	perky, green
2.	*Contains a voiceless alveolar stop*	about
3.	*Contains no stops*	man
4.	*Contains a velar stop*	perky, could, plaque, green
5.	*Contains a central vowel*	about, perky
6.	*Ends with a voiceless sound*	about, plaque
7.	*Begins with a voiced sound*	man, about, green
8.	*Contains a back vowel and a voiced stop*	could
9.	*Begins with a voiceless sound*	perky, could, plaque
10.	*Contains a front vowel and a voiceless stop*	perky, plaque

C.   ___ 1. table   ___ 6. uncle   ___ 11. pushin'   ___ 16. talkin'

       T 2. better   G 7. written   T 12. splatter   G 17. bitten

       ___ 3. errand   G 8. beaten   T 13. rotted   T 18. wedded

       ___ 4. listen   ___ 9. walked   G 14. sweatin'   G 19. rotten

       G 5. quittin'   ___ 10. Lincoln   T 15. bottle   T 20. fodder

D.   t 1. wished   t 6. danced   d 11. sailed   d 16. crabbed

      d 2. loaded   t 7. wrapped   t 12. leased   t 17. placed

      t 3. endorsed   d 8. hanged   t 13. reached   t 18. meshed

      d 4. endangered   t 9. hoped   d 14. toted   d 19. burned

      d 5. robbed   d 10. traded   t 15. wrecked   d 20. carved

E. 1. /kipət/   5. /pɝkt/   9. /pɝpət/   13. /tʊkɪ/

    2. /təkɪd/   6. /pækət/   10. /pɪkɪ/   14. /gækət/

    3. /ədɛbt/   7. /tɛpɪd/   11. /ətæk/   15. /dɛrbɪ/

    4. /paʊrɚ/   8. /taɪrɚ/   12. /tɔrkot/   16. /pipʔd/

F. 1. pottery
    2. puckered
    3. potato
    4. doctor
    5. target
    6. puppet
    7. guppy
    8. packing
    9. diapered
    10. paperboy
    11. daiquiri
    12. dieted

G. 1. direct   no error
    2. tighter   no error
    3. goaded   /goʊ(ɾ)əd/
    4. corker   no error
    5. Carter   /kɑɾɚ/
    6. partake   /pɑrteɪk/
    7. repeat   /ripit/ or /rəpit/
    8. poet   no error
    9. oboe   no error
    10. paper   /peɪpɚ/

H. 1. /kɪd/   kid
    2. /igɚ/   eager
    3. /tɛpɪd/   tepid
    4. /əbʌt/   abut
    5. /dɑkt/   docked
    6. /gɔdɪ/   gaudy

I. 1. /keɪp/
    2. /pɛrd/
    3. /dɔg/ or /dɑg/
    4. /taɪd/
    5. /kɛpt/
    6. /dɛt/
    7. /beɪk/
    8. /pɔr/
    9. /bɔrd/
    10. /pɔrk/
    11. /pit/
    12. /toʊp/
    13. /tʊk/
    14. /pʌt/
    15. /koʊt/
    16. /əpart/
    17. /gardəd/ or /garɾəd/
    18. /boʊɾɚ/
    19. /babɪ/
    20. /barɾɚ/
    21. /bɪgɚ/
    22. /bikɚ/
    23. /tubə/
    24. /kæbɪ/
    25. /pɪrd/
    26. /bækt/
    27. /pɝkɪ/
    28. /gɪrd/
    29. /dægɚ/
    30. /gɪdɪ/ or /gɪɾɪ/
    31. /kɑrpət/
    32. /dɑktɚ/
    33. /tɪkət/
    34. /dɛkt/
    35. /taɪəd/
    36. /bægbɔɪ/
    37. /dəbeɪt/ or /dibeɪt/
    38. /tɔrɪd/
    39. /pɛrət/
    40. /dɝɪ/

5.2—The Nasal Consonants

A. X 1. ring
    X 2. bomb
    ___ 3. pet
    ___ 4. stop
    X 5. tomb
    X 6. jasmine
    ___ 7. crease
    X 8. inside
    ___ 9. trait
    X 10. loaner
    X 11. moan
    X 12. spanking
    ___ 13. possible
    X 14. trench
    X 15. lung
    X 16. ripen
    X 17. unfair
    X 18. monkey
    ___ 19. lure
    ___ 20. failure

B. X 1. **angle**
    ___ 2. angel
    X 3. brink
    X 4. **mango**
    ___ 5. Angie
    X 6. **single**
    ___ 7. conjure
    ___ 8. singe
    ___ 9. ginger
    ___ 10. danger
    X 11. blinker
    X 12. **hanger**
    X 13. ringing
    X 14. **mingle**
    X 15. banging
    X 16. manx
    ___ 17. ingest
    X 18. singer
    X 19. **hunger**
    X 20. **jangle**
    ___ 21. congeal

C. See Exercise B directly above (**bold words**).

D.
___	1. hinge	___	7. ring	X	13. tango
X	2. bangle	___	8. drank	___	14. flange
___	3. wings	___	9. onyx	___	15. engine
X	4. single	X	10. tingle	X	16. English
___	5. wrong	___	11. bungee	___	17. tongue
X	6. mangle	X	12. kangaroo	___	18. dangerous

E.
___	1. pharynx	X	7. engine	X	13. ginger
X	2. England	___	8. flank	___	14. blanket
X	3. bungee	___	9. tingle	___	15. tongue
___	4. length	X	10. lunge	X	16. danger
___	5. lungs	___	11. strength	X	17. vengeance
___	6. jungle	___	12. tango	X	18. ranges

F.
1. *Contains an initial labial sound*	mutton, bank
2. *Contains a voiced initial sound*	good, mutton, bank, napped
3. *Ends with a stop*	good, bank, napped, code
4. *Contains a central vowel*	mutton, curving, taken, carton
5. *Ends with a voiceless sound*	bank, napped
6. *Contains a velar nasal*	curving, bank
7. *Contains a syllabic consonant*	mutton, carton
8. *Contains no nasals*	good, code
9. *Contains a low front vowel and a labial consonant*	bank, napped
10. *Contains a velar consonant and a back vowel*	good, carton, code

G.
1. /kæmp/	4. /pint/	7. /kræŋkɪ/	10. /bʌmpɪ/
2. /neɪm/	5. /tɪŋgə/	8. /kɔrn/	11. /pɪntoʊ/
3. /mɛlɪ/	6. /nɪŋgɪd/	9. /dænk/	12. /pɑrmɔɪ/

H.
1. nab	7. candy
2. conned	8. appoint
3. amass	9. cooking
4. anger	10. tumor
5. morning	11. tighten
6. bending	12. minded

I. 1. camper   no error
    2. adorn   no error
    3. duffer   /dʌfɚ/
    4. bunting   no error
    5. bingo   /bɪŋgoʊ/
    6. pecking   /pɛkɪŋ/
    7. Dayton   /deɪʔn̩/
    8. batter   /bærɚ/
    9. baking   /beɪkɪŋ/
    10. doorknob /dɔrnɑb/

J. 1. /kænd/   canned
    2. /mʌnɪ/   money
    3. /əteɪn/   attain
    4. /kɑŋgoʊ/   congo
    5. /bɝpt/   burped

K.
1. /mɪŋk/
2. /pɝt/
3. /tæn/
4. /kɪŋ/
5. /dʌn/
6. /nid/
7. /bæŋ/
8. /noʊm/
9. /mʌŋk/
10. /kɔɪn/
11. /ɝn/
12. /nut/
13. /taʊn/
14. /mud/
15. /naɪt/
16. /dʌm/
17. /kʊd/
18. /tɔrn/
19. /tʌŋ/
20. /gɔn/
21. /ʌndɚ/
22. /tæŋkɚd/
23. /pinʌt/ or /pinət/
24. /dændɪ/
25. /pɑrteɪk/
26. /mʌndeɪ/
27. /noʊmæd/
28. /bɑŋgoʊ/
29. /mædəm/
30. /gændɚ/
31. /omɪt/
32. /nəgeɪt/
33. /tunɪk/
34. /dɑŋkɪ/
35. /kəmænd/
36. /mɪrɚ/
37. /kaʊnʔn̩/or /kaʊntɪn/
38. /dɛrɪŋ/
39. /ɛmpaɪɚ/
40. /kaʊɚd/

5.3—The Fricative Consonants

A.   X 1. push   X 6. brazen   ___ 11. Montana   ___ 16. hombre
  X 2. thesis   X 7. cares   X 12. pleasure   X 17. leaks
  ___ 3. loom   ___ 8. burlap   X 13. leather   X 18. worthy
  X 4. happy   X 9. croissant   ___ 14. marrow   ___ 19. crouton
  X 5. caution   X 10. vender   X 15. other   X 20. rajah

B. ___ 1. mishap   ʃ 7. election   ʃ 13. friction   ʒ 19. allusion
    ʒ 2. usually   ___ 8. badge   ___ 14. juice   ___ 20. inject
    ʒ 3. decision   ʒ 9. lesion   ʃ 15. Sean   ʒ 21. Persia
    ___ 4. cheese   ʃ 10. lotion   ʃ 16. passion
    ___ 5. largest   ʒ 11. corsage   ʃ 17. ricochet
    ___ 6. reason   ___ 12. changed   ___ 18. college

C. ð 1. smoothly   ð 8. writhe   θ 15. oath   ð 22. smother
    θ 2. method   ð 9. lathe   ð 16. scathing   ð 23. bothers
    ð 3. other   θ 10. thought   ð 17. another   θ 24. atheist
    ð 4. those   ð 11. clothes   θ 18. anything
    θ 5. moth   ð 12. weather   θ 19. withstand
    ð 6. gather   θ 13. thimble   ð 20. wither
    θ 7. wrath   θ 14. booth   θ 21. author

D. 1. /mu___/   v, s, z   move, moose, moos
    2. /wɪ___/   f, θ or ð, z, ʃ   whiff, with (θ or ð), whiz, wish
    3. /ʌ___ɚ/   ð, ʃ   other, usher
    4. /lɛ___ɚ/   v, ð, s, ʒ   lever, leather, lesser, leisure
    5. /___ɛrɪ/   f, v, ʃ, h   fairy (ferry), very, sherry, hairy
    6. /ru___/   f, θ, z, ʒ   roof, Ruth, ruse, rouge
    7. /___aɪ/   f, v, θ, ð, s, ʃ, h   fie, vie, thigh, thy, sigh, shy, high (hi)
    8. /___ɪr/   f, v, s, ʃ, h   fear, veer, seer (sear), shear, here (hear)

E. 1. *Begins with a voiceless fricative*   hug, soon
    2. *Begins with a voiced obstruent*   them, beige, vend
    3. *Ends with a voiceless obstruent*   wreath, tape, cash
    4. *Contains a front vowel and a voiceless fricative*   wreath, cash
    5. *Contains an alveolar sound*   tape, soon, vend
    6. *Contains all voiced phonemes*   them, beige, vend
    7. *Contains a stop and a fricative*   beige, hug, cash, vend
    8. *Contains a nasal and a fricative*   them, soon, vend
    9. *Contains a fricative and a central vowel*   hug
    10. *Contains no fricatives*   tape

F. _z_ 1. babes   _z_ 7. bananas   _z_ 13. dramas

    _s_ 2. chafes   _s_ 8. drinks   _s_ 14. croaks

    _z_ 3. cars   _z_ 9. passes   _s_ 15. meats

    _s_ 4. books   _z_ 10. throws   _z_ 16. affairs

    _s_ 5. carpets   _z_ 11. loaves   _s_ 17. loafs

    _z_ 6. pushes   _s_ 12. roasts   _z_ 18. birds

G. 1. /ʃʊk/   5. /vɛrɪ/   9. /pɝs/   13. /feɪvɚ/
    2. /ʒɪŋ/   6. /ðaɪ/   10. /ʃark/   14. /kreɪzd/
    3. /zɔrt/   7. /θrʊ/   11. /ɪrðu/   15. /bɪʒɚ/
    4. /θɝd/   8. /vɔɪnz/   12. /ʃæku/   16. /hoʊðɚ/

H. 1. Asian   5. spared   9. serviced   13. fatten
    2. vortex   6. thanks   10. others   14. horror
    3. varnish   7. hearsay   11. frozen   15. gazebo
    4. bother   8. urban   12. shivered   16. birthdays

I. 1. bijou   /biʒu/   7. assure   no error; (or /əʃɝ/)
    2. neither   /niðɚ/   8. favored   /feɪvəd/
    3. verify   /vɛrɪfaɪ/   9. shining   /ʃaɪnɪŋ/
    4. hosed   /hoʊzd/   10. earthy   /ɝθɪ/
    5. Hoosier   no error   11. amnesia   no error
    6. panther   /pænθɚ/   12. unthinking   /ənθɪŋkɪŋ/

J. 1. /gɑrθ/   21. /θʌndɚ/
    2. /fɛns/   22. /hɛðɚ/
    3. /ʃɝ/, /ʃɔr/, or /ʃʊr/   23. /sæʔn̩/
    4. /doʊzd/   24. /ʃipɪʃ/
    5. /sɔrd/   25. /sɚaʊndz/
    6. /haɪvz/   26. /hɔrʔn̩/
    7. /ʃaʊt/   27. /θɝɾɪ/
    8. /θɔrnz/   28. /vɪʒən/
    9. /ðoʊz/   29. /fɛrɪŋks/
    10. /heɪst/   30. /θɝd beɪs/
    11. /pɚhæps/   31. /gɔɪɾɚ/
    12. /ʃɔrtɚ/, /ʃɔrɾɚ/   32. /tɛɾɚ/
    13. /pɚuzd/   33. /θaʊzənd/
    14. /ənvɝst/   34. /kɑ(ɔ)ntɔ(ʊ)r/
    15. /mʌðɚ/   35. /ʃɔrtkek/
    16. /kənsumd/   36. /vɛrid/
    17. /mɚaʒ/ or /mɚɑʒ/   37. /də(i)faɪz/
    18. /poʊʃənz/   38. /dɪ(ə)skʌst/
    19. /oʊʃt/   39. /ʃɔrthænd/
    20. /tɑrzæn/   40. /mʌrɚd/

5.4—The Affricate Consonants

A. ___ bon voyage   ___ fantasia   dʒ cabbage

    ___ barrage   tʃ touches   ___ exertion

    dʒ arrange   tʃ pasture   ___ sabotage

    tʃ charming   dʒ nitrogen   dʒ gender

    tʃ vulture   tʃ riches   ___ glacier

    ___ mushroom   ___ charade   dʒ eject

    dʒ gerbil   dʒ rigid   tʃ unchained

B. 1. /___ɛr/   f, ð, ʃ, h, tʃ   fair, there, share, hair, chair

  2. /___æt/   f, v, ð, s, h, tʃ   fat, vat, that, sat, hat, chat

  3. /___oʊ/   f, ð, s, ʃ, h, dʒ   foe, though, sew (so), show, hoe, Joe

  4. /___ɑrm/   f, h, tʃ   farm, harm, charm

  5. /___ɪn/   f, θ, s, ʃ, tʃ, dʒ   fin, thin, sin, shin, chin, gin

  6. /ri___/   f, θ, tʃ   reef, wreath, reach

  7. /bæ___/   θ, s, ʃ, tʃ, dʒ   bath, bass, bash, batch, badge

  8. /bi___/   f, z, tʃ   beef, bees, beach

C. 1. *Contains an initial voiced phoneme*   other, none, jeans, measure

  2. *Contains a fricative*   other, shrunk, jeans, hedge, measure

  3. *Contains affricate and front vowel*   jeans, hedge

  4. *Contains an affricate and a nasal*   jeans, churned

  5. *Contains a palatal obstruent*   shrunk, jeans, hedge, churned, measure

  6. *Contains an obstruent and a central vowel* other, shrunk, churned, measure

  7. *Contains a stop, nasal, and affricate*   churned

  8. *Contains all voiced sounds*   other, none, jeans, measure

D. 1. /skrʌntʃ/   5. /muʒd/   9. /oʊðən/   13. /fæʃtɚ/
  2. /pʊdʒɪ/   6. /kɪtʃən/   10. /dʒeɪd/   14. /gaʊtʃt/
  3. /tʃɔrz/   7. /moʊtʃ/   11. /hʌdʒ/   15. /dʒʌmpɪ/
  4. /hɑrʃɚ/   8. /ʃɑrm/   12. /tʃɝn/   16. /pɑrtʃt/

E. 1. chirped   5. adjoined   9. surely   13. mature
  2. junk   6. macho   10. jersey   14. chummy
  3. chit chat   7. garage   11. purchase   15. agitate
  4. wishbone   8. pasture   12. chocolate   16. jezebel

F.
1. major — /meɪdʒɚ/
2. March — no error
3. jumped — no error
4. Wichita — no error
5. wedged — /wɛdʒd/
6. usher — no error
7. sergeant — /sɑrdʒənt/
8. massage — no error
9. gorge — /gɔrdʒ/
10. manger — /meɪndʒɚ/

G.
1. /ʃɑkt/
2. /steɪʃən/
3. /bʊtʃɚ/
4. /nɪkɚz/
5. /ɛkstrə/
6. /tændʒənt/
7. /sʌðən/
8. /nɛktaɪ/
9. /kɔrsɑʒ/
10. /spɪrɪ(ə)ts/
11. /vɪvɪ(ə)d/
12. /ʃʌrɚ/
13. /ə(ɛ)ksaɪt/
14. /æksan/
15. /skaʊəd/
16. /kɑrvd/
17. /aʊtʃaɪn/
18. /dʒɛndɚ/
19. /kɛrləs/
20. /nɝtʃɚ/
21. /kæʒmɪr/
22. /tʃapɪŋ/
23. /kæʃbaks/
24. /dʒɛndɚz/
25. /tʃɑrmɪŋ/
26. /ʃarpənd/
27. /kæʃɪr/
28. /garbədʒ/
29. /ɔrkə(ɪ)dz/
30. /stræŋ(k)θən/
31. /ɛ(ə)gzɪsts/
32. /dʒɪndʒɚ/
33. /θɔrnɪ/
34. /idʒɪ(ə)pt/
35. /tʃaʊmeɪn/
36. /pɚvɝs/
37. /dʌtʃə(ɪ)s/
38. /æŋkʃə(ɪ)s/
39. /mɪstʃə(ɪ)f/
40. /kæp(t)ʃɚ/

5.5—The Approximant Consonants

A.
- w awkward
- 1 bellow
- w quick
- ___ today
- r torpedo
- r reasoned
- ___ towered
- ___ Jupiter
- 1 lazy
- r repaid
- w suede
- j fewer
- r, l peril
- w swiped
- j yawned
- w, 1 jonquil
- r screaming
- r, l barley
- j puny
- ___ fired

B.
- ___ tune
- ___ jealous
- X putrid
- ___ loop
- X fuel
- ___ keynote
- ___ hood
- ___ piano
- ___ maybe
- ___ jar
- ___ adjourn
- X Cupid
- ___ choosy
- X compute
- X usual
- X yours
- ___ daisy
- ___ boysenberry

C.
- ___ awesome
- X well
- X stalwart
- ___ how
- ___ showed
- ___ lower
- X why
- ___ awry
- ___ wrath
- ___ rowboat
- X reward
- ___ Howard
- X warrior
- X swept
- X quirk
- ___ borrowed
- ___ wrist
- X wayward

D.

___	lurk	___	surround	___	purchase
X	barter	X	rewritten	___	perfected
___	burgundy	___	tires	X	scorpion
X	unreal	X	fourth	___	flirtatious
X	guarded	X	spirited	X	grandiose
X	grasp	___	curvature	___	divert

E.
1. /dʒɛloʊ/
2. **/blaɪð/**
3. /riljə/
4. /ɚoʊlɚ/
5. /dʒɑr/
6. /sɝklz̩/
7. /fjɝt/
8. **/kwɔrl̩d/**
9. **/wʊln̩/**
10. /pjaɪd/
11. **/spjud/**
12. /walʃat/
13. **/swɪlz/**
14. ***/riwɝd/***
15. /poʊləs/
16. /fjunts/
17. /jɛlɪ/
18. **/skjud/**
19. /ɑkwɚd/
20. /riɚən/

F.
1. yellow
2. robust
3. warrior
4. yearned
5. beetles
6. grouched
7. repute
8. guava
9. liquid
10. tiled
11. curtailed
12. quarrel
13. luckily
14. Latin
15. fuchsia
16. question

G.
1. bowling   /boʊlɪŋ/
2. wrongful   /rɑŋfʊl/
3. warbled   no error
4. pewter   /pjurɚ/
5. quandary   /kwɑndrɪ/
6. regional   no error
7. lawyer   /lɔɪɚ/ or /lɔjɚ/
8. flurries   /flɝɪz/
9. fuming   no error
10. baloney   /bəloʊnɪ/
11. relish   /rɛlɪʃ/
12. confusion   /kənfjuʒən/

H.
1. /kwɪksænd/
2. /slaʊtʃt/
3. /dʒɝɪ/ or /dʒʊrɪ/
4. /əkweɪnt/
5. /ʃoʊldɚ/
6. /slɪðɚ/
7. /sɑrdʒənt/
8. /skjuɚ/
9. /kɔrdʒəl/
10. /jusfʊl/
11. /wɪθdru/
12. /wɝʃɪp/
13. /ɛ(ə)nʃraɪnd/
14. /fjumd/
15. /lʌn(t)ʃən/
16. /dʒunjɚ/
17. /ənskeɪðd/
18. /ʃrɪvl̩/
19. /jæŋkiz/
20. /kwɔrrɚ/
21. /bjugl̩/
22. /tʃɪzl̩/
23. /junə(ɪ)k/
24. /tʃɑrl̩z/
25. /bəlaŋ(g)ɪŋ/
26. /rubrɪ(ə)k/
27. /junik/
28. /bi(ə)kwɪð(θt)/
29. /kaɪæk/
30. /bɪljɚdz/

31. /aɪwɑ(ɔ)ʃ/
32. /lɪŋgwəl/
33. /kwɔrld̩/
34. /æŋgwɪ(ə)ʃt/
35. /aʊtwəd/

36. /rʌp(t)ʃɚ/
37. /ʃu wæks/
38. /kwoʊʃənt/
39. /stræŋglɚ/
40. /əlʊr/

Review Exercises

A. ?   1. writin'
    ɾ   2. rudder
    ?* 3. about
    ɾ   4. nutty
    np 5. harden

    ?   6. certain
    ɾ   7. crater
        8. winter
    ?   9. Martin
    np 10. sudden

*Possibly in coda position.

B.   1. wheel
    X   2. written
    X   3. regal
    X   4. Seton Hall
    X   5. candles

        6. pull
        7. contagious
    X   8. that'll
    X   9. grab 'em by the neck
        10. hold 'er by the tail

C. /k/   stop   velar   voiceless
   /r/   liquid   palatal   voiced
   /θ/   fricative   interdental   voiceless
   /ŋ/   nasal   velar   voiced
   /dʒ/ affricate   palatal   voiced
   /b/   stop   bilabial   voiced
   /ʃ/   fricative   palatal   voiceless
   /j/   glide   palatal   voiced
   /f/   fricative   labiodental   voiceless
   /n/   nasal   alveolar   voiced

D. Possible answers include:

1. deed, need
2. cone, cove
3. hum, thumb
4. hip, ship
5. rag, lag, nag

E.
1.	sin-sing	place
2.	jaw-raw	manner
3.	sue-shoe	place
4.	tin-tip	voice, manner, place
5.	clue-crew	place
6.	cop-mop	voice, manner, place
7.	choke-joke	voice
8.	pet-met	voice, manner
9.	done-gun	place
10.	even-Eden	manner, place
11.	Yale-rail	manner
12.	late-lake	place
13.	fame-shame	place
14.	cat-cad	voice
15.	pass-pad	voice, manner

F.
1.	jester	/dʒ/	voiced	prevocalic
2.	version			
3.	itchy	/tʃ/	voiceless	intervocalic
4.	cash			
5.	switched	/tʃ/	voiceless	postvocalic
6.	January	/dʒ/	voiced	prevocalic
7.	regime			
8.	mashing			
9.	crush			
10.	urgent	/dʒ/	voiced	intervocalic

G.
1.	<u>c</u>elery	/s/	voiceless	alveolar	fricative
2.	bree<u>ch</u>	/tʃ/	voiceless	palatal	affricate
3.	<u>ph</u>ase	/f/	voiceless	labiodental	fricative
4.	w<u>r</u>eck	/r/	voiced	palatal	liquid
5.	ca<u>ll</u>	/l/	voiced	alveolar	liquid
6.	me<u>th</u>od	/θ/	voiceless	interdental	fricative
7.	<u>y</u>es	/j/	voiced	palatal	glide
8.	cru<u>d</u>e	/d/	voiced	alveolar	stop
9.	<u>ch</u>asm	/k/	voiceless	velar	stop
10.	e<u>dg</u>e	/dʒ/	voiced	palatal	affricate
11.	<u>w</u>alk	/w/	voiced	labiovelar	glide
12.	cohe<u>s</u>ion	/ʒ/	voiced	palatal	fricative

H. 1. /bɝθmɑrks/
2. /kɑndʒɚɪŋ/
3. /bitʃkomɚ/
4. /ʌðɚwaɪz/
5. /dʒɔrdʒ buʃ/
6. /værɪkən/
7. /zɪŋk ɑksaɪd/
8. /hæŋkɚtʃɪf/
9. /ɛkspədaɪt/
10. /faʊndeɪʃən/
11. /ædmɪrəd/
12. /ðɛræftɚ/
13. /ɪndʒʌŋkʃən/
14. /kənvɝdʒəns/

15. /sæbətɑʒ/
16. /fəzɪʃən/
17. /bʌʔn̩ hol/
18. /dɪskɝədʒd/
19. /ivɑlvd/
20. /ɪndɪdʒənt/
21. /kɑzmos/
22. /tʃɪmpænziz/
23. /dɪskɑrdəd/
24. /prɛstidʒəs/
25. /tʃɑrmɪŋ/
26. /tɝkɪʃ bæθ/
27. /bɑðɚsəm/
28. /dʒæk naɪf/

29. /ɛnzaɪm/
30. /tuθ fɛrɪ/
31. /tʃɛrɪ paɪ/
32. /koɑθɚ/
33. /haɪəsɪnθ/
34. /ɛndʒɔɪmənt/
35. /fɑrməsɪst/
36. /ənwɝðɪ/
37. /wən hʌndrətθ/
38. /pæstʃɚaɪzd/
39. /fɪdʒɪrɪ/
40. /fɑðɚz deɪ/

I. 1. /eɔrrə/
2. /ɛrlaɪnɚ/
3. /kəndʒild/
4. /kɔkeɪʒən/
5. /vokeɪʃən/
6. /fjunɚl̩/
7. /rɛdʒɪstəd/
8. /jɛstɚdeɪ/
9. /novɛmbɚ/
10. /trʌbl̩səm/
11. /əphoʊlstɚd/
12. /ɪmpjudɪnt/
13. /tɔrɛntʃəl/
14. /dɪstrɪbjut/

15. /daɪəfræm/
16. /æpətaɪt/
17. /pɚsəvɪr/
18. /kɚeɪdʒəs/
19. /mʌskjulɚ/
20. /pəpaɪrəs/
21. /sikwɛnʃəl/
22. /pɔrtreɪl/
23. /θæŋksgɪvɪŋ/
24. /zaɪləfon/
25. /ɑrrɪtʃok/
26. /pɪdʒənhol/
27. /wɪljəmzbɚg/
28. /ʌndɚgroθ/

29. /hjuməəs/
30. /wɪrɪnəs/
31. /junɪ(ə)vɚs/
32. /əngædəd/
33. /mænjuskrɪpt/
34. /əbskjɝlɪ/
35. /nuklɪəs/
36. /kwɑdræŋgl̩/
37. /hɑrmənaɪz/
38. /rɛdʒɪstrɑr/
39. /pɑr bɔɪld/
40. /strʌkʃəl̩/

Chapter 6

Chapter Exercises

6.1 1. male
2. 250 Hz (1/0.004)
3. 0.0025 sec. or 2.5 msec. (1/400)

6.2

270	/i/	300	/u/	2290	/i/	870	/u/
390	/ɪ/	440	/ʊ/	1990	/ɪ/	1020	/ʊ/
530	/ɛ/	570	/ɔ/	1840	/ɛ/	840	/ɔ/
660	/æ/	730	/ɑ/	1720	/æ/	1090	/ɑ/

As the tongue lowers, the frequency of F_1 increases. As the tongue moves from front to back, the frequency of F_2 decreases.

6.3 Spectrogram *a* is "don" and spectrogram *b* is "dean." F_2 for *b* is above 2000 Hz, whereas F_2 for *a* is at a much lower frequency. Recall that the F_2 for /i/ is highest in frequency.

6.4 1. /t/, /d/
    2. /d/, /b/
    3. /p/, /t/
    4. /p/, /k/, /d/
    5. /g/

6.5 *a* = "bead" because it has the highest F_2; *b* = "bad" because it has no aspiration and must begin with a voiced stop; *c* = "pad" because aspiration is visible

6.6 *a* = "ban" because of a visible nasal formant; *b* = "bash" because the final phoneme is a fricative; *c* = "bat" because of the presence of a stop gap and the aspiration of the final phoneme

Review Exercises

A. 1. waveform
   2. 40
   3. *y; x*
   4. voiceless stops
   5. spectrum
   6. stop gap
   7. voice bar
   8. /h/
   9. /θ/

B. 1. d
   2. a
   3. f
   4. j
   5. b
   6. g
   7. h
   8. e
   9. c
   10. i

C. 1. F
   2. F
   3. F
   4. F
   5. T
   6. T
   7. T
   8. F
   9. T
   10. F
   11. T
   12. T

D. 1. rises
   2. lowers
   3. rises
   4. lowers
   5. F_1 and F_2 both lower

E. 1a. The spectrogram is of the word "knees" because it begins with a nasal consonant and ends with a voiced fricative (note the striations throughout the fricative).

   1b. The spectrogram is of the word "peace" because it begins with a voiceless stop (aspiration) and ends with a voiceless fricative (not vertical striations).

   2. Spectrogram *a* = "rain" and *b* = "lane"; note the low F_3 in spectrogram *a*, consistent with production of /r/.

3.

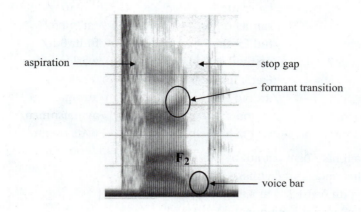

aspiration —————→   ←————— stop gap

————— formant transition

F$_2$

————— voice bar

Chapter 7

Chapter Exercises

7.1 1. /θ/
     2. /d/
     3. /t/
     4. /d/

     5. /t/
     6. /h/
     7. /v/
     8. /h/

7.2 1. noon   /nuən/   X
     2. pants   /pænts/   ___
     3. choose   /tʃjuz/   X
     4. friends   /frɛnz/   ___
     5. lamb   /læm/   ___
     6. straw   /strɔr/   X
     7. rinse   /rɪns/   ___
     8. milk   /mɛlk/   ___
     9. clam   /kəlæm/   X
    10. Wednesday   /wænzdeɪ/   ___

7.3 1. /mɪrəkl̩/   3. /ɑ(ɔ)θɚaɪz/   5. /məkænɪkl̩/
         /məækjələs/   /əθɔrəɾɪ/   /mɛkənɪstɪk/

     2. /əkjuz/   4. /dəmɑləʃ/
         /ækjəzeɪʃən/   /dɛməlɪʃən/

7.4 1. your mother   /jɔr mʌðɚ/   /jəmʌðɚ/
    2. right and left   /raɪt ænd lɛft/   /raɪʔn̩lɛft/
    3. food for thought   /fud fɔr θɑt/   /fudfɚθɑt/
    4. What will they do?   /wʌt wɪl ðeɪ du/   /wɚɭðedu/
    5. Thank him.   /θæŋk hɪm/   /θæŋkəm/
    6. as big as   /æz bɪg æz/   /æzbɪgəz/
    7. of mice and men   /ʌv maɪs ænd mɛn/   /əvmaɪsn̩mɛn/
    8. What is her name?   /wʌt ɪz hɝ neɪm/   /wʌtsəneɪm/

7.5 1. [aɪ bɛt ju aɪ kæn hɛlp ðɛm gɛt aʊt əv ðæt mɛs ‖]
       [aɪbɛtʃuaɪkənhɛlpm̩gɛtaʊrəðætmɛs ‖]
    2. [aɪ kat ju tʃiɾɪŋ an ðæt tɛst ‖ aɪ æm goʊɪŋ tu tɛl ðə titʃɚ ‖]
       [aɪkatʃutʃiɾɪŋanðæt tɛst ‖ aɪmgʊnətɛlðətitʃɚ ‖]
    3. [wʌt ɪz hɪz rizn̩ fɔr nat biɪŋ eɪbl̩tə kʌm tu ðə paɾɪ ‖]
       [wətsɪzriznfɚnatbiəneɪbl̩təkəmtə ðəpaɾɪ ‖]
    4. [wʌts ðə mærɚ wɪθ θɛlmə ‖ lɛt mi si ɪf aɪ kæn tʃɪr hɝʌp ‖]
       [wətsðəmærɚwɪθ θɛlmə ‖ lɛmɪsiəfaɪkəntʃɪrɚəp ‖]
    5. [wʌt dɪd ju du tu jɚ kar ‖ aɪ ʃʊd bi eɪbl̩tu gɛt ɪt goʊɪŋ ‖]
       [wədʒədurəjɚkar ‖ aɪʃədbiebl̩rəgɛtɪtgoən ‖]

7.6 1. ˌinˈtense   5. ˈteaˌbag   9. ˌeˈrode
    2. ˈfalseˌhood   6. ˈfrostˌbite   10. ˈhandˌshake
    3. ˈLuˌcite   7. ˌoˈbese   11. ˌreˈact
    4. ˌroˈsette   8. ˈenˌtree   12. ˈhouseˌhold

7.7 1. ˈleopard   5. ˈmurky   9. ˈscary
    2. ˈsweater   6. aˈnoint   10. ˈnaked
    3. ˈrhythm   7. ˈmagnet   11. exˈtreme
    4. conˈtend   8. beˈlief   12. paˈrade

7.8 1. ˈmeasuring   5. couˈrageous   9. soˈrority
    2. staˈtistics   6. ˈGermany   10. fraˈternity
    3. laˈryngeal   7. unˈbearable   11. ˈAlbuquerque
    4. ˈwarranted   8. Caˈnadian   12. dysˈphonia

7.9 1. ˌmyˈopic   5. ˌciˈtation   9. ˈaliˌmony
    2. ˈcyberˌspace   6. ˈcircumˌstance 10. comˈmuniˌcate
    3. ˈarchiˌtect   7. ˌbacˈteria   11. ˌeleˈvator
    4. ˌiˈdea   8. ˌefferˈvescent 12. ˌIndiˈana

7.10 The underlined words should be:
    1. matinee   4. uncle
    2. East   5. Mr.
    3. Flo

7.11 1. The girl's name was <u>Chris</u>.
Her name wasn't Pat.

2. Jared only forgot to get the <u>toothpaste</u> at the store.
Jared remembered to get everything else.

3. Why did they <u>walk</u> to the playground?
Why didn't they drive?

4. Why did they walk to the <u>playground</u>?
Why didn't they walk to the zoo?

5. <u>Mark</u> got a new blue bike for his birthday.
Valerie didn't get a new bike.

6. Mark got a new blue <u>bike</u> for his birthday.
He did not get a blue baseball cap.

7. Mark got a new <u>blue</u> bike for his birthday.
The bike wasn't green.

7.12 The answers are in bold.

Waitress:	Would you like something to **drink**?
Customer:	**Lemonade**, please. I would also like to **order**.
Waitress:	Would you like an **appetizer**?
Customer:	**No, thank you.**
Waitress:	Would you like to hear about our **specials**?
Customer:	**Please.**
Waitress:	We have **grilled salmon** and **fettuccine alfredo**.
Customer:	I'll have the **fettuccine**.
Waitress:	Would you like our **house dressing** on your **salad**? It's **Italian**.
Customer:	I would like to have **blue cheese**, please.
Waitress:	I'll also bring out some **fresh rolls**.
Customer:	**Thank you.**
Waitress:	**You're welcome.**

7.13 1. a. ˌSteve's ˈroommate is from ˌMinneapolis.
b. ˌSteve's ˌroommate is from Minneˈapolis.

2. a. ˌTim went ˌskydiving on ˈSaturday.
b. ˈTim went ˌskydiving on ˌSaturday.

3. a. The ˈanswer on the ˌexam was ˌ"false."
b. The ˌanswer on the ˌexam was ˈ"false."

4. a. ˌMary's ˌbirthday is next ˈTuesday.
b. ˌMary's ˈbirthday is next ˌTuesday.

5. a. ˈI'd like a ˌsteak for ˌdinner.
b. ˌI'd like a ˈsteak for ˌdinner.

6. a. ˌI went to New York ˈCity to see some ˌplays.
b. ˌI went to ˌNew York City to see some ˈplays.

7. a. ˌMy ˌprofessor ˌshaved his ˈmustache.
b. ˌMy ˈprofessor ˌshaved his ˌmustache.

8. a. ˌI need poˈtatoes from the ˌstore.
b. ˈI need ˌpotatoes from the ˌstore.

7.14 The answers are in bold.

1.	When will you leave?	Rising	**Falling**
2.	Is your brother home?	**Rising**	Falling
3.	I need to go the library.	Rising	**Falling**
4.	What's your favorite season?	Rising	**Falling**
5.	Did you get paid yet?	**Rising**	Falling
6.	The dog ran away.	Rising	**Falling**
7.	Sophie is my oldest friend.	Rising	**Falling**
8.	How did you know about that?	Rising	**Falling**
9.	Honest?!?	**Rising**	Falling
10.	I'm sure!!!	Rising	**Falling**

7.15
1. [piːz]
2. [liːv]
3. [ruːd]
4. [spɑː]
5. [læːg]
6. [tuː]

7.16
1. [raɪsːup]
2. [kaʔn̩ːɛrɪŋ]
3. [bɪgːʌnz]
4. [teɪlːaɪt]
5. [kɑ(l)mːɔrnɪŋ]
6. [bɑrːum]
7. [lifːaɪɚ]
8. [pʊʃːɛrɪ]

7.17
1. [I want hot dogs | ice cream | and cotton candy ‖]
2. [They left | didn't they ‖]
3. [The family | who lived next door | moved away ‖]
4. [What is her problem ‖]
5. [My uncle | the dentist | is 34 years old ‖]

Review Exercises

A.
1. [kæmːeɪk]	m/n	bilabial
2. /haʊʒɚ mʌðɚ/	ʒ/z+j	palatal
3. /dʒɪŋ geɪm/	ŋ/n	velar
4. [lɛb˺ paɪp]	b/d	bilabial
5. /hæʒ ʃeɪkn̩/	ʒ/z	palatal
6. [rɛg˺ gaʊn]	g/d	velar

B.
1. /bɛnz/
2. /wɪnɚ/
3. /lænmaɪn/
4. /kæn ə wɜˠmz/
5. /kaʊnɚ/
6. /twɛlfs/
7. /wəts ɚ prɑbləm/
8. /wɛp laʊdlɪ/

C. 1. [aɪ wɑnt tu goʊ hoʊm/‖]
    [aɪwɑnəgohom/‖]
 2. [lɛt mi si jɔr bʊk ‖]
    [lɛmɪsijɚbʊk ‖]
 3. [kʊd ju muv eɪ lɪtl̩ tu ðə raɪt ‖]
    [kʊdʒəmuvəlɪɾl̩təðəraɪt ‖]
 4. [dɪd dʒan ɛvɚ gɛt peɪd ‖]
    [dɪdʒanɛvɚgɛtpeɪd ‖]
 5. [waɪ dɪd ʃi liv soʊ ɝlɪ ‖]
    [waɪdʃilivsoɝlɪ ‖]
 6. [ɪt ɪz reɪnɪŋ kæts ænd dɑgz ‖]
    [ɪtsreɪnɪŋkætsn̩dɑgz ‖]
 7. [wɛn ɑr ju goʊɪŋ tu liv ‖]
    [wɛnɚjəgʊnəliv ‖]
 8. [ju hæv gɑt tu bi kɪdɪŋ ‖]
    [juvgɑɾəbikɪdɪŋ ‖]
 9. [hu ɪz goʊɪŋ tu reɪk ðʌ livz tunaɪt ‖]
    [huzgʊnərekðəlivztənaɪt ‖]
 10. [aɪ wɑnt tu wæks maɪ trʌk tumɑroʊ mɔrnɪŋ ‖]
    [aɪwɑnəwæksmaɪtrəktəmɑromɔrnɪŋ ‖]

D. 1. Did you ever go to the circus?
 2. When did she leave Georgia?
 3. My sister got a new boyfriend.
 4. Give me a day or two to decide.
 5. I am going to have to say "no" for now.
 6. I think it is going to rain either today or tomorrow.
 7. Would you ever think of doing that for me?
 8. Do you think that Susan took enough of them?
 9. I am sure that they are going to tell you what you need to do it.
 10. Try as he might, he just could not do what she wanted.

E. 1. cour'ageous
 2. 'terri,fied
 3. ma'jestic
 4. ,asth'matic
 5. 'Plexi,glas
 6. plur'ality
 7. 'manda,tory
 8. ,clan'destine
 9. ,flam'boyant
 10. ,cre'ation
 11. ,compu'tation
 12. ,cran'berry
 13. 'bulletin
 14. sur'rendered
 15. se'mantics
 16. co'lonial
 17. 'mercen,ary
 18. inde'pendent
 19. ,Oc'tober
 20. ,baller'ina

F.

			Reduced	Full
1.	/ˈɔrɪdʒɪn/	/əˈrɪdʒɪnˌet/	X	__
2.	/ˈmaɪkrəˌskop/	/ˌmaɪˈkrɑskəpɪ/	__	X
3.	/əˈrɪstəˌkræt/	/ˌɛrɪsˈtɑkrəsɪ/	__	X
4.	/ˈstrærədʒɪ/	/strəˈtidʒɪk/	__	X
5.	/ˈmeɪnɪˌæk/	/məˈnaɪəkˌl/	X	__
6.	/ˌhoˈmɑdʒənəs/	/ˌhoməˈdʒinɪəs/	__	X
7.	/ˈpɛrəˌlaɪz/	/pəˈræləsɪs/	__	X
8.	/ˈfɛlənɪ/	/fəˈloʊnɪəs/	__	X
9.	/pəˈspaɪɚ/	/pɚspəˈeɪʃn/	X	__
10.	/ˌriˈpit/	/ˌrɛpəˈtɪʃəs/	X	__

G.

		Rising	Falling
1.	I got a sweater for my birthday.	__	X
2.	Are you happy?	X	__
3.	The girls had spaghetti for supper.	__	X
4.	Are you positive?	X	__
5.	When you're finished, go to bed.	__	X
6.	Were you late for work today?	X	__
7.	Let me get back to you.	__	X
8.	Did you buy a new CD?	X	__
9.	What do you mean?	__	X
10.	Is that your idea of a joke?	X	__

H.
1. [If I want your help | you'll be the first to know ‖]
2. [Maybe I will | maybe I won't ‖]
3. [They bought a new house | didn't they ‖]
4. [The girls | who went swimming | all got a cold ‖]
5. [I can't really make up my mind ‖]
6. [I scream | you scream | we all scream | for ice cream ‖]
7. [When are you leaving on vacation ‖]
8. [Are your cousins coming for a visit | or not ‖]
9. [Do you have ants in your pants ‖]
10. [I quit my job | but only when I was sure I could get another ‖]

I.
1. [aɪkɔtmaɪkæt:ɑmbaɪðəteɪl ‖]
2. [wɪtʃ:æmpudɪʒubaɪætðəstɔr ‖]
3. [wʊdʒupʊtðəwaɪt:ebl̩klɑθanðəteɪbl̩pliz ‖]
4. [mɑm:aɪt:ekmɪʃɑpɪŋɪfaɪɡɛtgʊdgredz ‖]
5. [hævjufɪnɪʃt:epɪŋðətivispɛʃl̩jɛt ‖]

6. [wɪθːɛm | ɪtshɑrdtətɛlwətðɜrθɪŋkɪŋ ‖]

7. [plizgɪmijəfonːʌmbɚbifɔrjuliv ‖]

8. [klɛmːerə houmrʌnætðəbɪgːɛmlæstːuzdeɪ ‖]

9. [tɛrɪɱferl̩ ːʌvtupleautsaɪdwɪðːəwarɚsprɪŋklɚ ‖]

10. [aɪwontːekɛnɪmɔrəvðədʒʌŋkːɛnhænzaut ‖]

J. 1. [waɪkæntʃuɛvɚæktʃɚeɪdʒ ‖]
   [waɪkæntʃuɛvɚæktjɚeɪdʒ ‖]

2. [waɪ owaɪ | dɪdaɪɛvəlivaɪowə ‖]
   [waɪowaɪdɪdaɪɛvəlivaɪowə ‖]

3. [wɛndðeseðɜrflaɪtwəz ‖]
   [wɛndɪdðeseðɜrflaɪtwəz ‖]

4. [alprabligohomtəmarou ɔrðədeæftɚ ‖]
   [aɪwɪlprabligohoumtəmarou ɚ ɔrðədeæftɚ ‖]

5. [wɛrdʃiɛvɚgeʔn̩ aɪdiəlaɪkðæt ‖]
   [wɛrdɪdʃiɛvɚgetænaɪdiəlaɪkðæt ‖]

6. [jugarəbipʊlɪnmaɪlɛg ‖]
   [juvgatːəbipʊlɪŋmaɪlɛg ‖]

7. [maɪfrɛnz | ɛsbɪn̩deɪl | argʊnəpɪkmiəpətθri ‖]
   [maɪfrɛnz | ɛsbɪn̩deɪl | argouɪŋtəpɪkmiəpætθri ‖]

8. [waɪdʒuripɛntðəbarnalrɛrɪ ‖]
   [waɪdɪdʒuripɛntðəbarnalrɛrɪ ‖]

9. [ðɜrgʊnətɛljuwətʃənid ‖]
   [ðɜrgouɪŋtətɛljuwətjunid ‖]

10. [dɪdʃitɛktuəvəm ‖ næʃitʊkfɔr ‖]
    [dɪdʃitɛktuəvðəm ‖ naːʃitʊkfɔr ‖]

K. 1. a. The ˌclock is ˌrunning ˈslow.
   b. The ˈclock is ˌrunning ˌslow.

2. a. ˌAllison got ˌmarried in New ˈYork.
   b. ˌAllison got ˈmarried in New ˌYork.

3. a. Chrisˌtina ˈbought a new ˌbackpack.
   b. Chrisˈtina ˌbought a new ˌbackpack.

4. a. Dr. ˌMills is my ˌfavorite proˈfessor.
   b. Dr. ˈMills is my ˌfavorite proˌfessor.

5. a. The ˌreport is ˌdue in ˈfive ˌweeks.
   b. The ˌreport is ˌdue in ˌfive ˈweeks.

6. a. ˌRyan and ˌMindy went to Haˈwaii for their ˌhoneymoon.
   b. ˌRyan and ˌMindy went to Haˌwaii for their ˈhoneymoon.

7. a. ˈPatti's ˌfavorite ˌjeans are ˌripped in the ˌknees.
   b. ˌPatti's ˌfavorite ˌjeans are ˌripped in the ˈknees.

8. a. Did ˈyou ˌride the ˌnew ˌrollercoaster?
   b. Did ˌyou ˌride the ˈnew ˌrollercoaster?

9. a. ˌSid got ˌnew ˌskis for his vaˌcation in ˈUtah.
   b. ˌSid got ˌnew ˈskis for his vaˌcation in ˌUtah.

10. a. ˌI want to see that ˌmovie toˈnight at ˌ8.
    b. ˌI want to see that ˈmovie toˌnight at ˌ8.

Chapter 8

Chapter Exercises

8.1 _X_ 1. scissors   _X_ 5. today
     _X_ 2. baby   ___ 6. milk
     _X_ 3. banana   _X_ 7. mitten
     ___ 4. mama   ___ 8. lady

8.2 away 1. _____ _____   say   5. _____ _____
     cup   2. ___X___ /kʌ/   phone 6. ___X___ /foʊ/
     through 3. _____ _____   black 7. ___X___ /blæ/
     bread 4. ___X___ /brɛ/   stop 8. ___X___ /sta/

8.3 ___ 1. wagon   _X_ 4. pencil
     _X_ 2. children   _X_ 5. water
     ___ 3. jacket   ___ 6. yellow

8.4 _X_ 1. blue   _X_ 5. stop
     ___ 2. spot   _X_ 6. crayon
     ___ 3. path   _X_ 7. milk
     _X_ 4. spring   ___ 8. wish

8.5 ___ 1. shoe   ___ 5. comb
     _X_ 2. thank   _X_ 6. summer
     ___ 3. raisin   ___ 7. yellow
     _X_ 4. march   _X_ 8. shop

8.6 ___ 1. candy   _X_ 5. brush
     _X_ 2. rake   ___ 6. paper
     _X_ 3. bring   _X_ 7. goose
     ___ 4. clown   ___ 8. sing

8.7 ___ 1. shake   ___ 5. gem
     ___ 2. choose   _X_ 6. witch
     _X_ 3. Jack   _X_ 7. chalk
     ___ 4. mesh   _X_ 8. chase

8.8 ___ 1. soap   ___ 5. rice
     _X_ 2. leaf   ___ 6. yes
     _X_ 3. ring   _X_ 7. grow
     _X_ 4. lazy   ___ 8. free

8.9 <u>X</u> 1. middle   <u>X</u> 5. belt
     <u>X</u> 2. answer   ___ 6. telephone
     <u>X</u> 3. work   <u>X</u> 7. curtain
     ___ 4. could   ___ 8. bark

8.10 ___ 1. pie   <u>X</u> 5. boat
     <u>X</u> 2. tap   ___ 6. train
     ___ 3. lip   ___ 7. cause
     <u>X</u> 4. numb   <u>X</u> 8. big

8.11 <u>X</u> 1. pat   <u>X</u> 5. knife
     <u>X</u> 2. short   <u>X</u> 6. that
     ___ 3. Tom   <u>X</u> 7. phone
     ___ 4. tune   ___ 8. vat

8.12 <u>X</u> 1. turkey   <u>X</u> 5. bang
     ___ 2. kill   ___ 6. shook
     ___ 3. grass   <u>X</u> 7. cap
     <u>X</u> 4. fake   <u>X</u> 8. brag

8.13 <u>P</u> 1. pear   ___ 5. gone
     <u>D</u> 2. led   <u>D</u> 6. flag
     <u>P</u> 3. fair   <u>P</u> 7. shoe
     <u>D</u> 4. card   ___ 8. chair

8.14 1. chairs   initial consonant deletion
     2. letter   fricative replacing a stop
     3. witch   stop replacing a glide
     4. tape   backing
     5. bunny   initial consonant deletion; glottal replacement
     6. bad   backing; glottal replacement

8.15 1. ___ slack   5. <u>X</u> excuse
     2. ___ praised   6. ___ surprise
     3. <u>X</u> scorn   7. <u>X</u> stripe
     4. <u>X</u> despite 8. ___ smooth

8.16   1. X   skunk

2. X   snacked

3. ___   target   [tʰɑrgət̚]

4. ___   brave   [breɪv]

5. ___   toga   [tʰoʊgə]

6. X   guarded

7. ___   person   [pʰɝsən]

8. X   carefully

8.17   1. ___   mean   4. X   strung

2. X   boon   5. ___   slam

3. ___   buddy   6. X   thong

8.18   1. [kɛt̬l̩]   3. [wɑt̬ɚ]   6. [bæt̬l̩d]

8.19   1. [pj̊urɚ]   5. [hi dʌz̥]

2. [kl̥ɪrlɪ]   6. [rɪd̥ʒ strit]

3. [hiz̥ stʌbɚn]   7. [aɪ luz̥]

4. [beɪð̥ pæm]   8. [ðeɪ̥ pleɪd̥]

8.20   1. ___   could   4. ___   clam

2. X   kiss   5. X   keep

3. X   drop   6. ___   comb

8.21   1. /ɔ/   5. /ʊ/

2. /ɛ/   6. /æ/

3. /ɔ/   7. /ʊ/

4. /e/   8. /i/

8.22   1. [hʷʊd]   5.

2.   6.

3. [rʷuf]   7. [sʷwit]

4.   8. [dʷun]

8.23   1. ɔ   4. ɔ

2. c   5. c

3. c   6. ɔ

8.24   1. /ɤ/   4. /ɯ/

2. /œ/   5. /ø/

3. /ɒ/   6. /ʌ/

8.25   1. [æn̩θəm]   5. [mæθt̬aɪm]

2.   6. [wɛl̩θ]

3.   7.

4.   8. [pæn̩θɚ]

8.26 1. [ɪɱfɚɛntʃəl]   5. [əɱfrɛndlɪ]
      2.   6. [sʌɱflaʊɚ]
      3. [mɛɱfəs]   7.
      4.   8. [kɪɱfo(l)k]

8.27 1. _X_ lake   5. ___ scalding
      2. ___ mingle   6. _X_ liked
      3. _X_ loop   7. ___ hilly
      4. ___ beagle   8. _X_ lady

8.28 1. /x/   6. /k'/
      2. /pf/   7. /ʊ/
      3. /ʃ/   8. /ɗ/
      4. /β/   9. /ɣ/
      5. /ɬ/   10. /ɱ/

Review Exercises

A. 1. d   6. d
   2. c   7. b
   3. a   8. c
   4. b   9. d
   5. a   10. a

B. 1. c   6. d
   2. d   7. b
   3. a   8. c
   4. e   9. b
   5. a   10. e

C. 1. c   7. b, d, e
   2. b, d, e   8. a, c
   3. b   9. a
   4. b   10. a
   5. d, e   11. b
   6. a, c   12. b, d

D. 1. /sip/ or /lip/
    2. /græg/
    3. /dɑr/
    4. /wɛmən/ or /jɛmən/
    5. /beɪp/
    6. /ʒɛlɪ/
    7. /bʌv/
    8. /taɪn/
    9. /teɪm/
    10. /groʊ/

E. 1. reiterated articulation
    2. bidental median fricative
    3. velar nareal fricative
    4. labioalveolar plosive
    5. linguolabial median fricative
    6. whistled [s]
    7. interdental trill
    8. lateral + median voiced alveolar fricative

F. 1. [wɑb̥ster]
    2. /nɝs/
    3. /soʊldʒɚ/
    4. /æstrənat/
    5. /tɪtʃɚ/
    6. /trʌk draɪvɚ/
    7. /dɛntɪst/
    8. /frɪdʒɚerɚ/
    9. /tɛlfon/
    10. /wæmp/
    11. /tusbwəʃ/
    12. /bæftəb/
    13. /tɔɪwət/
    14. /hæmɚ/
    15. /warm kwak/
    16. /vækjum kwinɚ/
    17. /ɛlfənt/
    18. /taɪgɚ/
    19. /skwɝl/
    20. /paɪrɚ/
    21. /jaɪən/
    22. /dɑlfɪn/
    23. /kæŋgru/
    24. /ɑktəpʊs̥/
    25. /jɔɪjɚ/

G. 1. [tʃɛrɪz̥]
    2. [s̥ɛləi]
    3. [tʃiz̥]
    4. [s̥ɪrɪəl]
    5. [greɪps̥]
    6. [aɪs̥krim]
    7. [piz̥]
    8. [pænkeks̥]
    9. [ɛgz̥]
    10. [s̥paɪrɚ]
    11. [ɑktəpʊs̥]
    12. [s̥kwɝl̩]
    13. [s̥neɪk]
    14. [s̥kʌŋk]
    15. [dʒinz̥]
    16. [s̥wɛrɚ]
    17. [pədʒæməz̥]
    18. [s̥ændl̩z̥]
    19. [mɪʔn̩z̥]
    20. [s̥lɪpɚz̥]

    21. We went to Ben Franklin's and looked at the toys.
        [wiwɛntˀtubɛnfræŋklɪnz̥ | ænd lʊktætðətɔɪz̥ ‖]

    22. I saw some dolls that I liked.
        [aɪs̥ɑs̥əmdɑlz̥ðætaɪlaɪkt ‖]

23. They traveled to Maine from Nebraska.
    [ðeɪtræv̩ldtumeɪn | frʌmnəbraṣkə ‖]

24. We do spelling and math.
    [widuṣpɛlɪŋænmæθ ‖]

25. Sometimes we play mystery games.
    [ṣʌmtaɪmẓwipleɪmɪṣtrigeɪmẓ ‖]

H. 1. /frɑg/
    2. [ẓibrə]
    3. [kʊkɪẓ]
    4. /hæmbəgə/
    5. [ṣkʌŋk]
    6. [strɔbɛrɪẓ]
    7. /pɛəkit/
    8. [kɛatṣ]
    9. [ṣɪrɪəl]
    10. /hɑtdɑg/
    11. [pænkekṣ]
    12. [ṣɛlɚɪ]
    13. /dʒɚæf/
    14. [lɑmpṣtə]
    15. /ɚæbɪt/
    16. [ṣpaɪdə]
    17. /ɛləfənt/
    18. [aɪṣkrim]
    19. /bʌtʌ/
    20. [tʃɛrɪẓ]
    21. [ṣkwʌl]
    22. /ɑrəndʒ/
    23. [hɔṣ]
    24. /pəteɪtoʊ/
    25. /tʌtʊl/

I. 1. [pʰ]
    2. [u̞]
    3. [r̥]
    4. [gʷ]
    5. [zˡ or ʐ]
    6. [õ]
    7. [w̥]
    8. [k̚]
    9. [ŋ̊]
    10. [k̠]

J. Possible answers include:
    1. [st⁼ɔr]
    2. [m̃aɪ]
    3. [rʌb̚]
    4. [hɛn]
    5. [bɛtɚ]
    6. [tɛn̪θ]
    7. [dɹɪŋk]
    8. [kɑɫ]
    9. [ɪɱfɔrm]
    10. [kɪʔn̩]

K. 1. clue   [kʰlu]
    2. lymph   [lɪɱf]
    3. money   [mʌ̃nɪ]
    4. coop   [kʰupʰ]
    5. trial   [tʰɹaɪɫ]
    6. skunk   [sk⁼ʌ̃ŋkʰ]
    7. menthol   [mɛ̃n̪θɑɫ]
    8. sweet   [sʷw̥itʰ]

Chapter 9

Chapter Exercises

9.2   1. lid   [lɪ̞d]   4. caught [kɔ̞t] or /kɑt/ (if pronounced as /kɑt/)
      2. when   [wɛ̠n]   5. bag   [bæ̝g]
      3. rub   [rʌ̞b]

9.3   1. may   [me̞]   4. like   [laɪ̝k]
      2. lick   [lɪ̞k]   5. weed   [wi̞d]
      3. cat   [kæ̝t]

9.4 These vowels will vary, based on your dialect.

9.5   1. diphthongization   6. vowel merger
      2. ɪ/ə substitution   7. derhotacization
      3. laxing of vowels   8. monophthongization
      4. deletion of postvocalic /r/   9. tensing of vowels
      5. monophthongization   10. derhotacization

9.6   1. laxing of /u/   6. lack of vowel merger (lowering of /ɛ/)
      2. backing of /æ/   7. fronting of /ɑ/
      3. derhotacization   8. /r/ vocalization
      4. low back merger   9. rhotacization
      5. backing of /æ/   10. fronting of /ɑ/; /r/ derhotacization

9.7   1. [ræ̃ː]   6. /jɛlɪn/
      2. /wɪf/   7. /brʌvə/ or /brʌðə/
      3. /kɛʊl/   8. /haɪnd/
      4. /wiz/   9. /dɪnɪ/
      5. /wʌdn̩t/   10. /pɪkʊ/

9.8   1. cluster reduction   6. stopping
      2. ɑ/ʌ substitution   7. affrication
      3. deaffrication   8. stopping
      4. affrication   9. devoicing
      5. epenthesis   10. cluster reduction

9.9   1. Cantonese, Vietnamese, Korean, Japanese, Filipino
      2. Filipino
      3. Cantonese, Japanese
      4. Vietnamese
      5. Cantonese, Vietnamese, Japanese
      6. Japanese
      7. Vietnamese, Filipino
      8. Vietnamese, Korean, Japanese
      9. Korean
     10. Cantonese, Vietnamese

9.10   1. /mɜdʒd/   4. /əpɪə/
       2. /tʃɑns/   5. /ripɛə/
       3. /gəʊstlɪ/   6. [nɔːθstɑː]

9.11   1. fronting
       2. epenthesis of /ɪ/
       3. epenthesis of /ə/
       4. glide deletion
       5. gliding
       6. fronting
       7. regressive assimilation
       8. dentalization; aspiration
       9. retroflex stop; regressive assimilation
      10. retroflex /ɭ/ for /ɫ/

9.12   1. u/ʊ substitution   5. stopping
       2. gliding   6. dentalization; epenthesis
       3. devoicing; a/æ substitution   7. devoicing; a/ʌ substitution
       4. frication   8. fronting; i/ɪ substitution

9.13   _X_ 1. devoicing   _X_ 5. i/ɪ substitution
       _X_ 2. voicing   _X_ 6. devoicing
       ___ 3.   _X_ 7. epenthesis
       _X_ 4. deaffrication   ___ 8. win

Review Exercises

A. 1. /stɪl/   6. /fɔt/
    2. /stɪə/   7. [kɔːl]
    3. /fɛrɪ/   8. /trɛʒə/
    4. /diu/   9. /lanz/
    5. /meɪʃ/   10. /wɪn/

B. 1. lemon   7. heel
    2. sport   8. worthy
    3. precious   9. chair
    4. pure   10. stew
    5. wish   11. cart
    6. watch   12. carry

C. 1. /biwɛə/   6. /stɔə/
    2. [stɑːt/]   7. [skwɜːt]
    3. /hænə/   8. /glɛə/
    4. /səvɪə/   9. /dɑktə/
    5. [klɜːdʒɪ]   10. [kɑːbən]

D. 1. can't   6. explore
    2. broom   7. charter
    3. marrow   8. largest
    4. bath   9. demand
    5. parrot   10. conspire

E. 1. /mɑf/   6. /dɛm/
    2. /kʌz/   7. /mand/
    3. /ðɪn/   8. /weɪsəz/
    4. [kæ:]   9. /əlɛbn̩/
    5. /hɛʊld/   10. /skreɪt/

F. __X__   1. final stop deletion

    _____   2.

    __X__   3. deletion of unstressed initial syllable

    __X__   4. cluster reduction

    __X__   5. glottal stop substitution

    __X__   6. /ɛ/-/ɪ/ merger

    __X__   7. monophthongization

    __X__   8. /l/ (liquid) deletion

    _____   9.

    __X__ 10. fronting

    _____ 11.

    __X__ 12. final nasal deletion

G. 1. stopping   7. u/ʊ substitution
    2. i/ɪ substitution   8. dentalization
    3. deaffrication   9. affrication of a fricative
    4. a/ʌ substitution   10. stopping
    5. affrication and ɑ/ʌ substitution 11. stopping
    6. cluster reduction   12. epenthesis

H. 1. Korean, Japanese
    2. Cantonese, Japanese
    3. Vietnamese, Korean, Japanese, Filipino
    4. Cantonese, Vietnamese, Korean, Japanese, Filipino
    5. Korean
    6. Vietnamese, Filipino
    7. Cantonese
    8. Filipino
    9. Korean, Japanese
   10. Japanese

I.   1. Arabic   voicing   7. Russian   devoicing

    2. Russian   gliding   8. Arabic   epenthesis

    3. Russian   stopping   9. Russian   voicing

    4. both   u/ʊ substitution   10. Arabic   epenthesis

    5. both   a/ʌ substitution   11. both   r/ɹ substitution

    6. Russian   fronting   12. Arabic   pronouncing silent letters

J.   1. [ma | aɪ gɑɾə go ə ðəstɔː wɪθ pɔl tədeɪ ‖]

    2. [wərəju tɔkɪŋ əbaʊ? ‖ fəget əbaʊt ɪt ɔlɾɛdɪ ‖]

    3. [kɑːlɪ | waɪ dəju hæftə run ɛvrɪθɪŋ ‖]

    4. [aɪ hævə dɛntɪst əpɔɪ?mənt æt sɪks θɜːrɪ ‖]

    5. [rɔbət nidz təgoʊɾə ðə bɔbə | hɪz hɛrz tu lɔŋ ‖]

    6. [aɪ wɔkt ovətə ðə mɔl jestədeɪ æftənun tə getənu pɛɾə ʃuz ‖]

    7. [maɪ dɔg laɪks təɾən ɔl əraʊnd ðə jɑːd n̩ bɑːk ‖]

    8. [wɛn aɪ wəz pleɪŋ bæskətbɔl | aɪ ræn ɔlovə ðəkɔːt ‖]

    9. [aɪ gɑɾəgofudʃapən ‖ aɪ nid wɔɾəmɛlən | kɔn | n̩ soʊdə ‖]

  10. [maɪ frɛn mɛrizə wɪədoʊ | ʃidontwanəlimɪəloʊn ‖]

K.   1. [pak ðə ka ɪnðə gəɾaʒ ‖]

    2. [əmgoʊənə ðəmakət ɪn bɔstən ‖]

    3. [aɪ lʌvɾə ʃɔp havəd skwɪə ‖]

    4. [hæv juz gaɪz bɪnə ðəkeɪp ɔ maθədz vɪnjəd fə ðəsʌmə ‖]

    5. [doʊnt fəgɛɾəbrɪŋ jə pɔkətbʊk ‖]

    6. [danɚ lʌvztə drɪŋk tɔnɪk ‖]

    7. [kɪn ju wɪɾ jə dʌŋgəriz n̩ snɪkəz ‖]

    8. [gɛɾəfak fə ðæt judʒ hɛlpənə pastəŋgreɪvɪ ‖]

    9. [gəhɛdn̩gɪvmʌmɪ səm dʒɪmɪz fɚɚ bənænɚ splɪt ‖]

  10. [dʒɔn mɪlə ɪzə disənt jumən bɪən ‖]

L.   1. [ʃiz dravɪn tu luzɪænə təmaɾə mɔrnɪn ‖]

    2. [əmgʊnə bɔːl ədəzən ɛgz fɚ istɚ ‖]

    3. [læs naɪt aɪwəz takən təma frɛn mɛrɪlɪən ‖]

    4. [əmfɪksən təhævɾə ba səm tarz fəməkar ‖]

    5. [əmlʊkənfəma blu bal pɔɪ? peən ‖]

    6. [ju bɛɾə kʌvɚ ðæt brɔːlən pæn wɪθ əlumɪnəm fɔːl ‖]

    7. [weɪɾəmɪnətlɛrɪ | a nid ənə ðɚ mɪnət təmeɪkəpma mand ‖]

    8. [a lɛft ðə tʃɪkən aʊt ɑn ðə kaʊnɚ ænd ɪt spɔːld ‖]

    9. [ðə junɪvɚsərɪ əv tɛnəsi ɪz ɪn naksvəl ‖]

  10. [hɜ˞ɪkənz n̩ tɔrnaɪɾəz arboθ lardʒ dæmədʒɪn wɪnstɔrmz ‖]

M.   1. [də bɔɪ nid moʊ mʌnɪ ‖]

    2. [wi fɪksəntə gotudə stoʊ ‖]

    3. [hi bi pleɪən bal ætdəpark ‖]

    4. [ðɛr ar foʊ nu kɪːz ɪn maɪ klæs ‖]

    5. [maɪ sɪstə æn brʌvə wəzætdæt kansət ‖]

    6. [maɪ fæmlɪ goʊ tə tʃɜtʃ ɛrːɪ sʌndeɪ ‖]

    7. [joʊ maməkarɪnəmɪ̩əðəʃtriː? ‖]

    8. [ʃi faʊn faɪː kwoʊrəz ɪnə pɜs ‖]

    9. [kwanzə gat hə hɛr dən ‖]

    10. [ðə studənts hɛlpt dɛmsɛlvz tu brɛkfəs ‖]

N.   1. [pliʑ | pʊt dəflaʊəʑ ɪndə beɪs ‖]

    2. [ɪt wəs ə βɛrɪ əspɛʃɪəl okeɪzjən ‖]

    3. [ju sʊd kwɪt dʒɛlɪŋ æt jɔr marə ‖]

    4. [aɪ wəs nat suə | aɪ wʊt bi eɪbl̩tu hɛlp ‖]

    5. [maɪ feɪβəɪːitʃəʑ neɪmis mistə dʒɔnz ‖]

    6. [doʊnt lɛt jɔr dak pleɪ ɪn maɪ djart ‖]

    7. [waɪ doʊnt ju pʊt dis kloʊðz ɪn də gʌraʒ ‖]

    8. [jɛstədeɪ | aɪ wɛntːu ðə su | wɪθ dak ‖]

    9. [sɛlɪ pʊt ðə poteɪtoʊ tʃɪps an ðə loʊə sɛlf ‖]

    10. [aɪwəʑ bɛrɪ ɛksaɪrət əbaʊt winɪŋ də futbal geɪm ‖]

O.   1. [aɪ hæv wʌn jʌŋgə brʌzə ɪn maɪ fæməɪ ‖]

    2. [aɪwʊd raɪkə grɪld tʃiz sandwɪtʃ fɔrːʌntʃ priz ‖]

    3. [ɪt ɪz səpoʊs tu reɪn hɛvrɪ fɔr mʌtʃ əðəwik ‖]

    4. [zə rɪvə ɪz hɛvrɪ pʊrutəd ‖]

    5. [maɪ θɪstə kjoʊkoʊ wɪl bi twɛnɪsri jɪrʑold nɛksθɜsdeɪ ‖]

    6. [wʊdʒu raɪk tu goʊ ʃɔpɪŋ wɪsmi æftəaɪ gɛt af wɜk ‖]

    7. [wʊd jɔr ʌðə brʌzə hɛlp mi rɪft ðɪθ ‖ ɪts hɛvɪ ‖]

    8. [sæŋk ju bɛrɪ mʌtʃ fɔr zə bjutɪfʊl fraʊəz ‖]

    9. [aɪ hæv ə hard taɪm dɪstɪŋgwɪʃ bɪtˠwin zə sɪŋgjurə ænd prɜəl fɔrmʑ ‖]

    10. [ði oʊnrɪ konɛktɪŋ fraɪt ɪsːru pɔrtrənd ɔrəgɔn ‖]

P.   1. [taɪpɪŋ imeɪlʑ hɛlps mi fɪŋk ɪn ɪŋgrɪʃ ‖]

    2. [aɪ wɛnt tudə ʑu tu si də nu pændə bɪrs ‖]

    3. [wʌt duju θɪŋkəvdə nu tɛrəvɪʒn ʃoʊ ‖]

    4. [aɪ hæb tu ɔr θri frɛnz hu ar goʊɪŋ tu də sakə geɪm ‖]

    5. [juzəlɪ | si ɪs nat | so fɔrgɛtʰfʊl ‖]

    6. [aɪ bɛt ju dæt aɪ wɪl wɪn də reɪs ‖]

    7. [maɪ gɜlfrɛnd sɛnt mi fraʊəz last wik fɔr maɪ bɜfdeɪ ‖]

    8. [dɛr ar sɛvrəl pipəl aɪ nid tu gɛt tu noʊ ‖]

    9. [də leɪaʊt əʑ disːɪrɪ ɪs nat vɛrɪ kanvinɪənt ‖]

    10. [aɪ præn tu goʊ tu pədu fɔr maɪ mæstəʑ digri ‖]

Q. 1. [maɪ ɑntiz goʊɪŋ tu stʌdi ɔdɪə'lɔdʒɪ æt ðə juniwɝsɪɾɪ əv kæntəkɪ ‖]
2. [aɪ nid t̪u peɪ maɪ tjuɪʃən ɪn ðə bʊrsəz̥ ɔfɪs ‖]
3. [ðeɪ nid jɔr hɛlp ɪmidʒiətlɪ ‖]
4. [maɪ faɖɚ plæntəd hɝbz əraʊndɚ 'pɛrɪmɪtɚ əv maɪ gardən ‖]
5. [ðə kən'tɛnts əv ðə poʊʃən ɪnklud kælʃɪəm æn potæʃɪəm ‖]
6. [aɪ pʊt wɪnəgɚ æn ɔɪl ɔn maɪ təmeɪɾo ænd letɪus sæləd ‖]
7. [aɪ dʒəst gɑɾə baks əv tʃɔklət kʌvʊd kɛrəmɛlz ‖]
8. [maɪ ə'daləsənt kʌzɪn brʌɖɚ ɛksɛld æt ə'kædəmɪks ‖]
9. [ʃi ʃʊd skɛdjʊəl æn əpɔɪnːmənt wɪθə baɪo'lɔdʒɪ dɪpartmənt ‖]
10. [pliz rirɑɪt ðə læsːən'tæns əv ðə pɛrəgraf ‖]

R. 1. [aɪwʊd laɪk e wɔdkə ænd tɔnɪk pliz̥ ‖]
2. [pʊt de bʊks ovɚ dɛr ɑn də teɪbl̩ ‖]
3. [it wʌz difɪkʊlt fɔr mi tu lʊrn də kərɛkt pronaʊnseɪʃən ‖]
4. [aɪ hæv bɪn livɪŋ in də junaɪɾəd steɪts sins last ɔgəst ‖]
5. [xi xæz̥ mɛni prabləmz wɪθ hɪz vokæbələrɪ ‖]
6. [də rʌʃən ikɔnəmi dipɛnz ɔn də karənt praɪs əv ɔɪl ‖]
7. [maɪ jʌŋgɚ brʌðɚ aləgzandɚ ɪz stʌdɪŋ mɛtəlʊrdʒi æt mɔskoʊ steɪt junivɝsiti ‖]
8. [di aʊtɚ əv də bʊk wʊz e feɪməs raɪtʊr ‖]
9. [aɪ hɛd sɛvɔrəl wɪzɪtɚz frəm vʊrdʒinɪə last manθ ‖]
10. [haʊ mɛni ʌðɚ pipʊl nidəd tu teɪk di klɛs ‖]

S. 1. [bliz juz dæt wʊrd ɪn e sɛntəns ‖]
2. [aɪ nid ʃugɚ səbɪstɪtut fɔr maɪ kɔfi ‖]
3. [dʊktɚ kubɚ tɔld mi tu meɪk e kɔbi əv ðə hoʊmwɚk əsaɪnmənt ‖]
4. [ðɛr frɛnd robɪn gɑt mɛrɪd tu fɪktɔr maɪ nekst dɔr neɪbɔr ‖]
5. [aɪ wʌz diɓrest bikʊz wi hæv had soʊ mʌtʃ bæd weɖɚ ‖]
6. [bit gɔt ə prɛz̩ sɪntɪns bikʊz hi hɛd ðə polismɛn ‖]
7. [maɪ feɪfərɪt kɔtən ʃɝt ʃrʌŋk ɪn ðə lɔndərɪ ‖]
8. [bɪnɪ fɪzɪtəd hɝ fianseɪ ɑn fraɪdeɪ ‖]
9. [aɪ nid tu stʌdɪ ɪŋgəlɪʃ fonəloʊdʒɪ tu ɪmbruv maɪ pronaʊnzieɪʃən ‖]
10. [aɪ gru e bɪrd so ðæt aɪ wʊd əbɪr oʊldɚ ‖]

APPENDIX

Audio CDs to Accompany Fundamentals of Phonetics: A Practical Guide for Students, 4th Ed.

CD One

Track #	Chapter	Track Title	Text Page #
1	2	Intro. to Word Stress	26
2	2	Stress Word List 1	26
3	2	Stress Word List 2	27
4	2	Stress Word List 3	27
5	2	Stress Word List 4	27
6	2	Stress Word List 5	27
7	2	Stress Word List 6	27
8	2	Stress Word List 7	27
9	2	Stress Word List 8	28
10	2	Stress Word List 9	28
11	2	Stress Word List 10	28
12	2	Stress Word List 11	28
13	2	Stress Word List 12	28
14	2	Exercise 2.18	29
15	2	Exercise 2.19	29
16	2	Exercise 2.20	29
17	2	Review Exercise J	33
18	2	Review Exercise K	33
19	2	Review Exercise L	33
20	4	Review Exercise E	98
21	4	Review Exercise F	98
22	4	Review Exercise G	99
23	4	Review Exercise L	101
24	4	Review Exercise M	102
25	4	Assignment 4-1	103
26	4	Assignment 4-2	105
27	4	Assignment 4-3	107
28	4	Assignment 4-4	109

CD Two

Track #	Chapter	Track Title	Text Page #
1	5	Review Exercise H	156
2	5	Review Exercise I	157
3	5	Assignment 5-1	159
4	5	Assignment 5-2	161
5	5	Assignment 5-3	163
6	5	Assignment 5-4	165
7	5	Assignment 5-5	167
8	5	Assignment 5-6	169
9	5	Assignment 5-7	171
10	7	Exercise 7.4	211
11	7	Exercise 7.5	212
12	7	Exercise 7.6	214
13	7	Exercise 7.7	214
14	7	Exercise 7.8	215
15	7	Exercise 7.9	215
16	7	Exercise 7.11	217
17	7	Exercise 7.12	218
18	7	Exercise 7.13	220
19	7	Exercise 7.14	223
20	7	Exercise 7.16	225
21	7	Exercise 7.17	226

CD Three

Track #	Chapter	Track Title	Text Page #
1	7	Review Exercise C	227
2	7	Review Exercise E	229
3	7	Review Exercise G	230
4	7	Review Exercise H	230
5	7	Review Exercise I	230
6	7	Review Exercise J	231
7	7	Review Exercise K	232
8	7	Assignment 7-1	235
9	7	Assignment 7-2	237
10	7	Assignment 7-3	239
11	8	Review Exercise F	277
12	8	Review Exercise G	278
13	8	Review Exercise H	278
14	8	Assignment 8-2	283
15	8	Assignment 8-3	285
16	9	Review Exercise J	334
17	9	Review Exercise K	335
18	9	Review Exercise L	335
19	9	Review Exercise M	336
20	9	Review Exercise N	336
21	9	Review Exercise O	337
22	9	Review Exercise P	338
23	9	Review Exercise Q	338
24	9	Review Exercise R	339
25	9	Review Exercise S	339
26	9	Intro. Assign. 9-1	343
27	9	Assign. 9-1 #1 African Am.	343
28	9	Assign. 9-1 #2 Eastern Am.	343
29	9	Assign. 9-1 #3 Cantonese-Inf.	344
30	9	Assign. 9-1 #4 Spanish-Inf.	344
31	9	Assign. 9-1 #5 Southern Am.	344
32	9	Assign. 9-1 #6 Japanese-Inf.	345
33	9	Assign. 9-1 #7 Eastern Am.	345
34	9	Assign. 9-1 #8 Russian-Inf.	345
35	9	Assign. 9-1 #9 Arabic-Inf.	346
36	9	Assign. 9-1 #10 Asian Indian	346

Glossary

abduction movement of the vocal folds away from the midline (closed) position

accent modification treatment for a non-native speaker of English, designed to increase speech intelligibility without jeopardizing the integrity of the individual's first dialect

addition insertion of an extra phoneme in the production of a word, usually used in reference to disordered speech; also referred to as *epenthesis*

adduction movement of the vocal folds toward the midline (closed) position

affricate consonant characterized as having both a fricative and a stop manner of production (e.g., /tʃ and dʒ/)

African American English (AAE) dialect of English, spoken throughout the United States, traced back to the dialects of English spoken in Britain and brought to America by British settlers; previously referred to as Black English, Black English Vernacular, African American Vernacular English, and Ebonics

allograph differing letter sequences that represent the same phoneme (e.g., h<u>ea</u>t, k<u>ey</u>, and r<u>ee</u>d)

allophone variant production of a phoneme (e.g., [pʰ] and [p˺])

allophonic transcription *see* narrow transcription

alveolar referring to the alveolar ridge; a consonant produced with a constriction formed by the tongue apex or blade and the alveolar ridge (e.g., /t, d, n, s, z, and l/)

alveolar assimilation assimilatory phonological process that occurs when a non-alveolar consonant is produced with an alveolar place of production due to the presence of an alveolar phoneme elsewhere in the word

alveolar ridge gum ridge of the maxilla located directly behind the upper front teeth

antiformant negative resonance (brought about when the velum lowers during production of nasal sounds) that causes a decrease in the intensity of nasal and vowel formants

apex tip of the tongue

approximant consonant, such as a glide or liquid, produced with an obstruction in the vocal tract, less than that associated with the obstruents or nasals but greater than that associated with the vowels

articulation modification of the airstream by the speech organs in production of spoken language

articulation disorder difficulty in coordinating the articulators in production of a limited set of phonemes; difficulty with the motoric aspects of speech production

arytenoid cartilages paired cartilages of the larynx that attach to the superior portion of the cricoid cartilage; each vocal fold attaches to one arytenoid cartilage

aspiration production of a frictional noise (similar to /h/) following the release of a voiceless stop consonant

assimilation process by which phonemes take on the phonetic character of neighboring sounds due to coarticulation; refers to articulatory changes that result in the production of an allophone, or of a completely different phoneme

assimilatory processes phonological processes that involve an alteration in phoneme production due to phonetic environment

back (of the tongue); portion of the tongue body posterior to the front of the tongue; it lies inferior to the velum

Back Upglide Shift chain shift associated with the South; affects production of /ɔ/ and /aʊ/

Bernoulli effect drop in air pressure, created by an increase in airflow through a constriction; helps explain, in part, vocal fold adduction

bilabial phonemes produced with a constriction involving both lips (e.g., /p, b, m, and w/)

blade part of the tongue located just posterior to the tip

body (of the tongue); portion of the tongue posterior to the blade, making up the front and the back of the tongue

bound morpheme morpheme that must be linked to another morpheme in order to convey meaning (e.g., <u>pre</u>date and think<u>ing</u>)

broad transcription   phonemic transcription of speech indicated by the use of slash marks (virgules); diacritics are not used in broad transcription

bunched   one method of /r/ production in which the tongue apex is lowered as the tongue blade is raised to form one constriction with the palate, while the tongue root forms a second pharyngeal constriction

central incisor   any of the four front teeth, located in both the upper and lower jaws

chain shift   dialectal modification in the pronunciation of English vowels, reflecting an alteration in their place of production; the change in the articulatory target for one vowel has a relative effect on the targets for other vowels (e.g., Northern Cities Shift and Southern Shift)

citation form   pronunciation of a word as a single, isolated item

closed syllable   syllable with a consonant phoneme in the final position

close internal juncture   two syllables in the same intonational phrase with no transitional pause between them (e.g., /aɪskrim/)

cluster reduction   syllable structure phonological process that results in the deletion of a consonant from a cluster

coarticulation   articulatory process whereby individual phonemes overlap one another due to timing constraints and ease of production

coda   consonants that follow a vowel in any syllable; not all syllables have a coda

cognates   phonemes that differ only in voicing (e.g., /t/ and /d/)

complementary distribution   allophone production that is tied to a particular phonetic environment

connected speech   utterance consisting of two or more continuous words

consonant   phoneme produced with a constriction in the vocal tract; usually found at the beginning and end of a syllable; *generally* shorter in duration and having higher-frequency spectra than vowels

consonant cluster   two or three contiguous consonants in a syllable (e.g., strike, please, and leapt)

content word   word that contains the most salient information in an utterance (e.g., a noun, verb, adjective, or adverb)

creole   pidgin language that is passed on to a new generation of users

cricoid cartilage   the most inferior cartilage of the larynx, shaped like a class ring

damping   reduction in amplitude of energy (intensity) of a vibrating system

deaffrication   substitution phonological process that involves the replacement of a fricative for an affricate

denasality   *see* hyponasality

dental   referring to the teeth; a consonant produced with a constriction formed by either the tongue apex and the teeth (e.g., /θ and ð/) or by the lower lip and the upper teeth, or labiodental (e.g., /f and v/)

dentalization   production of an alveolar phoneme as linguadental, that is, with the tongue tip more forward than normal

derhotacization   loss of r-coloring of the central vowels /ɜ/ and /ɚ/, and postvocalic /r/

devoicing   assimilatory phonological process (voicing assimilation) that involves the replacement of a voiceless phoneme for a normally voiced, syllable-final consonant preceding a pause or silence

diacritic   specialized phonetic symbol used in narrow transcription to represent both allophonic production as well as suprasegmental features of speech

dialect   variation of speech or language based on geographic area, native language background, or social or ethnic group membership

diaphragm   major muscle that separates the abdomen from the thorax

digraph   pair of letters that represent one sound; the letters may be the same or different (e.g., look, think, and ear)

diphthong   single phoneme consisting of two vowel elements, the first termed the *onglide* and the second the *offglide*

diphthong simplification   *see* monophthongization

distortion   characteristic of disordered speech involving the production of an allophone of an intended phoneme

dorsum   body of the tongue, composed primarily of the front and back; also, the back of the tongue

Eastern American English   regional dialect of English spoken in the New England states and in New York, New Jersey, and Pennsylvania

Educated Indian English   a preferred method of English pronunciation adopted by educators in India; keeps the basic phonological concepts of received pronunciation, allowing for regional pronunciation; emphasis on correct usage of suprasegmental aspects of speech; also referred to as *Educated Indian Pronunciation*

Educated Indian Pronunciation   *see* Educated Indian English

ejective   non-pulmonic consonant produced with a large glottalic air pressure release; brought about by raising the larynx, causing a decreased area between the closed vocal folds and the constriction in the oral cavity

elision   omission of a phoneme from a word as a result of a historical change, or from coarticulation associated with connected speech

English Language Learner (ELL)   an individual who is attempting to master English as a second language; term adopted by the National Council of Teachers of English (NCTE)

epenthesis   addition of a phoneme to a word during speech production as a result of coarticulation, dialect, or a speech disorder

epiglottis   cartilaginous structure that protects the larynx from food and drink during swallowing

ethnolect   dialect associated with a particular ethnic group

external intercostal muscles   muscles located between the ribs that aid in inhalation; the external intercostals are superficial to the internal intercostals

external juncture   pause serving to connect two intonational phrases in connected speech

extIPA   extension to the IPA that has become the official diacritic set for the transcription of disordered speech; adopted by the International Clinical Phonetics and Linguistics Association in 1994

falling intonational phrase   fall, or declination, in the pitch of the voice across the length of an intonational phrase; usually associated with complete statements and commands, as well as wh-questions

final consonant deletion   syllable structure phonological process that involves the deletion of the final consonant in a syllable, resulting in an open syllable (CV)

formal standard English   the English of dictionaries, grammar books, and most printed manner; the idealized form of English used in teaching English

formant   resonant frequency of the vocal tract

formant transition   dynamic change in the resonant frequencies of the vocal tract over time, signaling modifications in the place of articulation of speech sounds (as seen on a spectrogram)

free morpheme   morpheme that can stand alone yet still carry meaning

free variation   refers to allophone production that is not tied to a particular phonetic environment

frequency   number of cycles a vibrating body completes in 1 second; usually indicated in Hz

fricative   consonant produced by forcing the breath stream through a narrow channel formed by two separate articulators in the vocal tract; (e.g., /s/ and /v/)

front   (of the tongue); the part of the tongue body anterior to the back of the tongue; it lies inferior to the (hard) palate

fronting   substitution phonological process that involves the replacement of an alveolar consonant for a velar or palatal consonant

function word   word that contributes little to the meaning of an utterance (e.g., a pronoun, article, preposition, or conjunction)

fundamental frequency   the basic rate of vibration of the vocal folds

General American English   sometimes used synonymously with *Standard American English* to denote a form of English devoid of any regional pronunciation; may be used when comparing regional or ethnic dialects to a national "standard"

given information   previous exchange of words, or shared world knowledge between two conversational participants

glide   consonant characterized by a continued, gliding motion of the articulators into the following vowel; also referred to as a semi-vowel (e.g., /j/ and /w/)

gliding   substitution phonological process that involves the replacement of a glide for a liquid

glottal   referring to the glottis; a phoneme produced at the level of the vocal folds (e.g., /h/)

glottal stop   allophonic variation of /t/ or /d/, produced when the release of the stop is at the level of the vocal folds instead of at the alveolar ridge (i.e., /ʔ/)

glottis   space between the vocal folds

grapheme   printed alphabet letter used in the representation of an allograph

habitual pitch   inherent fundamental frequency of a given individual

hard palate   structure, also known as the "roof of the mouth," that separates the oral and nasal cavities; also referred to as the *palate*

homorganic   two consonants sharing the same place of articulation (e.g., time and neck)

hyoid bone   "floating bone" that provides structural support for the larynx; attaches inferiorly to the larynx by a broad curtain-like ligament and superiorly to the tongue by muscle tissue

hypernasality   presence of excessive nasality accompanying the production of a non-nasal phoneme due to improper velopharyngeal closure

hyponasality   production of nasal phonemes with a raised velum; also referred to as *denasality*

idiolect   speech pattern unique to an individual, based on dialect and personal speaking habit

idiosyncratic process   phonological process that is not characteristic of the speech behavior of a typically developing child

implosive   non-pulmonic consonant produced with an ingressive glottalic airstream; brought about by lowering the larynx, causing an increased area between the vocal folds and the constriction in the oral cavity

impressionistic transcription   allophonic transcription of an unknown speaker or an unknown language

informal standard English   based on listener judgments of patterns of spoken English deemed to be acceptable or not

intensity   amplitude (magnitude) of energy associated with a particular sound; often indicated in decibels (dB)

interdental   phonemes produced by placing the tongue tip between the teeth (e.g., /θ and ð/)

internal intercostal muscles   muscles located between the ribs that aid in exhalation; the internal intercostals are deep to the external intercostals

International Phonetic Alphabet (IPA)   alphabet used to represent the sounds of the world's languages; created to promote a universal method of phonetic transcription

intervocalic   consonant located between two vowels (e.g., above)

intonation   modification of voice pitch associated with varying utterance types (such as a question or a statement), or associated with a speaker's particular mood

intonational phrase   changes in the fundamental frequency of the voice spanning the length of a meaningful utterance (a word, phrase, or sentence)

intraoral pressure   air pressure within the oral cavity, created by a constriction of the articulators during production of stop consonants

juncture   transitional pauses and breaks between syllables and words in speech production

labial   referring to the lips; consonant produced with a constriction formed at the lips (e.g., /f and v/); also used to refer to the bilabial phonemes /p, b, m, and w/

labial assimilation   an assimilatory phonological process that occurs when a non-labial phoneme is produced with a labial place of articulation due to the presence of a labial phoneme elsewhere in the word

labialization   addition of lip rounding to the articulation of a typically unrounded phoneme

labiodental   consonant produced with a constriction formed by the lower lip and upper central incisors (e.g., /f and v/)

language transfer   incorporation of native language (L$_1$) features into the target language (L$_2$) as the second language is being learned

larynx   cartilaginous and muscular structure that houses the vocal folds; responsible for phonation

lateral   manner of production in which the airstream is directed over the sides of the tongue (e.g., /l/)

lateralization   production of a nonlateral phoneme (any phoneme except /l/) with a lateral place of production (e.g., producing /s/ or /z/ as /ɬ/ or /ɮ/, respectively)

lax   description of a vowel produced with a reduction in muscular effort; a lax vowel does not appear in the final position of an open monosyllable (e.g., /ɪ, ɛ, æ, ʊ, ɚ, ʌ, and ə/)

lexical stress   *see* word stress

lingual   referring to the tongue; consonant produced with the tongue as the major articulator

liquid   generic label used to classify the two English approximant consonants /r/ and /l/

loudness   perceptual correlate of intensity

low back merger   dialectal variation reflecting a change in the articulatory targets for /ɔ/ and /ɑ/, so that no differentiation occurs in their production; characteristic of certain western and New England speakers

mandible   the lower jaw

manner of production   the way in which the airstream is modified as it passes through the vocal tract in production of consonants; English manners of production include stop, fricative, affricate, nasal, glide, and liquid

maxilla   the upper jaw

metathesis   transposition of phonemes in a word due to a speech error, dialectal variation, or speech disorder

minimal contrast   *see* minimal pair

minimal pair   pair of words that vary by only one phoneme (e.g., cook/book and passed/last); also referred to as *minimal contrast*

misarticulation   articulatory error, classically categorized as an omission, substitution, distortion, or addition

monophthong   vowel phoneme consisting of one distinct articulatory element (as opposed to a diphthong, which has two elements)

monophthongization   process of producing a diphthong as a monophthong (e.g., "fire" /fɑr/); also referred to as *diphthong simplification*

morpheme   smallest unit of language capable of carrying meaning

nares   the nostrils

narrow transcription   transcription of speech using diacritics to indicate allophonic production and/or suprasegmental aspects of speech; brackets, as opposed to slash marks, are used with narrow transcription; also referred to as *allophonic transcription*

nasal emission   audible escape of air through the nares due to improper velopharyngeal closure or to a cleft in the palate or the velum

nasal formant   first formant associated with nasal murmur; located around 250 to 300 Hz for the three nasal consonants

nasalization   production of an oral phoneme with accompanying nasal resonance, due to a lowered velum (e.g., [mɛ̃n])

nasal murmur   radiation of acoustic energy outward through the nasal cavity (due to a lowered velum) during production of nasal consonants

nasal phoneme   consonant produced with complete closure in the oral cavity along with a lowered velum to allow airflow through the nasal cavity; the only nasal phonemes in English are /m, n, and ŋ/

nasal plosion   release of a stop consonant through the nasal cavity, as opposed to the oral cavity, as in the word /sʌdn̩/

natural phonology   Stampe's theory that supports the idea that children are born with innate processes necessary for the development of speech

new information   exchange of words between two conversational participants that adds to the knowledge already shared

nonlinear phonology   method of phonological analysis that involves performing an inventory of a child's speech sound system on multiple levels including words, syllables, segments, and features; phonemes are identified without consideration of what is phonemic or contrastive in the target language (adult system), but rather which consonants and vowels are used contrastively in particular contexts in the child's system

non-resonant consonants (non-resonants)   *see* obstruent consonants

non-sibilant consonants   the fricatives /f, v, θ, ð, and h/; perceived as being less intense when compared to the sibilant consonants /s, z, ʃ, and ʒ/

Northern Cities Shift   ongoing change in the production of vowels, causing a shift from their standard place of articulation in the vowel quadrilateral; seen in the northern tier of the United States in cities such as Cleveland, Detroit, and Buffalo

nuclear accent   *see* tonic accent

nuclear syllable   *see* tonic syllable

nucleus   the part of a syllable with the greatest acoustic energy; usually, but not always, a vowel

obstruent consonants (obstruents)   class of sounds (with a noise source) including the stops, fricatives, and affricates; produced with a constriction in the oral cavity that results in turbulence in the airstream coming from the larynx; also referred to as *non-resonant consonants*

offglide   second element of a diphthong

omission   deletion of a phoneme in a word, usually related to disordered speech

onglide   first element of a diphthong

onset   all consonants preceding a vowel in any syllable; not all syllables contain an onset

open internal juncture   transitional pause between two syllables within the same tone group (e.g., /aɪ + skrim/)

open syllable   syllable with a vowel phoneme in the final position

oral phoneme   phoneme produced with a raised velum (velopharyngeal closure) so that the airstream is directed through the oral cavity; all English phonemes are oral except for /m, n, and ŋ/

palatal   referring to the hard palate; consonant produced with a constriction formed by the tongue blade and the hard palate (e.g., /ʃ, ʒ, tʃ, dʒ, r, and j/)

palate   *see* hard palate

palatoalveolar   consonant produced with a constriction formed by the tongue blade and the hard palate, slightly posterior to the constriction formed during production of alveolar consonants; often used to describe the place of production of /ʃ and ʒ/; also referred to as *postalveolar*

period   time course of one cycle of vibration; calculated by the formula $T = 1/f$, where T = time (in seconds) and f = frequency in Hz

pharynx   muscular tubelike structure that connects the larynx and the oral cavity; the throat

phonation   vibration of the vocal folds in creation of a voiced sound

phoneme   speech sound capable of differentiating morphemes

phonemic transcription   *see* broad transcription

phonetic alphabet   alphabet that contains a separate letter for each individual sound in a language (e.g., the IPA)

phonetics   study of the speech sounds, their acoustic and perceptual characteristics, and how they are produced by the speech organs

phonological disorder   difficulty in speech sound production resulting in multiple speech sound errors ultimately involving the sound system of a language; also used to describe articulation disorder

phonological processes   simplifications used by children not capable of producing adult speech patterns

phonology   systematic organization of speech sounds in the production of language; the study of the linguistic rules that specify the manner in which phonemes are organized and combined into syllables, words, and sentences

pidgin   a language that results when individuals speaking two different languages begin to communicate; typically characterized as having a reduced vocabulary and grammar

pitch   perceptual correlate of frequency

place of articulation   refers to the specific articulators employed in the production of a particular phoneme; the location of the constriction in the vocal tract in production of a consonant

plosive   *see* stop

point vowel   one of four extreme corner vowels of the vowel quadrilateral (i.e., /i, æ, u, and ɑ/)

postalveolar   *see* palatoalveolar

postvocalic consonant   consonant following a vowel (e.g., at)

prevocalic consonant   consonant preceding a vowel (e.g., me)

prevocalic voicing   assimilatory phonological process (voicing assimilation) that involves the voicing of a normally unvoiced consonant preceding the nucleus of a syllable

progressive assimilation   modification in the identity of a phoneme due to a previously occurring phoneme; left-to-right or perseverative assimilation

quality   perceptual character of a sound based on its acoustic resonance patterns; also referred to as *timbre*

r-colored vowel   speech sound consisting of the two elements: vowel + /r/ (e.g., /ɪr, ɛr, ʊr, ɔr, and ɑr/); also referred to as a *rhotic diphthong*

received pronunciation (RP)   originally a regional dialect of standard British English in southern England (historically referred to as BBC English) that became less regional and more a dialect of prestige and social class; regional variations exist today; the original form is now somewhat stigmatized

reduplication   a syllable structure phonological process that involves the repetition of a syllable of a word

regressive assimilation   modification in the identity of a phoneme due to a later occurring phoneme; right-to-left or anticipatory assimilation

resonance   vibratory properties of any sound-producing body

resonant consonants (resonants)   *see* sonorant consonants

retroflex   place of articulation that involves curling the tongue tip back so that it comes in contact with the area between the alveolar ridge and the hard palate; some English speakers produce /r/ with a retroflex articulation (postalveolar); some Asian Indian English speakers produce the plosives /t/ and /d/ with a retroflex articulation (i.e., / ʈ/ and /ɖ/, respectively)

rhotacization   production of a phoneme with an /r/ auditory quality (e.g., /r/, /ɝ/, or /ɚ/)

rhotic diphthong   *see* r-colored vowel

rhyme   syllable segment consisting of an obligatory nucleus (usually a vowel) and an optional coda

rising intonational phrase   general rise in the pitch of the voice across the length of an intonational phrase; usually associated with yes/no questions, tag questions, lists, and incomplete utterances

root   portion of the tongue that attaches to the anterior wall of the pharynx and to the mandible

rounded   rounded lip position during vowel production; the rounded English vowels include /u, ʊ, o, ɔ, ɝ, and ɚ/

sentence stress   added emphasis given to a specific word in a sentence due to the importance of that word in conveying meaning, or due to speaker intent; often found in association with the last word in a declarative utterance

sibilant   the alveolar and palatal fricatives /s, z, ʃ, and ʒ/, which are perceived as being louder than the other fricatives

sociolect   dialect associated with a particular social class

soft palate   *see* velum

sonorant consonants (sonorants)   class of sounds produced with resonance throughout the entire vocal tract (e.g., the nasals, glides, and liquids); they are produced with little constriction in the vocal tract and are therefore produced without much turbulence in the airstream coming from the larynx; also referred to as *resonant consonants*

Southern American English   regional dialect spoken in the southern and south Midland states

Southern Shift   ongoing change in the production of vowels, causing a shift from their standard place of articulation in the vowel quadrilateral; this shift is seen in the southern, middle Atlantic, and southern mountain states

spectrogram   graphic representation of the three major parameters that describe the acoustic characteristic of any sound: *time, frequency*, and *intensity*; time is indicated on the abscissa, frequency is indicated on the ordinate, and intensity is indicated by shading (more intense sounds are darker)

spectrum   frequency array, or energy pattern, characteristic of any sound

speech sound disorder   term used to refer to an individual with a phonological or articulation disorder

Standard American English (SAE)   form of English that is relatively devoid of regional characteristics; the English used in textbooks and by national broadcasters

sternum   the breastbone

stop   consonant characterized by (1) a complete obstruction of the outgoing airstream by the articulators, (2) a buildup of intraoral air pressure, and (3) a release; also referred to as a *plosive*; (e.g., /p/ and /g/)

stop gap   the time (in milliseconds) on a spectrogram that reflects increasing intraoral pressure prior to the release of a stop

stopping   substitution phonological process that involves the replacement of a stop for a fricative or an affricate

subglottal pressure   air pressure applied to the inferior surface of the vocal folds (glottis); the air pressure (from the lungs) necessary to blow the vocal folds apart

substitution   replacement of one phoneme by another in a syllable or word

substitution processes   phonological processes involving the substitution of one phoneme class by another (e.g., gliding, deaffrication, or fronting)

suprasegmental   feature of speech production, such as stress, intonation, and timing, that transcends the phonemic level

syllabic consonant   consonant that serves as the nucleus of a syllable (e.g., /l, m, and n/)

syllable   basic unit of speech production and perception generally consisting of a segment of greatest acoustic energy (a peak, usually a vowel) and segments of lesser energy (troughs, usually consonants); unit of speech consisting of an onset and/or a rhyme

syllable structure processes   phonological processes that generally simplify the production of syllables, creating a consonant–vowel (CV) pattern

tap   manner of consonant production involving a rapid movement of the tongue tip against the alveolar ridge resulting in the creation of a very brief phoneme (i.e., /ɾ/)

Telsur Project   telephone survey conducted by the University of Pennsylvania to study variation in vowel production across the United States

tempo   timing, or durational aspect, of connected speech

tense   description of a vowel produced with an increased muscular effort; a tense vowel can be located in the final position of an open monosyllable (e.g., /i, e, u, o, ɔ, ɑ, and ɝ/)

thoracic cavity (thorax)   part of the human body between the head/neck and the abdomen; the chest cavity

thyroid cartilage   the most anterior cartilage of the larynx to which the vocal folds attach; the notch of the thyroid cartilage forms the "Adam's apple"

timbre   *see* quality

time   (in acoustics); the duration of any particular sound

tongue advancement   term used to classify vowel production in relation to tongue position along the front/back dimension in the oral cavity

tongue height   term used to classify vowel production in relation to tongue position along the high/low dimension in the oral cavity

tonic accent   emphasis given to the tonic (nuclear) syllable in any particular intonational phrase; also referred to as *nuclear accent*

tonic syllable   syllable that contains the greatest pitch change in any particular intonational phrase; also referred to as *nuclear syllable*

trachea   tube, composed of cartilaginous rings embedded in muscle tissue, that connects the lungs with the larynx; windpipe

unreleased   stop consonant produced with no audible release burst

unrounded   spread or retracted lip position during vowel production (e.g., /i, ɪ, e, ɛ, æ, ɑ, ʌ, and ə/)

uvula   rounded, tablike structure located at the posterior tip of the velum

velar   referring to the soft palate (velum); consonant produced with a constriction formed by the back of the tongue and the velum (e.g., /k, g, and ŋ/)

velar assimilation   assimilatory phonological process that occurs when a non-velar phoneme is produced with a velar place of production due to the presence of a velar phoneme elsewhere in the word

velarization   backed production of an alveolar phoneme (such as /l/) so that the tongue is more posterior than normal (in the velar region): [rigɫ]

velar pinch   closeness in frequency between F_2 and F_3 during production of velar stop consonants

velopharyngeal closure   constriction formed by the velum and the rear wall of the pharynx, resulting in a diversion of the airstream into the oral cavity

velum   muscular structure located directly posterior to the hard palate; also referred to as the *soft palate*

vernacular dialect   variety of language spoken by a nonstandard speaker of a language

vocal cords   *see* vocal folds

vocal folds   elastic folds of tissue, primarily composed of muscle; also referred to as the *vocal cords*

vocalization   substitution of a vowel for postvocalic or syllabic /l/, postvocalic /r/, or the substitution of a non-rhotic vowel for the central vowels /ɚ/ and /ɝ/

vocal tract   network consisting of the larynx, pharynx, and the oral and nasal cavities

voice bar   low-frequency energy band as seen on a spectrogram (due to the vibrating vocal folds) that occurs during the stop gap phase of voiced stop consonants in non-initial position of words

voiced   phoneme produced with vocal fold vibration

voiceless   phoneme produced without vocal fold vibration

voice onset time (VOT)   time differential between the release of a stop consonant and the onset of voicing of the following vowel

voicing   participation of the vocal folds during phoneme production; all vowels are voiced, whereas only certain consonants are voiced

VoQS   voice quality symbols diacritic set; designed to be used in the transcription of individuals with voice disorders

vowel   phoneme produced without any appreciable blockage of airflow in the vocal tract

vowel merger   dialectal modification in which vowels with separate articulations fuse into one similar place of articulation (e.g., /ɑ/ and /ɔ/ both being produced as /ɑ/)

vowel quadrilateral   two-dimensional figure (representing tongue height and tongue advancement) that displays the relative position of the tongue during vowel production

vowel reduction   articulatory process associated with connected speech whereby the full form of a vowel is produced with less weight due to a more central production in the oral cavity, often similar to a mid-central vowel

waveform   graphic representation of sound that displays time on the abscissa and intensity on the ordinate

weak syllable deletion   syllable structure phonological process that involves the omission of an unstressed (weak) syllable either preceding or following a stressed syllable

word class   also known as "part of speech" (e.g., noun, verb, adjective)

word stress   production of a syllable with increased force or muscular energy, resulting in a syllable that is perceived as being louder, longer in duration, and higher in pitch; also known as word accent or *lexical stress*

Index